HEINEMANN DENTAL HANDBOOK

Heinemann Dental Handbook

Edited by
CHRISTOPHER J. BELL
BDS, MGDSRCS (Eng.)

*Teacher in Restorative Dentistry,
Bristol Dental School and Hospital
University of Bristol*

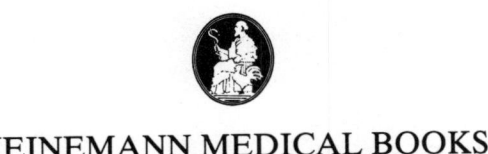

HEINEMANN MEDICAL BOOKS

Heinemann Medical Books
An imprint of Heinemann Professional Publishing Ltd
Halley Court, Jordan Hill, Oxford OX2 8EJ

OXFORD   LONDON   SINGAPORE   NAIROBI   IBADAN   KINGSTON

First published 1990

© Christopher J. Bell 1990
© of individual chapters retained by the contributors

British Library Cataloguing in Publication Data
Heinemann dental handbook.
  1. Dentistry
  I. Bell, Christopher J.
  617.6

ISBN 0 433 00104 6

Typeset and printed in Great Britain by
Redwood Press Limited, Melksham, Wiltshire

Contents

List of contributors ix

Preface xi

Part one Basic science

1 Oral biology and embryology 3
   D. ADAMS
2 Physiological topics in clinical dentistry 10
   S. J. W. LISNEY
3 Essential anatomy for general dental practitioners 23
   B. J. MOXHAM

Part two Child dental health

4 Interceptive orthodontics 43
   I. D. BROWN
5 Orthodontic cases to refer, treat yourself or leave alone 74
   I. D. BROWN
6 The use of fluoride in caries prevention 97
   R. J. ANDLAW
7 Fissure sealing and sealant restoration 100
   R. J. ANDLAW
8 Conservation of primary teeth 104
   R. J. ANDLAW
9 Trauma to children's teeth 110
   R. J. ANDLAW

Part three Restorative dentistry

10 The dental caries process 119
    R. J. ELDERTON
11 Caries in society and its preventive management 128
    R. J. ELDERTON

12	Restorative treatment: its problems and criteria for undertaking it R. J. ELDERTON	137
13	Essentials of rubber dam R. J. ELDERTON	148
14	Principles of cavity preparation R. J. ELDERTON	155
15	The way forwards with caries management in dental practice R. J. ELDERTON	175
16	Endodontics D. H. EDMUNDS	181
17	Elastic and non-elastic impression materials L. V. FOSTER and R. I. STEPHENSON	193
18	Pins in restorative dentistry L. V. FOSTER	205
19	Dental amalgam C. J. BELL and K. J. MARSHALL	209
20	Post crowns K. J. MARSHALL	217
21	Dental cements C. J. BELL	230
22	Enamel and dentine bonding agents C. J. BELL	234
23	Light-activated composite materials C. J. BELL	237
24	Castable ceramics C. J. BELL	242
25	Veneers S. M. HOOPER	244
26	Glass-ionomer cements C. B. G. JENKINS	254
27	Resin-bonded bridges C. B. G. JENKINS	262
28	Advanced tooth wear D. WILLIAMS	270
29	Occlusion in restorative dentistry A. C. WATKINSON	276
30	Complaints related to complete dentures A. HARRISON	282

31	Impression techniques A. HARRISON	286
32	Articulators A. C. WATKINSON	293
33	Design of partial dentures A. HARRISON	295
34	Duplication of full dentures C. J. BELL	304
35	Problems involving the oral mucosa with particular reference to prosthetics K. R. COWLES	306
36	Precision attachments A. C. WATKINSON	312
37	Implantology A. C. WATKINSON	315

Part four   Oral medicine, pathology and surgery

38	Pharmacology and therapeutics J. LUKER	321
39	The periodontium: diseases and treatment R. G. SMITH	335
40	Periodontal surgery S. L. MANTON and M. MIDDA	358
41	Conscious sedation C. SCULLY and M. J. GRIFFITHS	374
42	Dental local analgesia R. W. MATTHEWS	385
43	Mouth ulcers C. SCULLY	397
44	Lumps in the mouth C. SCULLY	408
45	Red, white and pigmented lesions C. SCULLY	415
46	Pain and neurological disease C. SCULLY	426
47	Emergencies in practice A. HILL	433
48	HIV infection S. R. PORTER	436
49	Oral surgery for the general dental practitioner J. W. ROSS	450

Part five   Examination techniques

50	General preparation C. J. BELL	475
51	The written papers C. J. BELL	476
52	The clinical case C. J. BELL	479
53	The 'viva' examination C. J. BELL	482
54	Causes of failure C. J. BELL	484
Index		485

List of Contributors

David Adams BSc MDS PhD
Reader in Oral Biology
University of Wales
Reginald J. Andlaw MSc PhD LDSRCS
Consultant Senior Lecturer in Child Dental Health
University of Bristol
Christopher J. Bell BDS MGDSRCS
Recognized Teacher in Restorative Dentistry
University of Bristol
Ian D. Brown BDS PhD DOrthRCS FDSRCS
Recognized Teacher in Child Dental Health (Orthodontics)
University of Bristol
Kenneth R. Cowles LDS
Special Lecturer in Prosthetic Dentistry
University of Bristol
David H. Edmunds BDS PhD FDSRCS
Consultant Senior Lecturer in Conservative Dentistry
University of Wales
Richard J. Elderton BDS PhD
Professor of Preventive and Restorative Dentistry
University of Bristol
Louise V. Foster BDS
Lecturer in Conservative Dentistry
University of Bristol
Mark J. Griffiths BDS MBBS FDSRCS
Clinical Lecturer in Oral Medicine and Oral Surgery
University of Bristol
Alan Harrison TD BDS PhD FDSRCS
Professor of Dental Care of the Elderly
University of Bristol
Anthony R. M. Hill BDS
General Dental Practitioner
Bristol
Susan M. Hooper BDS
Lecturer in Conservative Dentistry
University of Bristol

LIST OF CONTRIBUTORS

Clive B. G. Jenkins BDS MSD PhD FDSRCS
Consultant Senior Lecturer in Conservative Dentistry
University of Bristol

Stephen J. W. Lisney BSc BDS PhD
Senior Lecturer in Physiology
University of Bristol

Jane Luker BDS PhD FDSRCS
Associate Clinical Teacher in Oral Medicine, Surgery and Pathology
University of Bristol

Sarah L. Manton BDS PhD FDSRCS
Lecturer in Periodontology and Oral Medicine
University of Bristol

Kenneth J. Marshall BDS
Lecturer in Conservative Dentistry
University of Bristol

Robin W. Matthews PhD MDS BDS
Dental Clinical Dean and Senior Lecturer in Oral Medicine
University of Bristol

Marshall Midda BDS FDSRCS FFDRCSI
Clinical Lecturer in Periodontology
University of Bristol

Bernard J. Moxham BSc BDS PhD
Senior Lecturer in Anatomy
University of Bristol

Stephen R. Porter BSc BDS PhD FDSRCS and RCSE
Lecturer in Oral Medicine, Surgery and Pathology
University of Bristol

Jack W. Ross LDS FDSRCS
Clinical Lecturer in Oral and Maxillofacial Surgery
University of Bristol

Crispian Scully BSc BDS MBBS PhD FDSRCPS MRCPath MD MDS FFDRCSI
Professor of Oral Medicine, Surgery and Pathology
University of Bristol

Roger G. Smith BChD MDS FDSRCS
Consultant Senior Lecturer in Periodontology
University of Bristol

Richard I. Stephenson BDS
General Dental Practitioner
Alresford, Hants

Adrian C. Watkinson BChD MDS FDSRCS DRDRCS
Lecturer in Prosthetic Dentistry
University of Bristol

David R. Williams BSc BDS
Lecturer in Prosthetic Dentistry
University of Bristol

Preface

At all stages in a dental surgeon's career, the prospect of taking an examination can arise. For an undergraduate, such occurrences are a matter of course, but for a postgraduate dental surgeon there are now many opportunities to develop skills and knowledge, often resulting in some form of theoretical and clinical examination. The last part of this textbook strives to break new ground in that it will, it is hoped, assist both the undergraduate and postgraduate student by giving him or her advice about case presentation, 'viva' technique, and answering written questions.

The first parts combine texts drawn from the great talents in and around the University of Bristol Dental School. The subject matter of these varied contributions is based broadly on the University of Bristol MGDS Diploma course, and aims, as I have tried to do whilst running the course, to cover the important topics in dentistry, to guide candidates towards further updating their knowledge via reading and continuing education, and to leave them anxious to find out just a little more about the subjects covered—hence the references in 'Further Reading'.

It is very important to state at the outset that this book is not going to be all you need to pass every examination. Far from it! Rather, it is intended as a guide in which both undergraduate and postgraduate students may find indications of updated trends in dentistry 'all under one roof', using it as a revision course or as a starter for further reading. For simplicity, some chapters are presented in note form, and certain topics, for example radiology and cross-infection control, have been recently well-documented elsewhere.

For the undergraduate, the book will show the broad spectrum of dentistry. The practising dental surgeon, on reading even selected chapters, should be encouraged to attend courses and further increase his or her knowledge perhaps to the level of the MGDS.

The MGDS examination has become popular since the first year (1979) that it was held by the Royal College of Surgeons of England. With vocational training in general practice now established in many parts of the country, the need for trainer and trainee constantly to update their knowledge is paramount, which again is where this book comes in. Therefore, we all hope to cover a lot of ground within these pages, and if our work encourages both better understanding of dentistry, and helps a few people through some examinations, it will have been well worth the combined effort.

C. J. Bell, 1990

Part One
Basic Science

Chapter 1

Oral biology and embryology

FACIAL DEVELOPMENT

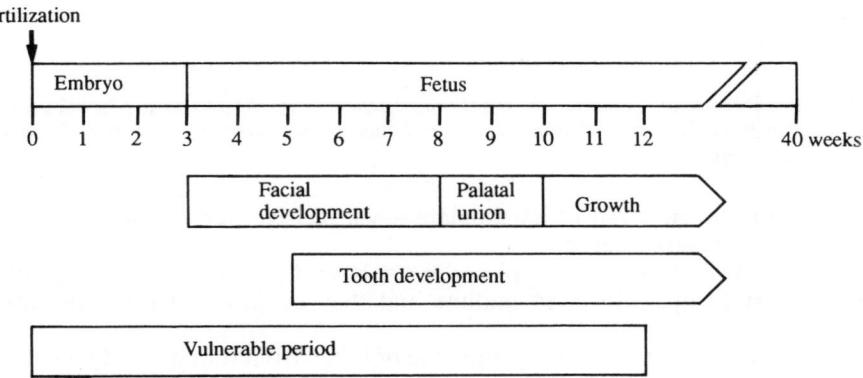

As early as the third week, mandibular arches form lower boundary of stomodeum — upper boundary is frontal process (Fig. 1.1). Frontal process has two nasal placodes — these divide the wide upper boundary into part lateral to placodes and part between the placodes.

Maxillary process arises from back part of mandibular arch, grows forward to form the upper boundary of primitive mouth. Meets, on its way, firstly lateral part of the frontal process, i.e. the part lateral to the nasal placode, then the central part of the frontal process, merging with it. How much this maxillary process contributes to the central part of the upper lip is debatable. In meeting the lateral nasal process, epithelial cells remain at this site and form the nasolacrimal duct as they run from eye to nose (Fig. 1.2).

Nasal placodes surrounded by proliferating mesenchymal tissue are connected to brain by olfactory nerves and appear to sink in. When maxillary process grows across below, the anterior nares are formed (Fig. 1.3). These end blindly at first but a breakdown of the tissue in the depths leads to formation of posterior nares.

Cleft lip results from failure of maxillary processes to fuse with the central part of frontal process — hence cleft runs into anterior nares (nostril).

Primary palate forms by union of maxillary process across the frontal process. The frontal process gives rise to (a) ala of nose; (b) tip of nose and front part of septum; (c) contributes to upper incisors and upper lip. It carries the

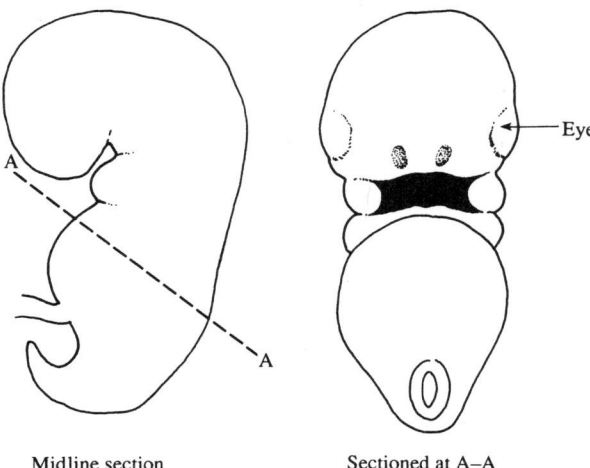

Fig. 1.1 *Embryo at 3.5 weeks: the frontonasal process with the two nasal placodes forms the upper boundary of the stomodeum and mandibular arches separate it from the pericardial region.*

innervation to the front of hard palate—via incisive nerve (continuation of long sphenopalatine nerve).

Initially eyes form as lens placodes on lateral part of head. Differential growth brings eyes closer to midline and they lie just above the primitive mouth.

Inside stomodeum, vertical projection of tissue from root partially divides it

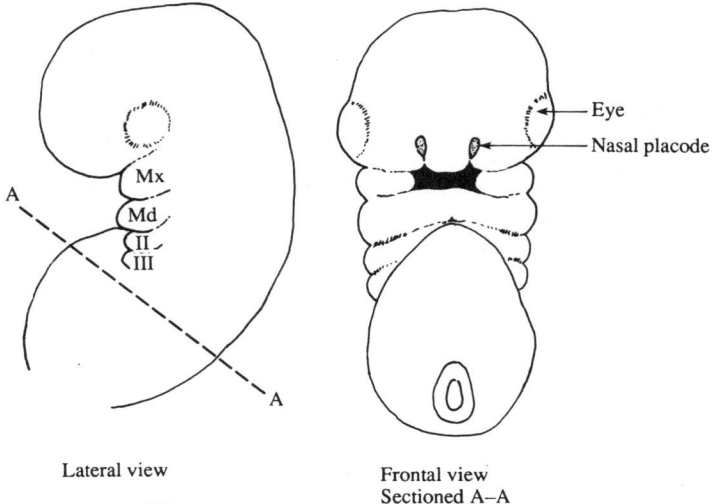

Fig. 1.2 *Embryo at 4 weeks: anterior nares are formed as the nasal placodes 'sink' by growth of surrounding tissue. Mx—maxilla; Md—mandible; II, III—second and third branchial arches.*

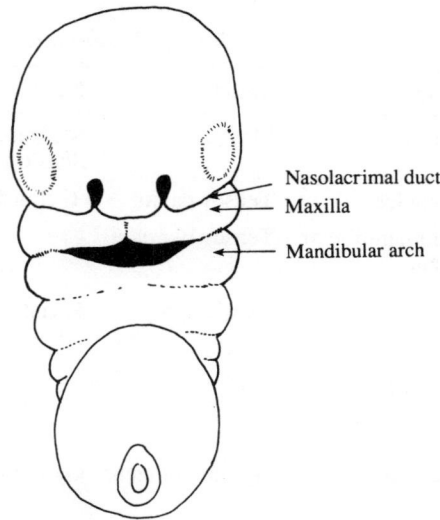

Fig. 1.3 *Embryo at 5 weeks: where the maxillary process meets the lateral part of the frontonasal process, the nasolacrimal duct is formed.*

into right and left halves. From sides, horizontal shelves grow in, meet the tongue, and are directed downwards alongside it. Tongue later descends, about 8–10 weeks, allowing palatal shelves to assume a horizontal position, where they meet and fuse with the vertical projection (nasal septum). Thus the stomodeum becomes left and right nasal cavities and oral cavity. Closure of palate starts about one-third of way back from the primary palate (Fig. 1.4). Zips up front and back from here.

It is interesting to note that the epithelium on the processes at the point of union appears to be 'programmed to die' when union occurs, thus allowing mesenchyme to meet and fuse. Cleft palate may occur by failure of processes to meet or a poor union which subsequently breaks down.

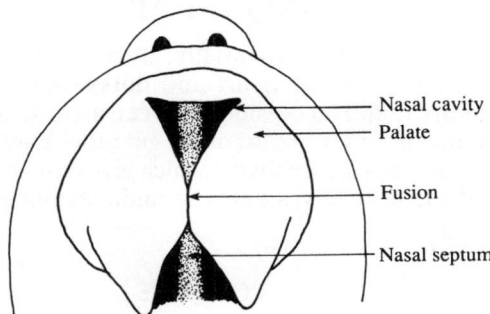

Fig. 1.4 *Fetus at 8 weeks: when the tongue moves out of the way the palatal shelves come together as shown, and union occurs forwards and backwards from the point of fusion.*

Table 1.1
Branchial arch derivatives

Arch	Cartilage	Muscles	Nerve	Pouches
1st	Meckel's	Mastication	Mandibular division V	Auditory tube
	Ear ossicles	Tensor palati	+ chorda tympani	Middle ear
	Sphenomandibular ligament	Tensor tympani		
2nd	Reichart's	Expression	Facial	Tonsil
	Ear ossicles			
	Part hyoid			
	Styloid process			
3rd	Remainder hyoid	Stylopharyngeus	Glossopharyngeal	Inferior parathyroid
				Thymus
4th	Thyroid	Pharynx constrictors	Vagus + cranial accessory	Superior parathyroid
		Soft palate		
6th	Cricoid	Laryngeal muscles	Recurrent laryngeal(X)	
	Arytenoid			

Palatal union occurs at 8–10 weeks. This is a critical period and any circumstance which prevents descent of tongue, e.g. insufficient amniotic fluid to allow neck to 'unbend', may be a predisposing factor in cleft palate.

BRANCHIAL ARCHES

Series of arches developing sequentially, as neck elongates, to contain the arterial vessels connecting the heart and dorsal aorta. First arch becomes mandible. Clefts are found on outside, between arches, and pouches are found on the inside, lining the anterior part of the gut tube. Each arch has an artery, is served by a nerve and has mesenchyme which gives rise to muscle and cartilage. A knowledge of the derivatives helps in understanding the anatomy of this region (Table 1.1).

TONGUE

Anterior two-thirds from a swelling on floor of mouth in midline between the mandibular arches (tuberculum impar) and from adjoining parts of the mandibular arch.

Posterior third—forms from third arch material (cupola) which overgoes the second arch in midline to meet the anterior part.

Hence anterior part is supplied by lingual nerve—from the mandibular division of V—the nerve of first arch. Posterior part supplied by glossopharyngeal nerve—nerve of third arch.

Chorda tympani subserves taste function, in anterior two-thirds (part of VIIth nerve, the nerve of the 'buried' second arch).

Taste from the circumvallate papillae is transmitted via IXth nerve, even though these are in front of line of junction between anterior two-thirds and the part derived from third arch.

Thyroid gland comes from a cord of ectoderm which originates in midline where anterior and posterior parts of tongue meet—foramen caecum. Cord passes into neck region in front of hyoid bone, and pulls with it the parathyroid material (see Table 1.1).

ANOMALIES OF DEVELOPMENT

The major anomalies are:

1. *Cleft lip*—lack of fusion of maxillary process and frontal process. May be uni- or bilateral.
2. *Cleft palate*—ranges from divided uvula to complete cleft involving alveolus, between the incisor and canine teeth. May be bilateral, and can occur independently of cleft lip.
3. *Mandibular facial dysostosis* (Treacher-Collins syndrome)—mainly a deficiency of mandibular arch growth.
4. *Midline cleft of mandible*—rare, caused by breakdown of tissues in midline due probably to poor blood supply.
5. Other *rare abnormalities* include macrostomia, where mandibular and maxillary processes fail to merge at angles of mouth, and oblique facial cleft in line of lacrimal duct.

TOOTH DEVELOPMENT

Initiation probably from mesoderm underlying ectoderm in a band around developing jaws. This mesoderm in reptiles has been shown to migrate from the neural crest region and is sometimes called ectomesenchyme or mesectoderm.

Under the influence of the underlying mesoderm the epithelium over the ridges grows down and branches into an outer sheet (which will form the cleavage plane between lips and cheek on the outer side and the alveolar part of the jaws on the inside) and an inner sheet—dental lamina.

Tooth buds appear on the inner sheet, at first four in each quadrant; then, by backward extension, a fifth; and later the buds for the permanent molars in succession.

Tooth buds undergo cap and bell stages with the enamel organ (epithelium-derived) surrounding the papilla (mesoderm-derived).

Enamel organ is made up of stellate reticulum, the internal enamel epithelium and the external enamel epithelium — the outermost layer. Internal enamel epithelial cells become ameloblasts (enamel-forming cells). There is also a layer of flat cells between stellate reticulum and the ameloblasts, an intermediate layer — stratum intermedium. Enamel laid down by ameloblasts. Initially crystallites of hydroxyapatite form and make up prisms with inorganic content about 30%. Amelogenesis starts at highest part of future amelodentinal junction (ADJ). Maturation or secondary mineralization occurs when full width of enamel is reached at tip of crown. Gradual increase in mineral to 96% — soluble organic 'amelogenins' squeezed out leaving 'enamelin' as organic framework.

Maturation almost complete prior to eruption but enamel remains relatively 'porous' and ions from oral environment may be adsorbed.

Fluoride can be adsorbed to greatest extent immediately after eruption, into the surface layer. May reach 500 p.p.m. in this region. Can increase in concentration slowly with age but porosity declines as more 'foreign' ions are adsorbed into surface layers.

Dentine production — starts by induction of odontoblasts by the inner enamel epithelium, at future ADJ. Dentine production starts just prior to initiation of enamel formation. Odontoblasts retreat leaving a cell process behind and laying down collagen and mineral around it — dentinal tubules. Always a layer of predentine — non-mineralized — between odontoblasts and dentine.

Side branches of odontoblasts join up dentinal tubules especially at periphery — may be responsible for spread of caries.

Mineral content of dentine is about 70% by weight. Tubules bend first towards future root apex then follow sigmoid course inward — called primary curves of tubules. Dentine formation slows after eruption but continues throughout life. Stimulation of odontoblasts, e.g. by attrition, slow caries or cavity preparation, induces accelerated production of dentine — at pulpal ends of affected tubules.

ROOT FORMATION

Crown formation reaches its full extent and is followed by an extension of its epithelial component into the underlying tissue, in form of tube — 'sheath of Hertwig'.

This is made up of inner and outer layers of the enamel organ — no stellate reticulum. The outermost cells of developing pulp are induced to become odontoblasts under influence of inner 'enamel' epithelium, just as in the crown.

As root elongates, Hertwig's sheath higher up breaks down into a network of epithelial strands.

From the follicle around tooth cementoblasts differentiate and lay down cement on the root, incorporating the fibres of the developing periodontal ligament.

The attachment of the collagen fibres to the cement and through it to dentine occurs under conditions that we seek to reproduce in the treatment of periodontal disease (re-attachment). Hence root planing, acidic treatment of the root surface and antimicrobial therapy are designed to result in a clean, healthy dentine surface with possibly collagen fibres exposed, upon which fibres will adhere either by incorporation of cement or by chemical bonding to the existing fibres.

When the root is two-thirds formed, eruption occurs. Tables of eruption dates can be found in most dental anatomy texts. Generally speaking the deciduous teeth erupt between 6 months and 30 months. There is a mixed dentition period — 6–11 years — and the permanent 'stable' dentition is present at about 12 years, with the exception of the third molars. Root completion takes approximately a year after eruption in the deciduous teeth, and approximately 2 years in the permanent teeth.

The crowns of deciduous teeth all are in the process of mineralization at birth, so all have a neonatal line (presumably due to an interruption of nutrition at birth) as does the first permanent molar if its mineralization has started over the primary cusp. The neonatal line can only be detected when normal enamel–dentine formation resumes, since only then does the 'defect' become apparent. This is a useful point in forensic cases, where one has to determine whether a child died at or just after birth — an absent neonatal line indicates that survival after birth was unlikely.

ERUPTION PROCESS

When the developing tooth is ready to erupt the crown, covered with the remnants of the enamel organ, approaches the base of the overlying epithelium. Proliferation of both the overlying epithelium and the reduced enamel epithelium result in a thick layer of epithelial cells above the tooth and through which the tooth passes to reach the oral cavity. Thus the tooth has a bloodless, epithelium-lined pathway. When the opposing tooth is met, guidance occurs by the inclined planes of the interdigitating cusps. Position also depends on muscle forces of tongue on lingual side and cheeks and lips on the other.

Passive eruption may occur with attrition of crown, and the occlusal plane may shift with growth of alveolar processes.

Abnormalities of tooth position may be due to:

(a) imbalance of the muscles on lingual and buccal sides;
(b) early loss of deciduous teeth — no guidance mesially or distally;
(c) abnormal external forces e.g. thumb sucking;
(d) discrepancies in size relationship between upper and lower jaws;
(e) crowding due to discrepancies between size of jaw and size of teeth;
(f) crowding due to supernumerary teeth;
(g) early or late eruption of neighbouring teeth;
(h) malpositioned tooth germ.

Chapter 2

Physiological topics in clinical dentistry

INTRODUCTION

Physiology is the study of normal body function and so it is the cornerstone to recognizing, understanding, preventing and treating abnormality and disease in all their various guises. This chapter deals with some situations that crop up in dental practice and briefly describes the physiological mechanisms and changes that underlie them.

WHY DO PEOPLE FAINT?

The brain depends critically upon an adequate supply of oxygen and should this be compromised, either by a reduction in the amount of oxygen being carried in the blood or by a reduction in cerebral blood flow, then a feeling of faintness (syncope) follows. Sometimes the oxygen lack is severe enough for there to be a transient loss of consciousness. Normally, mechanisms operate to keep the oxygen content of the blood and the cerebral blood flow relatively constant but these are not foolproof and when they are found to be wanting a faint occurs. The two most common causes of fainting are strong emotional responses and changes in posture.

Emotional faint (vasovagal faint, vasovagal syncope)

The thought or sight of surgical instruments, blood, etc. sometimes triggers two physiological responses which together can lead to a dramatic fall in systemic arterial blood pressure and hence a decreased cerebral blood flow. They occur simultaneously and they are:

1. A dilatation of blood vessels in skeletal muscle mediated by an increase in activity of certain sympathetic nerve fibres supplying muscle arterioles (the *vaso* component). This produces a drop in the resistance of the vasculature and hence a lowered blood pressure.

2. A fall in heart rate mediated by an increase in activity of parasympathetic nerves travelling to the heart in the vagus nerves (the *vagal* component). The lower heart rate results in a drop in cardiac output and this contributes further to the fall in blood pressure.

The neural connections that link the initial emotional response and these two cardiovascular changes are unknown but they seem to be unique to man.

Postural faint (postural syncope)

After getting up from the supine position there is a redistribution of blood in the venous side of the circulation. As blood shifts to the gravitationally dependent parts of the body, especially the large veins of the legs, venous return to the heart falls and the consequence is a drop in cardiac output. In those with sluggish cardiovascular reflexes — this particularly includes the elderly — the compensation for these changes is slow and the drop in cardiac output is enough to cause blood pressure, and hence cerebral perfusion, to fall below adequate levels.

Recovery from such faints is normally quite quick and uneventful and the appropriate first-aid measures are well known. For a small proportion of people, however, fainting may be a sign of an underlying cardiac condition, an arrhythmia or infarction, for example, so anyone with a history of repeated fainting episodes should be referred for specialist investigation.

MORE ON THE NEED FOR OXYGEN

Hypoxia is a term used to describe any situation where there is a lack of oxygen at the tissues in general, and not just the brain. It can have many causes including a low partial pressure of oxygen (low PO_2) in the air being breathed, heart or lung disease, and anaemia. In clinical dentistry it is important to be able to recognize and distinguish between different types of hypoxia, namely hypoxic hypoxia, anaemic hypoxia and stagnant hypoxia, because the immediate treatment for each is different. A fourth type of hypoxia, histotoxic hypoxia, caused when the cellular mechanisms of oxygen utilization by cells are poisoned (e.g. by cyanide), is extremely rare and need not be considered any further. A sign that can give warning of hypoxia is cyanosis.

Cyanosis

The colour of the skin and mucous membranes is partly dependent on the level of blood flow in the underlying vessels and on the state of the haemoglobin in those vessels. Oxygenated haemoglobin is red, giving the tissue a pink-red tinge, but the deoxygenated form is a dark blue-purple. Abnormally high amounts of deoxygenated haemoglobin in the blood make skin and mucous membranes appear a bluish-grey colour and this is cyanosis. The strict definition of cyanosis is that it occurs when the local concentration of deoxygenated haemoglobin is 5 g/100 ml of blood or more (the normal adult haemoglobin concentration is about 15 g/100 ml blood). These colour changes are most obvious in the nail beds, ear lobes, lips and mucous membranes, but they will be harder to see in people with darkly pigmented skin. Cyanosis may be restricted to just a few parts of the body, the hands and face of someone who has been out in the cold, for example, or it can be generalized, and it is important to make a distinction between the two (see below).

Hypoxic hypoxia

Oxygen is transported around the body in the blood where large amounts of it are combined reversibly with haemoglobin. The haemoglobin molecules are contained within the red blood cells (RBCs, erythrocytes). Because of a biochemical subtlety of the haemoglobin molecule the relationship between oxygen uptake by haemoglobin and the level of oxygen in the alveolar air in the lungs (expressed as the partial pressure, PO_2, rather than the concentration) is not straightforward. Each molecule has four O_2-binding sites and when the first is occupied by an O_2 group there is a small shape change in the haemoglobin complex which makes it easier for the next one to bind. This effect continues as each successive O_2 molecule latches onto haemoglobin and the net effect is that it is 700 times easier for the fourth one to bind compared with the first. At a PO_2 partial pressure of 100 mmHg, the sort of value found in the pulmonary alveoli under normal conditions, haemoglobin becomes fully saturated. In other words, all the O_2-binding sites on the haemoglobin in blood leaving the pulmonary capillaries are occupied. Anything that causes a reduction in the pulmonary alveolar PO_2 will affect oxygen uptake. A variety of circumstances can cause this, and those that could occur in a dental surgery include:

(a) breathing air with a low PO_2 — e.g. breathing from an anaesthetic machine when there is too little oxygen in the gas mixture;

(b) inadequate ventilation of the lungs — e.g. in a patient going through an acute asthmatic attack; a patient with an object lodged in the airway; inadequate artificial ventilation.

Hypoxic hypoxia can also arise if the thickness of the barrier between air in the pulmonary alveoli and blood in the adjacent capillaries is increased. Normally the alveolar/capillary barrier is very thin, consisting of just a film of alveolar fluid, the alveolar epithelium, the capillary endothelium, and the basement membrane sheet that separates these two cell layers. In patients with pneumonia or pulmonary oedema the thickness of the barrier is increased and consequently gas movement is hindered. Even though the alveolar PO_2 may be at its normal value of 100 mmHg, blood does not remain in the pulmonary capillaries long enough for the haemoglobin to become fully saturated and the outcome is hypoxia.

Generalized cyanosis may accompany hypoxic hypoxia and when it does it is a sign that the cause of the hypoxia needs to be identified and the appropriate action taken without delay.

Anaemic hypoxia

The blood of normal healthy adults contains about 15 g of haemoglobin per 100 ml, and each gram is capable of carrying 1.35 ml of O_2. Thus it follows that the total oxygen-carrying capacity of 100 ml of fully saturated arterial blood is just over 20 ml (only a negligible amount is carried directly in solution). If the amount of haemoglobin available to combine with O_2 falls by half, the amount of oxygen that can be carried is also going to be halved; there is no possibility of compensation of any sort in the oxygen transport mechanism because the haemoglobin is already fully saturated with O_2.

The anaemias are diseases where the oxygen-carrying capacity of blood is reduced, either because of decreased numbers of red blood cells or because of a decrease in their haemoglobin content. They include iron deficiency anaemia, pernicious anaemia (Vitamin B_{12} or folic acid deficiency), sickle cell disease, and a variety of less common haemolytic anaemias. A form of 'functional anaemia' can occur when there is the normal amount of haemoglobin in the blood but not all of it is able to combine with oxygen. An example of this is carbon monoxide poisoning. Carbon monoxide reacts with haemoglobin to form carbonmonoxyhaemoglobin (carboxyhaemoglobin), and this is incapable of taking up O_2. The affinity of carbon monoxide for haemoglobin is 250 times that of O_2 and, once formed, carbonmonoxyhaemoglobin dissociates only very slowly. The combined effect of these two facts is that small amounts of carbon monoxide can have a significant influence on oxygen transport. Cigarette smokers may have 5% or more of their haemoglobin combined with carbon monoxide, with a corresponding decrease in their oxygen-carrying capacity.

Cyanosis does not occur in anaemic hypoxia because of the low haemoglobin concentration and so other signs have to be taken as clues, e.g. pallor (particularly noticeable in the nail beds and mucous membranes), tiredness, feeling faint, being short of breath on exertion.

Stagnant hypoxia

If the circulation is sluggish the blood may not be able to deliver enough oxygen to the tissues, even though the haemoglobin concentration and the PO_2 are within normal limits. As progressively more oxygen dissociates from haemoglobin and the concentration of deoxyhaemoglobin rises, cyanosis develops. Stagnant hypoxia can be confined to just part of the body, as would be the case if the venous outflow from a limb was blocked, or it can be generalized: this is likely to happen in cardiac failure or peripheral circulatory failure (shock). The pattern of cyanosis in the two is different, being confined to the affected limb in the first instance and involving the whole body in the second.

Stagnant hypoxia and an accompanying cyanosis sometimes occur in patients with abnormally high numbers of circulating red cells (polycythaemia). Here the extra cells cause the viscosity of the blood to be increased and this leads to a slower circulation through peripheral vascular beds.

Tissue susceptibility to hypoxia

Sudden hypoxia from situations such as blockage of the airway (acute hypoxic hypoxia) or heart failure (acute stagnant hypoxia) presents a very real and immediate threat to the body. The brain is especially sensitive to interruption of its blood supply — and hence its oxygen supply. Normal brain function is impaired 4 s after stoppage of the cerebral circulation and consciousness is lost after about 8 s. If the blood supply is cut off for 1 min there is likely to be full recovery but it takes at least 15 min. The recovery time gets longer with increased periods of cerebral ischaemia and it may take days for the brain to return to normal after a 4-min episode. With times longer than this, up to a limit of 8–10 min, it is still possible for the brain to recover but there is a high risk of irreversible damage. The respiratory centre in the brain stem, which coordinates all the neural activities involved in breathing, is among the most sensitive regions of the brain to oxygen lack.

The heart is similarly sensitive. Whereas a resting heart can be successfully revived after several hours, a fact that makes it possible to take a donor heart from one part of the country to another for transplant surgery, an active heart can only tolerate a 3–4 min interruption of its blood supply. After this the recovery period becomes progressively longer and during this time the heart is unable to maintain an adequate blood pressure for normal perfusion of its own tissue, let alone the brain and the rest of the body.

Other organs are more tolerant and the liver and kidneys can be resuscitated after 3–4 h of ischaemia, although it may be several days before recovery is complete. The picture is similar for skeletal muscle.

THE MECHANISMS OF HAEMOSTASIS

In the normal course of events, bleeding from a wound stops within minutes of the injury. Three interconnected sets of events — the response of the damaged vessels, the responses of platelets, and the blood coagulation reactions — all contribute to stopping the bleeding.

The vascular response

The walls of damaged small arteries and arterioles contract in direct response to trauma and to chemicals released from platelets at the injury site (see below); this reduces the calibre of the vessels and hence the blood loss. Damaged capillaries may be sealed by movements of the endothelial cells that make up their walls.

Platelets

Platelets make several contributions to normal haemostasis. Wherever a blood vessel is injured collagen fibres in the underlying supporting connective tissue are exposed and these are an attractant to circulating platelets. When they contact the collagen their properties change and they become sticky, reinforcing their attachment to the damaged vessel wall and also attracting other platelets. As well as this they release chemicals, among them serotonin, ADP, and phospholipids, which further increase platelet adhesion and also trigger platelet contraction. All these events lead to the formation of a 'platelet plug' that helps to stop the loss of blood. Incidentally, aspirin inhibits synthesis of certain of the phospholipids produced by platelets and hence it has an anti-haemostatic action.

Blood coagulation

Neither of the two responses already described is stable and it needs the blood coagulation process to occur before bleeding is truly stopped. Blood coagulation involves a cascade of biochemical reactions in which various circulating factors interact to finally bring about the conversion of soluble fibrinogen into a network of insoluble fibrin strands. The initiating events in this series of reactions are the contact of a particular clotting factor (factor XII) with exposed collagen fibres at the injury site, and the release of tissue thromboplastin, a protein–phospholipid complex, from damaged cells. The fibrin mesh builds up in and around the platelet plug, trapping more platelets and also red blood cells, and in doing so forms a clot. The various factors involved in the coagulation process have been identified and a deficiency of any one can result in a failure of clot formation (e.g. haemophilia A — lack of factor VIII).

Anticoagulant therapy

Occasionally patients with cardiovascular disease are prescribed anticoagulants as part of their treatment. Heparin and coumarin derivatives are the two most commonly used.

Heparin acts by potentiating the action of antithrombin III; this circulating plasma protein inhibits thrombin and this in turn is required for the conversion of fibrinogen to fibrin.

Coumarin-like substances ('warfarin', dicoumarol) are Vitamin K analogues and they interfere with the synthesis of clotting factors in the liver (II [prothrombin], VII, IX, X).

Bleeding disorders

Disturbance of any one of the three sets of events that contribute to haemostasis can result in abnormal bleeding. For example, increased capillary fragility will lead to bleeding into the skin and mucous membranes. It is not uncommon to see these petechial haemorrhages in elderly people (senile purpura); here the cause is thought to be an age-related change in the properties of the capillary endothelial cells. Similar haemorrhages can be found in people with vitamin C deficiency. Shortage of platelets (thrombocytopenia) may have several causes and, like deficiencies in the blood coagulation system, calls for proper haematological testing.

THE WAY LOCAL ANAESTHETICS WORK (see also Chapter 42)

Information in the nervous system is transmitted by trains of frequency-coded impulses (action potentials) conducted along individual nerve fibres (also called axons). Each impulse consists of a momentary reversal in the electrical potential that exists across the nerve fibre membrane; this change in potential of about 100 mV comes about through the movement of ions, principally Na^+ and K^+, across the membrane. Under resting conditions the nerve cell membrane is relatively impermeable to these ions and the transmembrane potential is maintained at a steady, constant level. During an action potential, however, the membrane permeability changes for just a few milliseconds, first to Na^+ and then to K^+, and these changes allow small amounts of Na^+ and K^+ to move down their concentration gradients. The Na^+ ions move into and K^+ out of the cell, and these movements constitute an action potential. The permeability changes that are the key to each impulse are imagined to be associated with the opening and closing of channels (also referred to as 'pores' or 'gates') in the membrane. These channels are ion-specific, i.e. there are distinctly separate Na^+ and K^+ channels, but the precise details of their physical structure are still to be worked out.

Action potentials are conducted along nerve fibres in two ways. In the very small ones, the unmyelinated fibres, impulses are propagated along their length as a wave of potential change, in much the same way as a ripple spreads along a trough of water. Ion channels throughout the length of the fibres are involved. In the larger, myelinated fibres, where the axon is covered by a sheath of fatty, insulating myelin, the action potentials occur only at the gaps in the myelin sheath, the so-called nodes of Ranvier. The impulses are often described as 'jumping' from node to node.

The family of pharmacological agents collectively known as local anaesthetics have their action by 'blocking' the Na^+ channels; the exact mechanism is not yet known. By doing so they prevent movement of Na^+ ions across the nerve membrane and so action potentials cannot be generated. In this way the passage of impulses and the coded information they represent is stopped. The interaction between local anaesthetic and Na^+ channels is readily reversible, impulse conduction being restored to normal as the concentration of anaesthetic in the immediate neighbourhood of the nerve fibres falls.

DIFFICULTIES IN BREATHING

During normal quiet breathing about 500 ml of air moves in and out of the lungs with each breath and 12 such breaths are taken every minute. This amounts to an average resting pulmonary ventilation rate (pulmonary minute volume) of 6 l/min, enough to replenish the 250 ml of O_2 consumed by the body each minute and to remove the 200 ml CO_2 produced. Taking these breaths requires a certain amount of muscular effort. Expansion of the thorax, which is the beginning of inspiration, comes about because (a) the diaphragm contracts and hence moves downward; and (b) the external intercostal muscles contract, causing the rib cage to move upwards and outwards. By way of contrast, expiration is a purely passive event, occurring by virtue of the elastic recoil of the lungs and chest wall. Healthy people are largely unaware of the muscular activity associated with breathing but this is not necessarily the case for those with disease affecting the airways and lungs. While these people can usually cope while in the upright position, if they lie down—in a dental chair, for example—breathing can become difficult and it requires more effort. Why should this be so? There are three reasons.

1. Lying on a firm surface impedes movement of the rib cage. Consequently the external intercostal muscles have to do more work to move the ribs enough for them to make their normal contribution to expansion of the chest during inspiration.

2. Movement of the diaphragm accounts for three-quarters of the change in thoracic volume during resting breathing. While standing up the diaphragm has relatively little work to do when it contracts and displaces the underlying abdominal contents because gravity is tending to pull them downwards anyway. When lying down, however, gravity does not offer the same assistance and so the diaphragm has to do more work in order to achieve the usual increase in thoracic volume.

3. Changing from being upright to lying down causes a change in the distribution of blood in the venous side of the circulation, the pattern of which is dictated by gravity. This redistribution includes an increase in the volume of blood in the large veins of the thorax, and so potential space there that previously accommodated expansion of pulmonary alveoli now becomes taken up by blood. A greater change in thoracic volume is needed to get the same movement of air in and out of the lungs and this means more work for the respiratory musculature.

This explanation for a common observation serves as a simple reminder that it is very much kinder to treat patients with breathing difficulties sitting up rather than lying down.

THE MANDIBULAR REST POSITION

Being able to determine the mandibular rest position of a patient has some clinical value, for example, when deciding the vertical height of a new set of full dentures or when investigating temporomandibular joint dysfunction. In some instances it can be difficult to judge just when the lower jaw is in the so-called rest position and so attempts have been made to get some understanding of the physiological mechanisms underlying it.

Role of tonic muscle activity

One view is that the mandible is held in its rest position by low levels of on-going, tonic activity in the jaw elevator muscles (masseter, temporalis and medial pterygoid). On top of this, muscle spindles — length receptors in the muscles themselves — provide continuous feedback to the elevator motoneurons so that the level of on-going activity can be reflexly modulated to compensate for any length changes that happen. By this simple negative-feedback loop the rest position can be maintained with just a minimal amount of muscle activity.

There is no doubt that the neural circuitry for this mechanism exists but it is another matter to show that this is how the rest position is controlled. One way of doing so would be to demonstrate the presence of on-going activity in the jaw elevators: although some claim to have done this, using recordings of the electrical events in muscle that accompany contraction (electromyographs; EMGs,), others have pointed out the limitations of the technique. The general consensus is that EMGs are inappropriate for deciding whether or not the jaw muscles are active when the mandible is in its rest position, and so for now this explanation has to be left in limbo because it cannot be properly tested.

Tissue elasticity

An alternative view is that the lower jaw is held in its rest position simply by passive forces and that muscle activity is not involved at all. In its simplest terms this idea proposes that the weight of the mandible is balanced by the inherent elastic properties of the elevator muscles. Of course, other factors have to be taken into account, such as the elastic forces exerted by the depressor muscles and the skin, but the overall concept of an equilibrium in which all the various passive forces are in balance still holds true. There is experimental evidence in favour of this idea.

Although research has given a clearer picture of the physiology of the mandibular rest position it has not come up with any easy ways of determining it in patients. The only tool that could be of use is electromyography but because of the technical drawbacks this is impracticable so far as routine clinical use is concerned.

THE SENSITIVITY OF DENTINE

Nobody needs to be reminded that stimulation of exposed dentine in a patient who has not been given a local anaesthetic is very likely to lead to them feeling pain. There are two long-standing puzzles associated with dentine sensitivity. The first is, how is it that a wide range of stimuli, including hot, cold, gentle touching, drying with a pledget of cotton wool or a stream of warm air, and contact with concentrated solutions, all evoke the same sensation? The second is, why is it that dentine at the amelodentinal junction (ADJ) seems to be the most sensitive? Many suggestions have been made to explain the sensitivity of dentine but only three have any substance to them.

Nerves in dentine

Sensory nerves supply the dental pulp, so if it could be shown that terminal branches of some of these nerves extend into dentinal tubules we would have the beginnings of an explanation. Experimental studies on both human and animal teeth have failed to demonstrate anything more than a scanty innervation of dentine. Only a fraction of the tubules contain a nerve process and in those that do the process only passes about a third of the way up the tubule, well short of the ADJ. This is not enough to account for all the clinical and experimental observations on dentine sensitivity.

Odontoblasts as sensory receptors

Most, if not all, of the tubules in healthy dentine contain an odontoblast process, so it is easy to appreciate how these cells came to be thought of as candidates for the job of sensory receptor. Two things, however, stand against the idea. The first is that, except in young teeth, the processes do not appear to traverse the whole length of the tubules and so it is hard to explain the sensitivity of outer dentine and particularly that near the ADJ. The second is that if such an arrangement is to work there has to be some kind of functional link between the odontoblasts and sensory nerve fibres; this is so excitatory signals can pass from the one to the other. Although a link of this sort is known to exist in other situations (between chemosensory cells and nerves in taste buds, for example), there is no evidence of it being present between odontoblasts and pulpal nerves.

The 'hydrodynamic mechanism'

Each dentinal tubule with its odontoblast process and non-cellular tubular material could be thought of as a miniature hydraulic system. The tubule acts as the cylinder, the odontoblast process is the piston, and the non-cellular tubular contents are the equivalent of the hydraulic fluid. Movement of the tubular contents will cause displacement of the odontoblast process and this in turn would be expected to mechanically excite nerve endings in the predentine and/or odontoblast layer where they mingle with the odontoblasts. All the stimuli described before would be expected to cause movement of the tubular contents in one direction or the other, and experiments have shown that some of the stimuli do indeed bring about fluid movement between dentine and pulp of extracted human teeth. While much of the evidence fits, so making the hydrodynamic mechanism an attractive proposition, it may not be the whole story. Intradental nerves that discharge impulses after application of a hot stimulus to a tooth respond in a way that suggests they may be being activated directly, rather than indirectly by odontoblast movement. The site of activation is probably in the inner dentine, where most intradentinal nerves are found, or in the pulp.

Thus it seems possible that two intradental sensory mechanisms are operating, one particularly sensitive to heating and the other less discriminating, responding to a wide range of stimuli.

HOW DOES SWELLING COME ABOUT?

Under normal physiological conditions there is a fine balance between the movement of water out of capillaries into the tissue space and vice versa, but if this is upset, fluid collects in the tissues and a puffy swelling (oedema) develops. In any particular capillary bed, several factors interact with each other to determine this balanced, two-way flux of water. These are:

1. The difference in hydrostatic pressure between blood in the capillaries and fluid in the interstitial space. Interstitial fluid pressure is normally low and to all intents and purposes negligible, leaving capillary hydrostatic pressure as the more important of the two. This in its turn is dependent on the systemic arterial blood pressure and the vascular resistance (mainly from arterioles) upstream of the capillary bed. Its value is higher at the arteriolar end of the bed than at the venular end.

2. The difference in osmotic pressure between the capillary and interstitial fluid. The difference that exists comes about because there are proteins in the blood — the plasma proteins — that are not found in the interstitial space; the permeability of the capillary walls is such that these proteins normally remain confined to the circulation. The plasma protein osmotic pressure, or oncotic pressure, is more or less constant from one end of the capillary bed to the other.

3. The permeability of the capillaries.

At the arteriolar end of a typical capillary bed the hydrostatic pressure tending to force water out is greater than the oncotic pressure drawing it back in, so the overall effect is loss of water, i.e. there is net filtration. The situation is reversed in the venular half of the capillary bed, where the oncotic pressure exceeds the hydrostatic pressure, and so here there is net water reabsorption. The amount of water moving out on the arteriolar side and that moving in on the venular side do not quite balance; only about 18 of the 20 l of water filtered each day in the body are reabsorbed. The other 2 l do not remain in the interstitial space, however, but eventually drain into the lymphatic system, so becoming lymph, and return to the circulation via that route.

When tissue is damaged, as with injury or during surgery, this balanced state of affairs is perturbed. Nervous reflexes triggered by the trauma lead to arteriolar dilatation in the vicinity of the injury; this lowers the resistance offered by these arterioles and this in turn leads to an increase in hydrostatic pressure in the capillaries downstream. Consequently there is a shift towards greater filtration and water starts to collect in the interstitium. Tissue damage also results in release of histamine from mast cells and this affects capillaries by increasing their permeability. Plasma proteins are now able to leak out into the tissue space, thus reducing the plasma protein osmotic pressure, and so again filtration is favoured. The combined effect of these two things is localized oedema around the injury site. Excessive build-up of fluid, however, is prevented by concomitant changes in factors that allow lymphatic flow to increase.

Oedema also occurs in other situations — for example, after standing up for a long time. Here the tilting of the balance towards greater net filtration is caused by the increased venous pressure that follows stagnation of blood in the large veins of the lower legs. Walking about from time to time pumps blood out of the veins and so helps to stop oedema from developing.

RECOVERY AFTER HAEMORRHAGE

Severe haemorrhage is fortunately a rare event in a dental surgery but it may not be so rare to have to treat people who are at various stages in the recovery from significant blood loss. It is unlikely that patients will be encountered who are in the earliest phase of recovery but some appreciation of the events that are taking place then helps in understanding the problems that will last for weeks after the haemorrhage.

The immediate threat posed by major blood loss comes from the reduction in circulating volume. The knock-on effect of this is a fall in venous return to the heart and therefore a fall in the amount of blood it can pump out again; inevitably this leads to a drop in systemic arterial blood pressure. Various cardiovascular reflex responses then come into play to bring about some compensation for these changes. These include an increase in heart rate and in the force of contraction of heart muscle in order to increase cardiac output; constriction of veins to reduce the amount of blood in this side of the circulation; and vasoconstriction in some tissues. The distribution of this vasoconstriction is selective and serves to divert what cardiac output there is away from less crucially important tissues, such as skin, muscle and the abdominal viscera, to more vital organs, e.g. the heart, lungs and brain. In these ways the blood pressure and perfusion of vital organs are maintained at adequate levels but these responses only provide a short-term solution. In the long term recovery can only begin if the loss of circulating volume can be made up in some way.

Restoring circulating volume

The reduced blood pressure and the arteriolar constriction just mentioned cause a lowering of capillary hydrostatic pressure in tissues such as skin, muscle and the viscera, so in these places the balance of water movement in and out of capillaries is shifted in favour of net reabsorption (see previous section). By this mechanism about 500 ml of fluid can be restored to the circulation in the first 15 min after a severe haemorrhage; after this the rate of fluid transfer declines so that after an hour 1 l will have been moved from the interstitial space into the plasma. Over the next few hours another mechanism operates to make a further contribution to the restoration of circulating volume. The amount of Na^+ reabsorbed in the kidneys is increased and as a consequence water is also retained. The rise in plasma Na^+ also triggers the sensation of thirst and so more water is added to the body through drinking.

If these various mechanisms fail there is the danger of hypovolaemic shock. With a blood loss of 10% of circulating volume (500 ml — the sort of amount taken from a blood donor) it is hard to detect evidence of these compensatory mechanisms and recovery is uneventful. With a 20–30% loss, heart rate is significantly elevated, the pulse pressure becomes smaller, and blood pressure is also measurably lower. Vasoconstriction in skin and muscle occurs. Even without medical intervention there will usually be a full recovery. If the blood loss reaches 40% of circulating volume (2–3 l) all these changes are present but are more pronounced; there may be a complete shunting of blood flow away from skin, muscle and the viscera. Renal blood flow may also be compromised. Without treatment there is a strong likelihood of shock. A blood loss of 50% or more will probably be fatal unless intensive medical treatment is given.

Restoring other blood constituents

While restoration of the circulating volume removes the immediate threat, the dilution of the blood that goes with it results in a lowered plasma oncotic pressure and a lowered red blood cell count (anaemia). If the plasma protein concentration is not returned to normal, the water added to the circulation would soon be lost back to the interstitium. It takes 3–6 days for the liver to synthesize enough protein to do this but very little is known about the control mechanisms involved. It goes without saying that anyone with chronic liver disease will show a delayed or impaired recovery.

It takes longer still, 4–6 weeks, for the numbers of red blood cells to return to normal. The rate at which new red blood cells are formed is controlled by a hormone, erythropoietin, the main source of which is the kidneys. Renal hypoxia, as would occur in anaemia, triggers release of erythropoietic factor, which combines with a circulating plasma protein from the liver to give erythropoietin. This travels via the blood stream to bone marrow where it accelerates the rate of differentiation of new red blood cells from precursor stem cells. Disease of the kidneys, liver or bone marrow will affect the chances of a full recovery of erythrocyte numbers after haemorrhage.

FURTHER READING

Bradley R. M. (1981). *Basic Oral Physiology*. New York: Year Book Medical Publishers.

Bray J. J., Cragg P. A., Macknight A. D., Mills R. G., Taylor D. W. (1989). *Lecture Notes on Human Physiology*, 2nd edn. Oxford: Blackwell Scientific.

Emslie-Smith D., Paterson C. E., Scratcherd T., Read N. W. (1988). *Textbook of Physiology*, 11th edn. Edinburgh: Churchill Livingstone.

Ganong W. F. (1989). *Review of Medical Physiology*, 14th edn. Connecticut: Appleton and Lange.

Chapter 3

Essential anatomy for general dental practitioners

Although many general dental practitioners claim that their knowledge of anatomy is weak, it is only the incorrigible dilettante who denies the importance of the subject. Take for example the following case history:

An inferior alveolar nerve block was given to a patient within the right infratemporal fossa prior to dental treatment. After several minutes, the patient complained of blurred vision and the dentist noticed that there was a squint of the right eye.

While this may not be a common event following an inferior alveolar nerve block, it presents a very frightening experience for the patient, which is aggravated if the dentist is unable to give a rational and reassuring explanation. The visual defects suggest that the anaesthetic solution could have entered the orbit, possibly by way of the inferior orbital fissure, which lies near the antero-superior corner of the infratemporal fossa. Vascular spasm may provide another explanation since in some people the orbit is supplied by the middle meningeal artery, which is a branch of the maxillary artery in the infratemporal fossa. Fortunately, these visual complications are transient, passing away with the disappearance of anaesthesia.

Good arguments could be levelled for including in this chapter virtually all the regions/systems within the head and neck, but perhaps many would agree that the following topics are amongst the most 'essential'.

1. The sensory innervation of the oral cavity
2. The lymphatic drainage of orodental structures
3. Tissue spaces around the jaws and their importance in the spread of infection
4. The maxillary air sinus

THE SENSORY INNERVATION OF THE ORAL CAVITY

The oral mucosa receives its sensory innervation primarily from the maxillary and mandibular divisions of the trigeminal nerve (the Vth cranial nerve). The trigeminal nerve also supplies the teeth and their supporting tissues. Thus, there is no need to dwell here on the importance of this cranial nerve to clinical dentistry. It seems appropriate to begin this section by describing the general course and distribution of the maxillary and mandibular nerves and then to provide details concerning the specific innervation to the various structures/regions of the mouth.

(a)

(b)

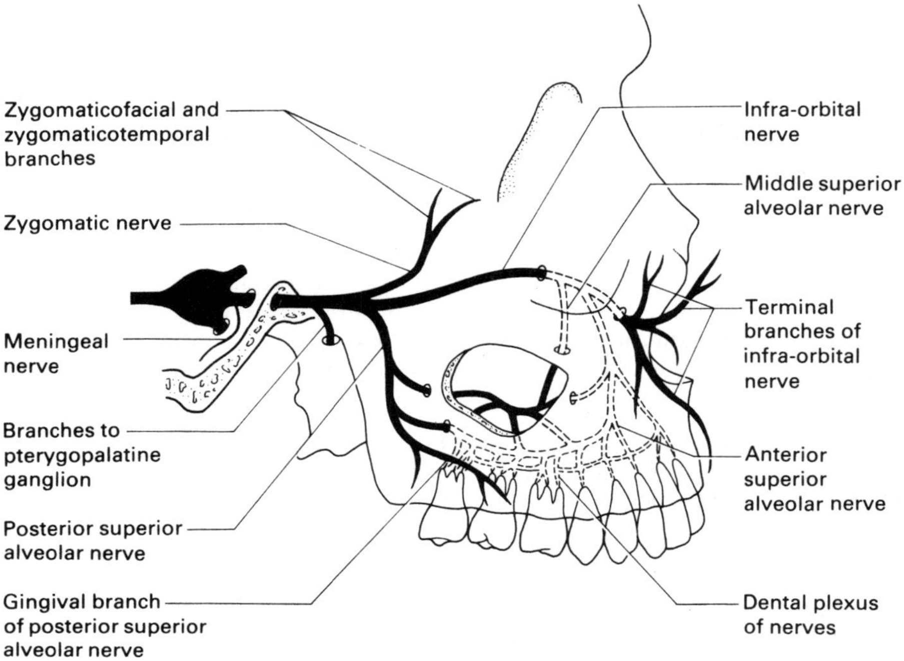

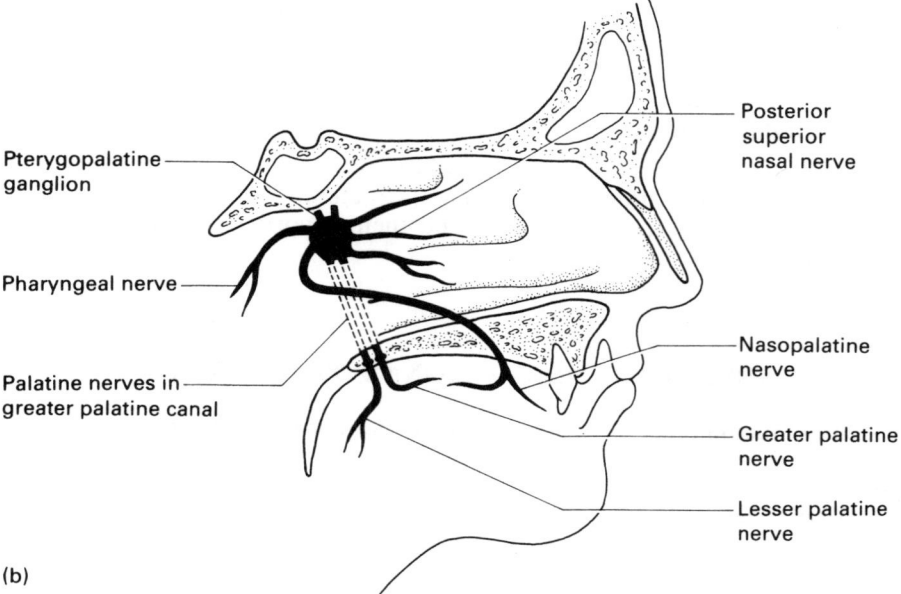

Fig. 3.1 *(a) The maxillary nerve. (b) Branches of the pterygopalatine nerve.*

The maxillary nerve (Fig. 3.1)

This division of the trigeminal nerve contains only sensory fibres. It supplies the maxillary teeth and their supporting tissues, the hard and soft palate, the maxillary air sinus, much of the nasal cavity, and the skin overlying the middle part of the face.

The maxillary nerve exits the cranial cavity (middle cranial fossa) at the foramen rotundum to emerge into the pterygopalatine fossa. It is in this fossa that most of the branches of the maxillary nerve are derived. The branches can be categorized into those that arise directly from the maxillary nerve, and those that are derived indirectly from the pterygopalatine parasympathetic ganglion.

The branches from the main nerve trunk are:

(a) meningeal nerve;
(b) ganglionic branches;
(c) zygomatic nerve —
   (i) zygomaticotemporal nerve,
   (ii) zygomaticofacial nerve;
(d) posterior superior alveolar nerve;
(e) infraorbital nerve —
   (i) middle superior alveolar nerve,
   (ii) anterior superior alveolar nerve.

The branches associated with the pterygopalatine ganglion are:

(a) orbital nerve;
(b) nasopalatine nerve;
(c) posterior superior nasal branches;
(d) greater palatine nerve;
(e) lesser palatine nerve;
(f) pharyngeal branch.

The **meningeal nerve** is the only branch from the main trunk of the maxillary nerve that does not originate in the pterygopalatine fossa (arising within the middle cranial fossa before the foramen rotundum). It runs with the middle meningeal artery and innervates the dura mater lining the middle cranial fossa.

The **ganglionic branches** (usually two in number) connect the maxillary nerve to the pterygopalatine ganglion. These branches contain sensory fibres (which pass through the pterygopalatine ganglion without synapsing) and postganglionic autonomic fibres from the ganglion (which are destined for the lacrimal gland in the orbit).

The **zygomatic nerve** leaves the pterygopalatine fossa through the inferior orbital fissure. It then passes along the lateral wall of the orbit before dividing into zygomaticotemporal and zygomaticofacial branches. These pass through the zygomatic bone to supply overlying skin. The zygomaticotemporal nerve also gives a branch to the lacrimal nerve. This carries autonomic fibres to the lacrimal gland.

The **posterior superior alveolar nerve**(s) is one of three superior alveolar nerves that supply the maxillary teeth. The middle and anterior superior alveolar nerves are branches of the infraorbital nerve (see below). The three superior alveolar nerves form a plexus just above the roots of the maxillary

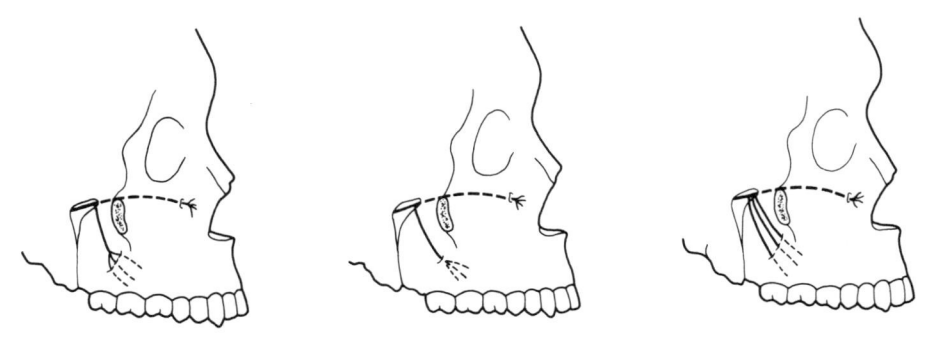

Fig. 3.2 *Variations in the extrabony course of the posterior superior alveolar nerve.*

teeth. Indeed, it is difficult to trace the precise innervation of the teeth from a specific superior alveolar nerve. As a general rule, however, the incisors and canines are supplied by the anterior nerve, the molars by the posterior nerve and the premolars by the middle nerve. The posterior superior alveolar nerve(s) leaves the pterygopalatine fossa through the pterygomaxillary fissure. Thence, it runs on the tuberosity of the maxilla and eventually enters the bone to supply the maxillary molar teeth and the maxillary sinus. Before entering the maxilla, the nerve provides a gingival branch which innervates the buccal gingiva around the maxillary molars. The extrabony course of the posterior superior alveolar nerve is variable (Fig. 3.2). The nerve can subdivide into several branches just before or just after it enters the maxilla. Alternatively, it may arise as several distinct branches at the main trunk of the maxillary nerve.

The **infraorbital nerve** can be regarded as the terminal branch of the maxillary nerve proper. It leaves the pterygopalatine fossa to enter the orbit at the inferior orbital fissure. Initially lying in a groove in the floor of the orbit (the infraorbital groove), the infraorbital nerve runs into a canal (the infraorbital canal) and passes on to the face at the infraorbital foramen.

The middle and anterior superior alveolar nerves arise from the infraorbital nerve in the orbit. The middle superior alveolar nerve is found in about 70% of the population. Occasionally, it arises not from the infraorbital nerve but from the maxillary nerve in the pterygopalatine fossa. The nerve may run in the posterior, lateral or anterior walls of the maxillary air sinus. It terminates in the region of the premolar teeth. The anterior superior alveolar nerve arises within the infraorbital canal, generally as a single nerve but sometimes as two or three small branches. The nerve runs down the anterior wall of the maxillary sinus in a narrow, sinuous canal (the canalis sinuosus) to reach the maxillary incisor teeth. Near the anterior nasal spine, the anterior superior alveolar nerve gives off a small nasal branch which innervates the nasal mucosa around the nostril.

The terminal branches of the infraorbital nerve arise as the nerve emerges through the infraorbital foramen on to the face. Palpebral branches supply skin of the lower eyelid. Nasal branches innervate skin overlying the side of the external nose (also part of the septum between the nostrils). Labial branches supply the skin and oral mucosa of the upper lip, the labial gingiva of the anterior teeth in the upper jaw, and the skin overlying the anterior part of the cheek covering the body of the maxilla.

The branches of the maxillary nerve that arise with the pterygopalatine parasympathetic ganglion contain not only sensory fibres from the maxillary nerve, but also autonomic fibres from the ganglion (to be distributed to glands) and sympathetic fibres, which supply blood vessels.

The **orbital nerve** passes from the pterygopalatine ganglion into the orbit through the inferior orbital fissure. It supplies periosteum and, via sympathetic fibres, the orbitalis muscle of the eyeball. The orbital nerve can also pass through the posterior ethmoidal foramen to innervate posterior ethmoidal air cells and the sphenoidal air sinus.

The **nasopalatine nerve** (once called the long sphenopalatine nerve) runs from the pterygopalatine ganglion into the nasal cavity through the sphenopalatine foramen. It passes across the roof of the nasal cavity to reach the back of the nasal septum. The nasopalatine nerve then passes downwards and forwards (within a groove on the vomer) to supply the postero-inferior part of the nasal septum. It terminates by passing through the incisive canal on to the hard palate to supply oral mucosa around the incisive papilla (see Fig. 3.6).

The **posterior superior nasal nerve** (once termed the short sphenopalatine nerve) enters the back of the nasal cavity through the sphenopalatine foramen. It divides into lateral and medial branches. The lateral branches supply the posterosuperior part of the lateral wall of the nasal fossa. The medial branches cross the roof of the nasal fossa to supply the nasal septum overlying the posterior part of the perpendicular plate of the ethmoid.

The **greater palatine nerve** (alternatively called the anterior palatine nerve) passes downwards from the pterygopalatine ganglion, through the greater palatine canal, and on to the hard palate at the greater palatine foramen. Within the greater palatine canal, it gives off nasal branches that innervate the postero-inferior part of the lateral wall of the nasal fossa. On the palate, it runs forwards at the interface between the palatine process and the alveolar process of the maxilla to supply much of the mucosa of the hard palate and palatal gingiva (except around the incisive papilla) (see Fig. 3.6).

The **lesser palatine nerve**(s) (alternatively termed the posterior palatine nerve) passes downwards from the pterygopalatine ganglion, through the greater palatine canal, and on to the palate at the lesser palatine foramen (or foramina) (see Fig. 3.6). It runs backwards to supply the soft palate.

The mandibular nerve (Fig. 3.3)

This is the largest division of the trigeminal nerve and is the only one to contain motor as well as sensory fibres. Its sensory fibres supply the mandibular teeth and their supporting structures, the mucosa of the anterior two-thirds of the tongue and the floor of the mouth, the skin of the lower part of the face (including the lower lip) and parts of the temporal region and the auricle of the ear. Its motor fibres supply the four 'muscles of mastication' and the mylohyoid, anterior belly of digastric, tensor veli palatini and tensor tympani muscles.

The mandibular nerve is formed in the infratemporal fossa by the union of the sensory and motor roots immediately after they leave the skull at the foramen ovale. At this point, the nerve lies on the tensor veli palatini muscle and is covered by the lateral pterygoid muscle. After a short course, the nerve divides into a small anterior trunk and a larger posterior trunk. Before this division, the main trunk gives off two branches—the meningeal branch and the nerve to medial pterygoid. The anterior trunk of the mandibular nerve is mainly motor, the posterior trunk mainly sensory.

The branches of the mandibular nerve are:

(a) meningeal branch (nervus spinosus),
(b) nerve to medial pterygoid;
(c) anterior trunk—
    (i) masseteric nerve,
    (ii) deep temporal nerves,
    (iii) nerve to lateral pterygoid,
    (iv) buccal nerve;
(d) posterior trunk—
    (i) auriculotemporal nerve,
    (ii) lingual nerve,
    (iii) inferior alveolar nerve.

The **meningeal branch of the mandibular nerve** (nervus spinosus) arises from the main trunk of the mandibular nerve. It is a 'recurrent nerve' as it runs back into the middle cranial fossa through the foramen spinosum. It supplies the dura mater lining the middle cranial fossa and the mucosa of the mastoid antrum and mastoid air cells.

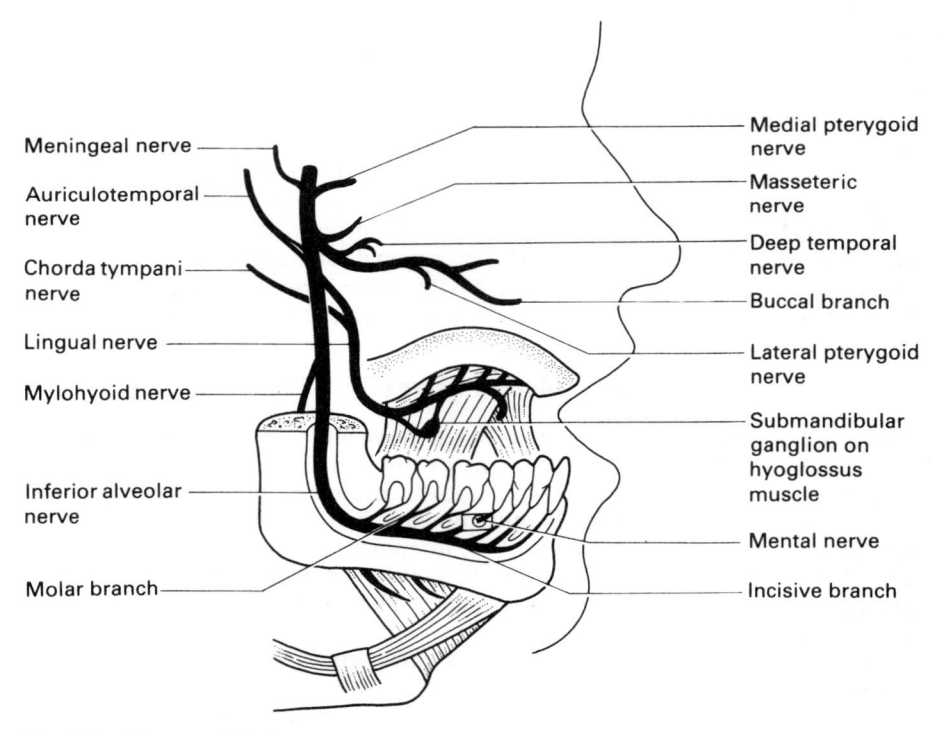

Fig. 3.3 *The mandibular nerve.*

The **nerve to the medial pterygoid muscle** enters the deep surface of the muscle and also gives slender branches which pass uninterrupted through the otic parasympathetic ganglion to supply the tensor tympani and tensor veli palatini muscles.

The **masseteric nerve** is usually the first branch of the anterior trunk of the mandibular nerve. It passes above the upper border of the lateral pterygoid muscle and crosses the mandibular notch (between the condylar and coronoid processes) to be distributed into the masseter muscle. It also gives an articular branch to the temporomandibular joint.

The **anterior** and **posterior deep temporal nerves** also pass above the lateral pterygoid muscle. They subsequently enter the deep surface of the temporalis muscle.

The **nerve to the lateral pterygoid muscle** may arise separately or may run with the buccal nerve before entering the deep surface of the lateral pterygoid muscle.

The **buccal branch of the mandibular nerve** (sometimes referred to as the long buccal nerve) is the only sensory branch of the anterior trunk of the mandibular nerve. On emerging between the heads of the lateral pterygoid muscle, it passes downwards and forwards across the lower head to contact the medial surface of the temporalis muscle as it inserts on to the coronoid process of the mandible. It then clears the ramus of the mandible to lie on the lateral surface of the buccinator muscle in the cheek. At this point, it is close to the retromolar fossa of the mandible. It now gives branches to the skin of the cheek, before piercing buccinator to supply its lining mucosa, the buccal sulcus, and the buccal gingiva related to the mandibular molar and premolar teeth. It may also carry secretomotor fibres to minor salivary glands in the buccal mucosa (these being postganglionic fibres from the otic ganglion).

The **auriculotemporal nerve** is the first branch of the posterior trunk of the mandibular nerve. It is essentially sensory but it also distributes autonomic fibres to the parotid gland derived from the otic parasympathetic ganglion. It arises as two roots that encircle the middle meningeal artery and unite behind the artery. The nerve then runs backwards under the lateral pterygoid muscle to lie beneath the mandibular condyle (between the condyle and the sphenomandibular ligament). On entering the parotid region, it turns to emerge superficially between the temporomandibular joint and the external acoustic meatus. From the upper surface of the parotid gland, the auriculotemporal nerve ascends on the side of the head with the superficial temporal vessels, passing over the posterior part of the zygomatic arch. It gives several branches along its course:

1. Ganglionic branches which communicate with the otic parasympathetic ganglion.
2. Articular branches which enter the posterior part of the temporomandibular joint; these carry proprioceptive information important in mastication.
3. Parotid branches which convey parasympathetic secretomotor fibres and sympathetic fibres to the parotid gland; these fibres are related to the otic ganglion. Sensory fibres from the auriculotemporal nerve supply the gland (with the exception of the capsule, which is innervated by the great auricular nerve).

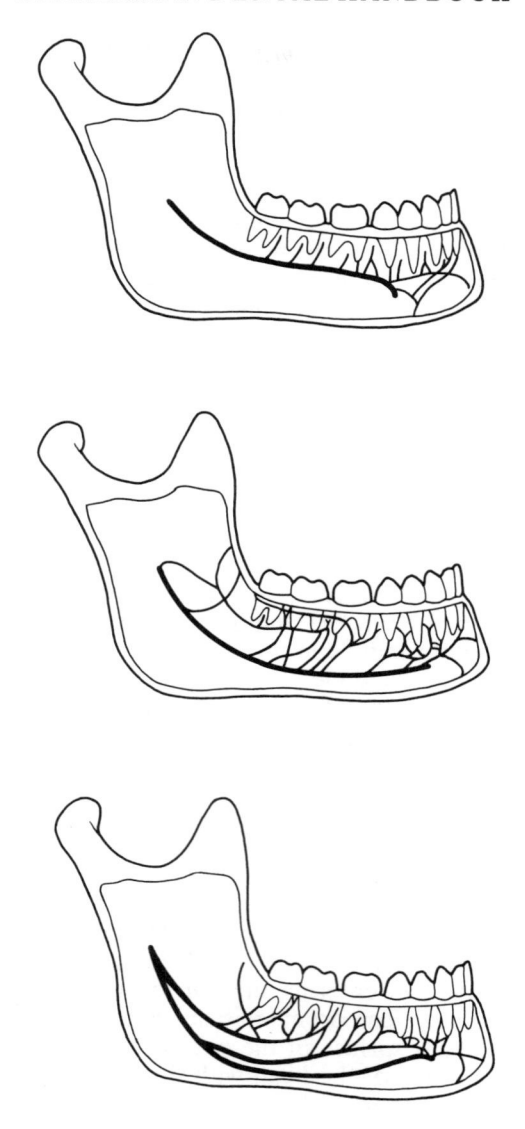

Fig. 3.4 *Variations in the course of the inferior alveolar nerve (modified after Carter R. B., Keen E. N. (1971). J. Anat.,* **103***, 433).*

4. Auricular branches (usually two) which supply the tragus and crus of the helix of the auricle, part of the external acoustic meatus, and the outer (lateral) surface of the tympanic membrane.

5. Superficial temporal branches which are cutaneous nerves supplying part of the skin of the temple.

The **lingual nerve** is the second branch of the posterior trunk of the mandibular nerve. It is essentially a sensory nerve but, following union with the chorda tympani branch of the facial nerve, it also contains parasympathetic fibres. Initially, the nerve lies on the tensor veli palatini muscle deep to the lateral pterygoid muscle. Here, the chorda tympani nerve (which has entered the infratemporal fossa via the petrotympanic fissure) joins the posterior surface of the lingual nerve. Emerging from the inferior border of the lateral pterygoid muscle, the lingual nerve curves downwards and forwards in the space between the ramus of the mandible and the medial pterygoid muscle (the pterygomandibular space). At this level, it lies anterior to, and slightly deeper than, the inferior alveolar nerve. This completes the course of the nerve in the infratemporal fossa. It then runs towards the floor of the mouth, passing downwards and forwards to lie close to the lingual alveolar plate of the mandibular third molar tooth. Before curving forwards into the tongue, the nerve is found above the origin of the mylohyoid muscle and lateral to the hyoglossus muscle. On the superficial surface of the hyoglossus muscle, the lingual nerve twists twice around the submandibular salivary duct, first on the lateral side of the duct and then on the medial side. It enters the tongue behind the sublingual salivary gland. Suspended from the lingual nerve as it runs across the hyoglossus muscle is the submandibular parasympathetic ganglion.

The lingual nerve itself supplies the mucosa covering the anterior two-thirds of the dorsum of the tongue (see Fig. 3.5), the ventral surface of the tongue, the floor of the mouth, and the lingual gingiva of the mandibular teeth.

The **chorda tympani branch of the facial nerve** is distributed through the lingual nerve and has two types of fibres. Sensory fibres are associated with taste to the anterior two-thirds of the tongue. Preganglionic, parasympathetic fibres pass to the submandibular parasympathetic ganglion in the floor of the mouth. Postganglionic fibres are secretomotor to the submandibular and sublingual glands.

The **inferior alveolar nerve** is the third branch of the posterior trunk of the mandibular nerve. Although it is essentially a sensory nerve, it also carries motor fibres which are given off as the mylohyoid nerve. Indeed, the mylohyoid nerve contains all the motor fibres of the posterior trunk of the mandibular nerve. The inferior alveolar nerve descends deep to the lateral pterygoid muscle, posterior to the lingual nerve. Here, it is crossed by the maxillary artery. On emerging at the inferior border of the muscle, it passes between the sphenomandibular ligament and the ramus of the mandible to enter the mandibular foramen.

The mylohyoid nerve is given off just before the mandibular foramen. It pierces the sphenomandibular ligament and runs in a groove (the mylohyoid groove) which lies immediately below the mandibular foramen. The mylohyoid nerve supplies the mylohyoid muscle and the anterior belly of the digastric.

The main distribution of the inferior alveolar nerve is to the mandibular teeth and their supporting structures but the course of the nerve through the mandible is variable (Fig. 3.4). The molar branches to the premolar and molar teeth come either directly from the inferior alveolar nerve in the mandibular canal by short or long branches, or indirectly from the nerve outside the mandibular canal by a series of alveolar branches. The mandibular canal may be closely related to the roots of the mandibular molars, even to the extent of occasionally perforating a root.

Table 3.1
Sensory innervation of the teeth and gingiva. The teeth are numbered according to their position along the tooth row

Maxilla	Nasopalatine nerve	Greater palatine nerve			Palatal gingiva
	Anterior superior alveolar nerve	Middle superior alveolar nerve		Posterior superior alveolar nerve	Teeth
	Infraorbital nerve	Posterior superior alveolar nerve and buccal nerve			Buccal gingiva
	1 2 3	4 5	6 7 8		
Mandible	Mental nerve	Buccal nerve and perforating branches of inferior alveolar nerve			Buccal gingiva
	Incisive nerve	Inferior alveolar nerve			Teeth
	Lingual nerve and perforating branches of inferior alveolar nerve				Lingual gingiva

The main trunk of the inferior alveolar nerve divides near the premolars into mental and incisive nerves. The mental nerve runs for a short distance in a mental canal before leaving the body of the mandible at the mental foramen to emerge on to the face. It supplies the skin and mucosa of the lower lip, and labial gingiva of the mandibular anterior teeth. The incisive nerve runs forwards in an incisive canal. This nerve usually innervates only the incisor and canine teeth, but occasionally it supplies the first premolar.

The sensory innervation of the teeth and gingiva (Figs. 3.1–3.4)

The dentition of the upper jaw is innervated almost entirely by branches of the maxillary nerve. The teeth are supplied by the anterior, middle and posterior superior alveolar branches. The palatal gingiva is innervated by the nasopalatine and greater (anterior) palatine branches via the pterygopalatine ganglion. The labial and buccal gingiva are supplied by the infraorbital and the posterior superior alveolar branches.

The dentition of the lower jaw is innervated by the mandibular nerve. The teeth receive their nerve supply from the molar and incisive branches of the inferior alveolar nerve. The lingual gingiva is supplied mainly by the lingual branch of the mandibular nerve. The labial gingiva is innervated by the mental branch of the inferior alveolar nerve and the buccal gingiva by the buccal branch of the mandibular nerve.

Table 3.1 summarizes the nerve supply to the teeth and gingiva.

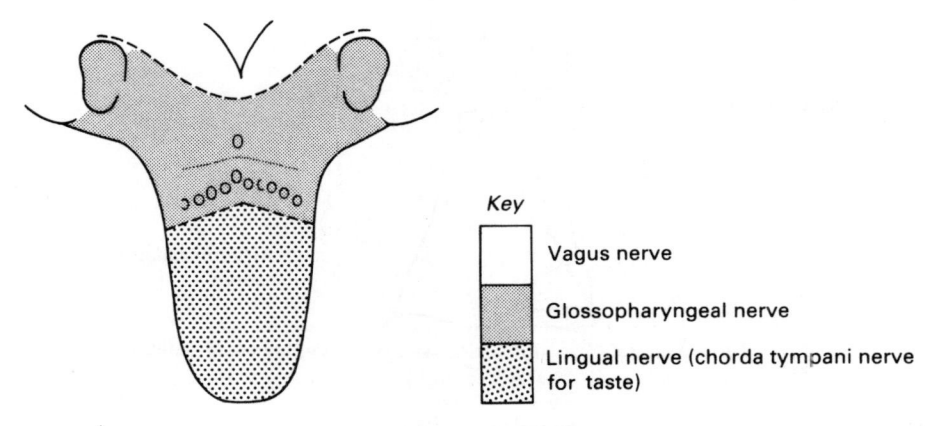

ESSENTIAL ANATOMY FOR GENERAL PRACTITIONERS 33

Fig. 3.5 *Sensory innervation of the dorsum of the tongue.*

Anaesthetic 'escape' may be the result of 'aberrant' innervations of the teeth. Indeed, there are reports that cervical spinal nerves or even the nerves to the musculature of the jaws may contribute to the dental nerve supply.

The sensory innervation of the lips and cheeks

The mucosa of the upper lip is supplied by the infraorbital branch of the maxillary nerve. The lower lip is innervated by the mental branch of the mandibular nerve.

The mucosa of the cheek is innervated by the buccal branch of the mandibular nerve.

The sensory innervation of the tongue and the floor of the mouth (Fig. 3.5)

Concerning general sensation (i.e. excluding taste), three distinct nerve fields can be recognized on the dorsum of the tongue. The anterior part of the tongue in front of the circumvallate papillae is supplied by the lingual branches of the mandibular nerves. Behind, and including, the circumvallate papillae, the tongue is innervated primarily by the glossopharyngeal nerves. Small areas on the posterior part of the tongue around the epiglottis are supplied by the superior laryngeal branches (internal branches) of the vagus nerves. Concerning taste, the anterior part of the tongue is innervated by the chorda tympani branches of the facial nerves. These are distributed through the lingual nerves. The posterior part of the tongue, including the circumvallate papillae, has a similar innervation for taste as that for general sensation.

The mucosa on the ventral surface of the tongue and on the floor of the mouth is supplied by the lingual branches of the mandibular nerves.

The sensory innervation of the palate (Fig. 3.6)

The sensory supply to the palate is derived mainly from branches of the maxillary nerve via the pterygopalatine ganglion. A small area behind the

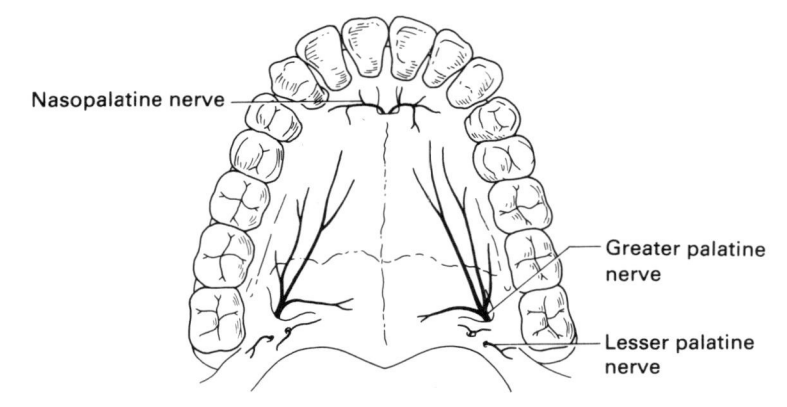

Fig. 3.6 *Sensory innervation of the palate.*

incisor teeth is supplied by the nasopalatine nerves. The remainder of the hard palate is innervated by the greater palatine nerves. The soft palate is supplied by the lesser palatine nerves. There is evidence to suggest that some areas supplied by the lesser palatine nerves may also be innervated from the facial nerves. The posterior part of the soft palate and the uvula may be supplied by the glossopharyngeal nerves.

THE LYMPHATIC DRAINAGE OF THE MOUTH (Fig. 3.7)

The lymphatic system consists of groups of lymph nodes connected by fine (capillary-like) lymph vessels. The system has two significant functions. First, it is an important component of the immunological system. Second, it provides a means whereby tissue fluid which has not returned to the circulation via the tissue's capillary bed can return via the lymphatic vessels. Knowledge of the lymphatic drainage of the mouth is of value clinically for an appreciation of the possible mode of spread of infections and tumours.

The principal sites of drainage of lymphatic vessels from the oro-dental tissues are the submental, submandibular, and jugulodigastric lymph nodes.

The submental nodes lie immediately beneath the chin, between the anterior bellies of the digastric muscles and on the mylohyoid muscle. Vessels from these nodes drain into either the jugulo-omohyoid group of the deep cervical chain of lymph nodes near the root of the neck or into the submandibular nodes.

The submandibular nodes are found close to (sometimes within) the submandibular salivary glands. Efferent vessels pass into the deep cervical lymph nodes.

The jugulodigastric nodes are a prominent group of nodes belonging to the deep cervical chain of lymph nodes. This chain is located on the carotid sheath of the neck and deep to the sternocleidomastoid muscle. As indicated by the name, the jugulodigastric part is situated close to the digastric muscle.

The lymph vessels from the teeth usually run directly into the submandibular lymph nodes on the same side. However, lymph from the mandibular anterior teeth drains into the submental lymph nodes. Occasionally, lymph from the molars may pass directly into the jugulodigastric group of nodes.

The lymph vessels of the labial and buccal gingiva of the maxillary and mandibular teeth drain into the submandibular nodes, although for the labial regions of the mandibular incisors they may drain into the submental lymph nodes. The lingual and palatal gingiva drain into the jugulodigastric group of nodes either directly, or indirectly through the submandibular nodes.

Lymphatics from the bulk of the palate terminate in the jugulodigastric group of nodes. Vessels from the posterior part of the soft palate terminate in pharyngeal lymph nodes.

Lymphatics from the anterior two-thirds of the tongue may be subdivided into two groups of vessels: marginal and central vessels. The marginal lymphatics drain the lateral third of the upper surface of the tongue and the lateral margin of its lower surface. The remaining regions drain into the central vessels. The marginal vessels pass to the submandibular lymph nodes of the same side. The vessels at the tip of the tongue pass to the submental lymph nodes. Central vessels behind the tip drain into ipsilateral and contralateral submandibular lymph nodes. Some marginal and central lymph vessels pass directly to the jugulodigastric group of nodes (or even the jugulo-omohyoid nodes). Lymphatics from the posterior third of the tongue drain into the deep cervical group of nodes, vessels centrally draining both ipsilaterally and contralaterally.

The reader must keep in mind that the above description of the lymphatic drainage of the mouth is only a consensus view of what in reality is a very variable system. Indeed, in a clinical situation all manner of modes of drainage and of interconnections between groups of lymph nodes are possible.

Protecting the entrance of the pharynx at the back of the mouth and nose is a

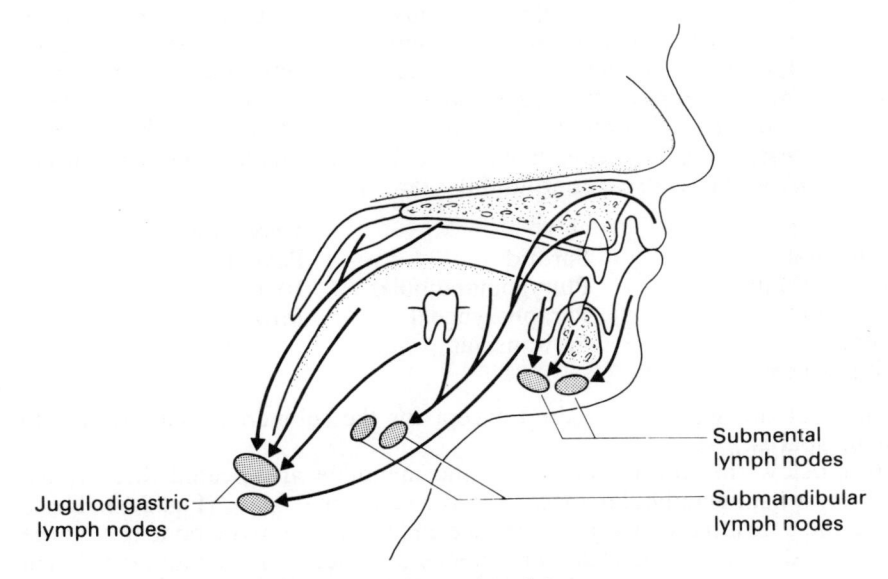

Fig. 3.7 *The lymphatic drainage of the orodental tissues.*

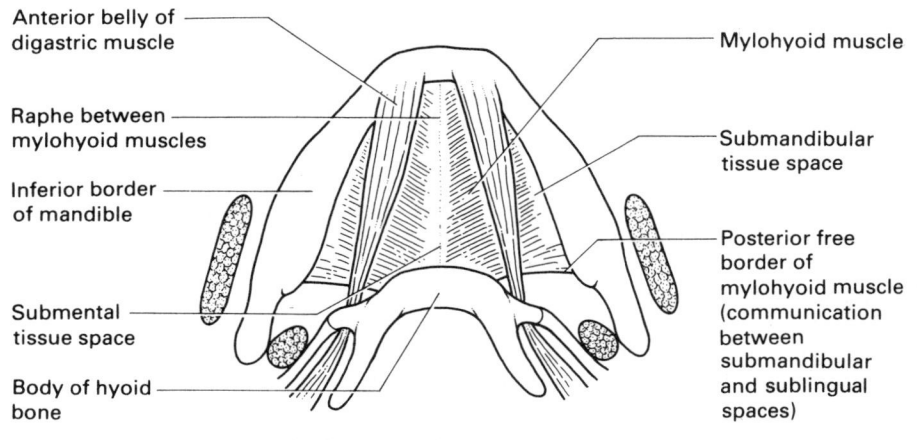

Fig. 3.8 *Tissue spaces in the floor of the mouth.*

ring of lymphoid tissue known as Waldeyer's tonsillar ring. At the oropharyngeal isthmus lie the palatine tonsils between the pillars of the fauces, and the lingual tonsils on the pharyngeal surface of the tongue. At the nasopharynx are the tubal tonsils and adenoids (pharyngeal tonsils).

THE TISSUE SPACES AROUND THE JAWS

The dissemination of infection in soft tissues is influenced by the natural barriers presented by bone, muscle and fascia. Around the jaws, however, the tissue spaces are primarily defined by muscles (principally the mylohyoid, buccinator, masseter, medial pterygoid, superior constrictor and orbicularis oris muscles). None of the 'spaces' are actually empty and they should be regarded merely as potential spaces which are normally occupied by loose connective tissue. It is only when such things as oedema, pus, bleeding or tumours destroy the loose connective tissue that a definable space is produced.

The potential tissue spaces around the jaws are:

Lower jaw		*Upper jaw*
Submental	Parotid	Palatal
Submandibular	Pterygomandibular	Facial
Sublingual	Parapharyngeal	Infratemporal
Buccal	Peritonsillar	
Submasseteric		

(Note that the spaces are paired except for the submental, sublingual and palatal spaces.)

Just below the inferior border of the mandible are located three tissue spaces: two submandibular spaces and the submental space (Fig. 3.8). These spaces lie beneath the mylohyoid muscle and above the hyoid bone (i.e. in the suprahyoid region of the neck). The submental space is found under the chin in the midline, between the mylohyoid muscles and the investing layer of deep cervical fascia. It is bounded laterally by the two anterior bellies of the digastric muscles. The submental space communicates posteriorly with the two submandibular spaces. The submandibular space is situated between the anterior and posterior bellies of the digastric muscle. It communicates with the sublingual space around the posterior free border of the mylohyoid muscle. Inflammation can spread into the submental and submandibular spaces from any of the mandibular teeth but for this to occur requires that the dental abscess lies below the attachment of the mylohyoid muscle on the mandible (the mylohyoid or internal oblique line). Should the abscess lie above the attachment of the muscle, it will spread into the sublingual space of the floor of the mouth. Spread of infection across the suprahyoid region is virtually unhindered but direct spread into the lower parts of the neck is to some extent prevented by the attachment of the investing layer of deep cervical fascia to the hyoid bone. Should the inflammation track backwards from the suprahyoid region, however, it may then spread to other parts of the neck by way of the pharyngeal spaces.

The sublingual space lies in the floor of the mouth, above the mylohyoid muscles. It is continuous across the midline and communicates with the submandibular spaces over the posterior free borders of the mylohyoid muscles. Thus, a sublingual abscess can spread directly from the mouth into the upper part of the neck. Note that the mylohyoid muscle is a barrier between the sublingual and suprahyoid (submental and submandibular) spaces and that the mode of spread of a dental abscess from a mandibular tooth depends upon the relationship between the root apex and the line of attachment of the muscle to the mandible.

The buccal space is located in the cheek, on the lateral side of the buccinator muscle (a region normally occupied by the buccal pad of fat). Thus, the buccinator muscle delineates the buccal space from the oral vestibule. Consequently, a dental abscess spreading externally from a posterior tooth (upper or lower) is quite likely to be restricted by the buccinator muscle to the buccal sulcus of the vestibule. Furthermore, the muscle has to be penetrated before a buccal/facial abscess appears. Alternatively, a more direct mode of spread into the buccal space will occur if the root apex of the tooth with an abscess lies beyond the attachments of the buccinator muscle on to the jaws.

Many of the tissue spaces around the jaws are situated in the retromandibular regions (Fig. 3.9). Should a dental abscess from a mandibular molar spread posteriorly towards the ramus of the mandible, it may track into the submasseteric spaces, the pterygomandibular space, the parotid space, or the para- and retropharyngeal spaces. If the abscess tracks within the pharynx (between the constrictor muscle layer and the mucosa), it can reach the peritonsillar space.

Between the lateral surface of the ramus of the mandible and the masseter muscle is a series of spaces called the submasseteric spaces. These spaces are formed because the fibres of the masseter muscle have multiple insertions on to the lateral surface of the ramus. For this reason, abscesses within the submasseteric spaces may present problems with respect to the attainment of proper drainage.

Between the medial surface of the ramus of the mandible and the medial pterygoid muscle lies the pterygomandibular space. This space is therefore

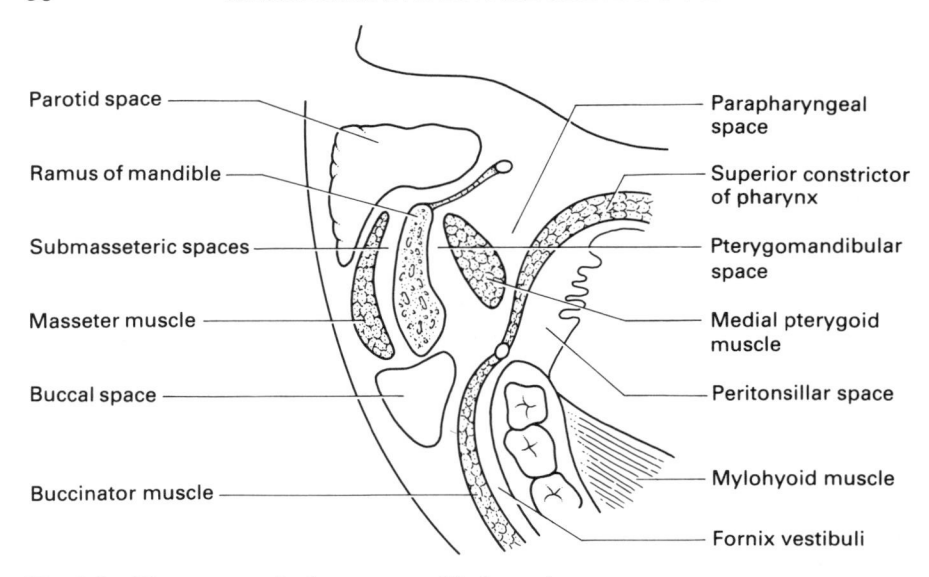

Fig. 3.9 *Tissue spaces in the retromandibular region.*

within the infratemporal fossa. A dental abscess from a molar spreading posteriorly into the infratemporal fossa can either track into the pterygomandibular space and/or into the pharyngeal spaces around the superior constrictor muscle of the pharynx (see below). The pterygomandibular space is delimited inferiorly from the upper part of the neck by the attachment of the medial pterygoid muscle to the inner surface of the angle of the mandible.

The parapharyngeal space is particularly prone to receiving infections from the jaws and teeth. It is found within the deep part of the infratemporal fossa, between the superior constrictor of the pharynx and the medial surface of the medial pterygoid muscle. (It is bounded superiorly by the base of the skull.) The parapharyngeal space, however, is not restricted to the infratemporal fossa of the head but continues inferiorly into the upper part of the neck. It also communicates with the retropharyngeal space behind the pharynx. It is the retropharyngeal space which continues down into the lower part of the neck and the thorax (by way of the retrovisceral space).

Beyond the ramus of the mandible and the infratemporal fossa is located the parotid space (in and around the parotid gland).

The peritonsillar space lies around the palatine tonsil between the pillars of the fauces. It is part of the intrapharyngeal space and is bounded by the inner surface of the superior constrictor of the pharynx and its mucosa. Infections in the peritonsillar space (quinsy) usually spread up or down the intrapharyngeal space, although it is possible for there to be spread through the wall of the pharynx and into the parapharyngeal space externally.

Around the upper jaw, the muscles of facial expression define a number of very small tissue spaces in the face. One such space is the canine fossa. This is located between the levator labii superioris muscle and the zygomaticus muscles.

There is no true tissue space in the hard palate as the mucosa there is firmly bound to the periosteum. However, inflammation can strip away some of this periosteum to produce a well-circumscribed palatal abscess.

The so-called infratemporal space is the upper extremity of the pterygomandibular space. It is closely related to the maxillary tuberosity and therefore the upper molars.

THE MAXILLARY PARANASAL AIR SINUSES

The paranasal air sinuses are invaginations from the lateral wall of the nose extending into the surrounding bones. There are four sets of paired paranasal sinuses: frontal, ethmoidal, sphenoidal and maxillary. The sinuses are lined by respiratory epithelium. There is considerable variation in the morphology of the sinuses from individual to individual, and between the sinuses of each side. The precise function of the paranasal sinuses is unknown, although some believe that they lighten the skull and add resonance to the voice. It is conceivable, however, that they simply reflect the considerable growth of the bones in which they are situated.

The maxillary air sinuses are the largest of the paranasal sinuses. They are situated in the bodies of the maxillary bones. Clinically, the root apices of some of the posterior maxillary teeth are closely related to the sinuses. Thus, extraction of a maxillary tooth may produce an oro-antral fistula through the floor of a sinus or a tooth fragment (possibly even a whole tooth) may be pushed into the sinus. A further clinical feature relates to the fact that the maxillary teeth share a sensory innervation with the mucosa of the maxillary sinus. Consequently, discomfort/pain associated with sinusitis may be referred to the teeth.

The maxillary sinus is pyramidal in shape. The base (medial wall) forms part of the lateral wall of the nose. The apex extends into the zygomatic process of the maxilla. The roof of the sinus is part of the floor of the orbit. The floor of the sinus is formed by the alveolar process and part of the palatine process of the maxilla. The anterior wall of the maxillary sinus is the facial surface of the maxilla and the posterior wall is the infratemporal surface of the maxilla. The sinus may be partially divided by incomplete bony septa.

The medial wall of the maxillary sinus has the opening (ostium) of the sinus. The roof has the infraorbital nerve and vessels within the infraorbital canal. The floor of the sinus lies below the level of the floor of the nose and is related to the roots of the cheek teeth. As the size of the sinus varies considerably, this relationship will also vary. Usually, at least the second premolar and first molar are related to the floor of the sinus. However, the sinus may extend anteriorly to the first premolar (and sometimes even to the canine) and posteriorly to the third molar tooth. The anterior superior alveolar nerve and vessels (which arise from the infraorbital nerve and vessels near the midpoint of the infraorbital canal) pass downwards in a fine canal (canalis sinuosus) in the anterior wall of the maxillary sinus, to be distributed to the anterior teeth. The posterior superior alveolar nerve and vessels pass through canals in the posterior surface of the sinus.

In an isolated maxillary bone, the ostium of the maxillary sinus is large. However, the ostium in an intact specimen is considerably reduced by portions of the adjacent bones (namely the perpendicular plate of the palatine bone, the uncinate process of the ethmoid bone, the inferior nasal concha and the lacrimal bone) and by the overlying nasal mucosa. The ostium lies high up at the back of the medial wall of the maxillary sinus, being unfavourably situated for drainage. It usually opens into the middle meatus of the lateral wall of the nose (via the posterior part of the ethmoidal infundibulum at the hiatus semilunaris). An accessory ostium is sometimes found behind the major ostium.

The innervation of the maxillary sinus is derived from the maxillary nerve via its infraorbital and posterior, middle and anterior superior alveolar branches. The arterial supply to the sinus is derived chiefly from the maxillary artery (via its posterior superior alveolar, anterior superior alveolar, infraorbital and greater palatine branches). The veins draining the sinus correspond to the arteries and pass to the facial vein or the pterygoid venous plexus.

Part Two
Child Dental Health

Chapter 4

Interceptive orthodontics

When the permanent incisors have erupted, at around 8–9 years of age, it will be possible for the dental practitioner to classify the occlusion on the basis of the incisor relationship and to estimate the degree of crowding present. At this stage a child may be diagnosed as having a class II, division 2 malocclusion with crowding in both arches, for example, which may prompt the question as to whether any measures could have been taken previously to prevent this from arising.

WHY DO TEETH ERUPT INTO THE POSITIONS THEY DO?

The crowns of erupted teeth are in a position of balance with respect to forces exerted by the lips and cheeks on the outside of the dental arch and by the tongue on the inside. Their apical position is determined by the basal bones of the jaws. Whether there is crowding or not will depend upon the combined mesiodistal widths of the teeth with respect to the length of the dental arch. These factors — the size, shape and relationship of the basal bones of the jaws and of the surrounding soft tissues — are, together with tooth size, genetically determined. The fact that a patient presents as having a class II, division 2 malocclusion with crowding in both arches, for example, was therefore decided at the moment of conception.

DOES MALOCCLUSION HAVE TO BE TREATED?

The reasons for treating malocclusion can be grouped under aesthetic and functional considerations.

Aesthetic considerations

Straight teeth look better than crooked teeth. This is the commonest reason for treating malocclusion. Parents like their children to have straight teeth and this attitude may well be more prevalent in some social groups and geographical locations than in others. However, are well aligned teeth likely to be more resistant to periodontal disease and caries? The evidence is contradictory. The Todd Report[1] on English and Welsh schoolchildren noted significantly more dental caries and gingival inflammation in children with crowded dentitions.

However, Dickson[2] found that loss of teeth, from whatever cause, is little affected by the degree of crowding when he compared a group of dentate over-65-year-olds with younger age groups.

Functional considerations

There are some relatively rare functional reasons for advising orthodontic treatment. The following conditions should be looked for:

1. *Traumatic overbite*. This condition arises in some class II, division 1 and division 2 cases when the overbite is deep enough to result in the gingival tissues being bitten into by opposing incisors and periodontal breakdown occurs. As periodontal destruction does not happen in every case and may not be apparent for several years it is better to advise parents that potentially traumatic overbites may not remain symptom-free and that treatment should be considered to eliminate the risk.

2. *Mandibular displacement on closure*. In most individuals the mandible remains in centric jaw relationship as it closes from the rest position into the intercuspal position. In a few individuals, however, one or more teeth erupting into abnormal positions interfere with this path of closure so that the mandible is subconsciously displaced to permit a more comfortable occlusion.

Intercuspal positions such as these are termed 'bites of convenience' or 'bites of accommodation' and the abnormal tooth contacts producing them are described as premature or initial contacts. A typical example of a bite of accommodation would be an individual having a narrow maxillary dental arch with respect to the mandibular and who instead of occluding the teeth in a cusp-to-cusp position displaces the mandible to one side to achieve a bite of accommodation in which a cusp-to-fossa occlusion is produced. The individual concerned would show mandibular displacement towards the side of the crossbite (Fig. 4.1).

Another commonly seen situation would be when an instanding maxillary lateral incisor, for example, erupts into an edge-to-edge position and where, in order to avoid contact with this tooth, the mandible displaces forwards so that when in occlusion the lateral incisor is seen to be in crossbite (Fig. 4.2).

The significance of displacement of the mandible on closure is that if left untreated it may lead to temporomandibular joint problems in later life.[3] In fact, whenever a tooth is seen to be in crossbite the patient should be carefully checked to see if there is mandibular displacement on closure. It is certainly possible to have a crossbite without associated displacement in which case there is no functional reason to treat the malocclusion. An anterior crossbite of this type should still be treated for aesthetic reasons though, but a posterior crossbite could be left alone.

THE TIMING OF ORTHODONTIC TREATMENT TO REDUCE AN OVERJET AND/OR RESOLVE CROWDING

The space required for these objectives will have to be provided for by the extraction of permanent teeth. First premolars are often the preferred choice as these teeth provide space close to where it is required. As maxillary canines need to be retracted first of all to provide space for incisor alignment it follows that treatment cannot start until first premolars and maxillary canines have erupted, at about 11–12 years of age.

THE IMPORTANCE OF RADIOGRAPHIC SCREENING IN THE EARLY MIXED DENTITION

First premolars would not be extracted for orthodontic purposes if other permanent teeth were developmentally absent, of abnormal form, grossly

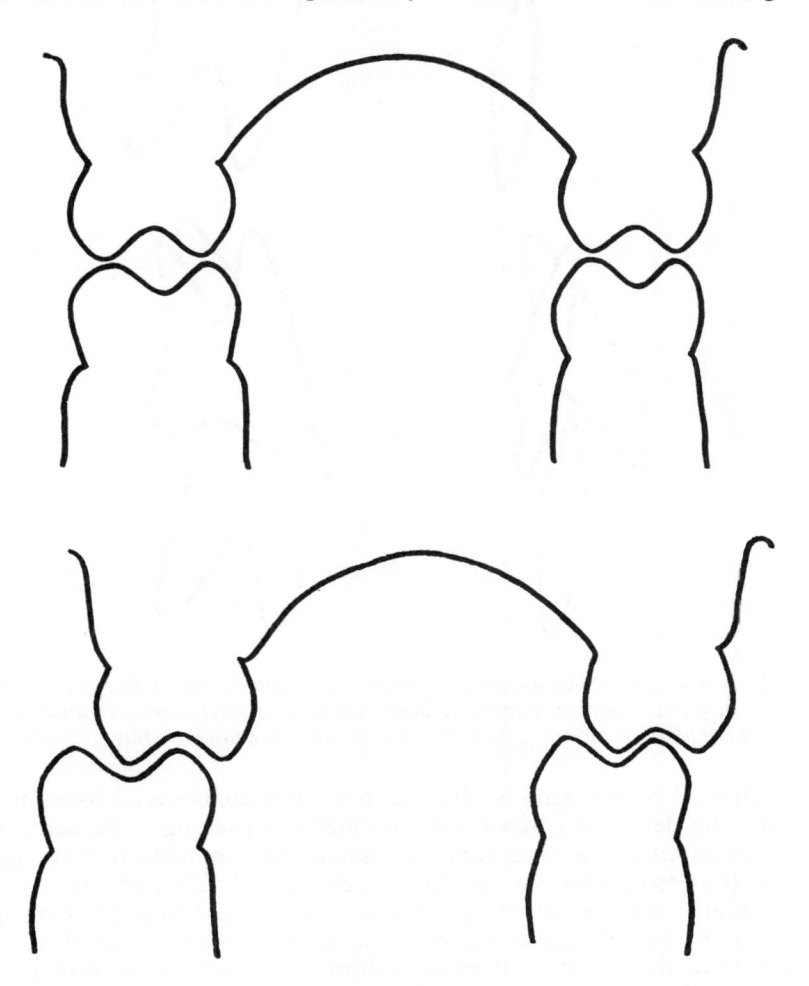

Fig. 4.1 *Top: Coronal section of a symmetrically narrow maxillary arch in which there is a 'cusp-to-cusp' occlusion at initial contact on closure from the rest position. Bottom: The mandible deviates to the right in order to produce a 'cusp-to-fossa' occlusion.*

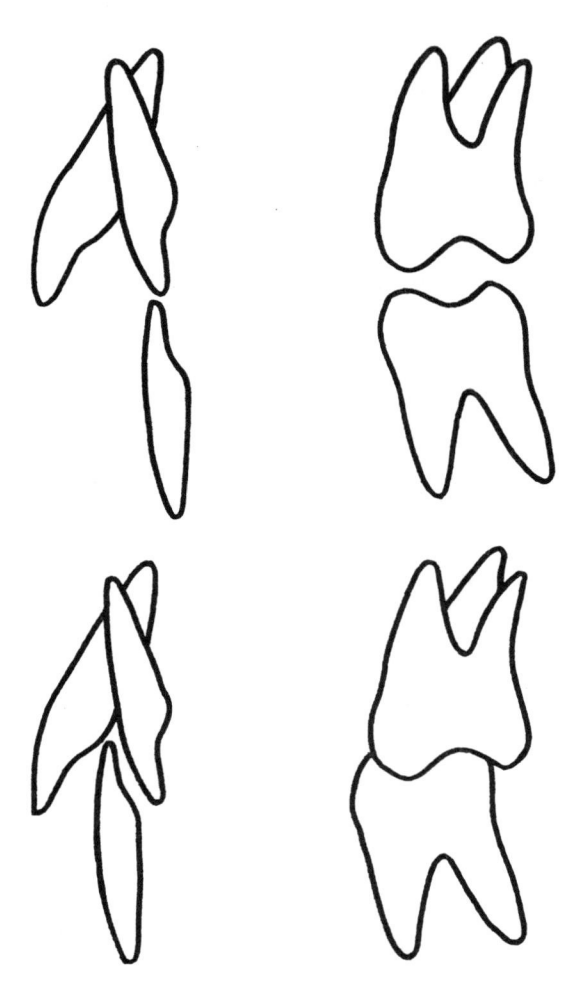

Fig. 4.2 *A palatally placed incisor gets in the way of the normal path of closure of the mandible. Bottom: The mandible is displaced forward to avoid this initial contact with the result that the affected incisor is now in crossbite when the jaws are fully occluded.*

displaced or of poor prognosis. 'Interceptive' orthodontics is all about making sure that the dentition is developing normally and taking steps, such as referring for advice at the correct time, if it is not. The dental practitioner is in the ideal position to monitor the developing dentition of child patients.

The number of permanent teeth present should be checked at 8 years of age by means of radiographs as a routine screening procedure. At this age all permanent teeth, with the exception of third molars, should be present in the jaws. The radiographs taken should be:

(a) orthopantomogram (OPG) or left and right lateral obliques;
(b) nasal occlusal.

The nasal occlusal radiograph is necessary because OPGs and lateral oblique radiographs cannot be relied upon to give accurate representation of the anterior teeth.

Radiographic examination must also be combined with clinical examination so that aberrations in dental development can be identified and acted on where appropriate. The more common aspects of interceptive orthodontics, as it affects the dental practitioner, will now be considered.

THE DECIDUOUS DENTITION

Clinical examination may reveal the presence of supplemental deciduous incisors or their developmental absence. Nothing need be done about these anomalies other than warning the parents that the same situation may arise in the permanent dentition and that this can be dealt with later.

If deciduous incisors are extracted because of caries then there is no need to undertake balancing extractions. In the case of unilateral loss of a deciduous canine or molar, however, then it is usual to 'balance' by also removing the contralateral tooth in order to preserve symmetry of crowding. This subject will be covered in greater detail in a later section.

THE MIXED DENTITION

This is the time when the dental practitioner must be on guard that the dentition is developing normally. As has been mentioned previously, routine radiographic screening should be undertaken at 8 years of age to check the number of permanent teeth present. The various regions of the mouth will now be covered.

1. Incisor region

(A) Non-eruption of maxillary permanent central incisors

It is useful to remember that the laterals are the last of the maxillary permanent incisors to erupt, at about 8–9 years of age. The clinician should therefore be suspicious if one or both deciduous central incisors are still present when the permanent lateral incisors have erupted. It is extremely rare for maxillary permanent central incisors to be developmentally absent but much more common for them to fail to erupt for the following reasons:

(i) *Presence of an unerupted blocking supernumerary tooth.* A nasal occlusal radiograph will reveal the presence of an unerupted, usually tuberculate, supernumerary in association with the crown of the unerupted incisor. Referral should be made so that a full orthodontic assessment can be carried out as teeth other than the supernumerary frequently need to be removed. For example, if there is insufficient space within the arch to accommodate the unerupted incisor then extraction of the two maxillary deciduous canines can also be carried out. Failure to do this will often result in the incisor remaining unerupted even though the blocking supernumerary has been removed.

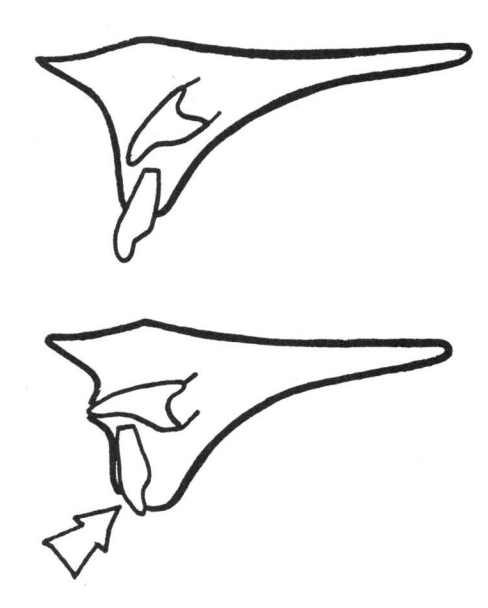

Fig. 4.3 *Top: At 4–6 years of age the crowns of the developing permanent maxillary central incisors are situated just superior to the apices of the deciduous incisors. Bottom: Trauma to the deciduous incisors at this stage that results in their intrusion may also produce dilaceration of the permanent incisors.*

Providing sufficient eruptive force remains and the tooth is not deeply placed then the blocked central incisor often erupts spontaneously following removal of the supernumerary. Prompt referral at 8 to 9 years of age is therefore beneficial. In older patients, or when the unerupted incisor is more deeply placed, an orthodontic appliance will need to be considered so as to bring the incisor down using gentle traction.

(ii) *Dilacerated maxillary central incisors.* Such teeth show an abnormal angulation between crown and root or within the root. The condition is usually consequent on trauma which succeeds in intruding the associated deciduous incisor into the alveolar process. The deciduous tooth may then re-erupt but the developing permanent incisor remains damaged (Fig. 4.3). Dilacerated incisors usually fail to erupt. Very rarely, where the deformation is minimal, these teeth can be brought down into the arch by orthodontic means. In the majority of cases, however, they need to be removed surgically. Refer for advice at 8 to 9 years of age.

(B) Avulsed maxillary central incisors

Re-implantation can be successful providing it is done quickly. Such teeth will need to be splinted for about 10 days and endodontic treatment undertaken if required. Check also, clinically and radiographically, that the neighbouring teeth haven't been damaged too.

Even if root resorption occurs, the re-implanted tooth may last for several years and act as a space maintainer until it has to be replaced by a partial denture or a bridge.

If the re-implanted tooth becomes ankylosed it will not be possible to move it by orthodontic means. Should orthodontic treatment be required later, to reduce an overjet, for example, then refer the patient for advice at that stage, as the extraction of the tooth concerned will have to be considered as part of an overall treatment plan.

(C) Traumatic loss of maxillary central incisors

Careful observation and questioning are essential.

1. Is there any chance that the tooth could have been inhaled? Refer for radiography of the chest if concerned.
2. Could any tooth fragments be embedded in an associated lip injury?
3. Has only the crown been lost and yet the root remains in situ?
4. Have any other teeth been damaged?

When an incisor has been traumatically lost a decision has to be made on whether the space should be maintained by a partial denture or allowed to close down.

For aesthetic reasons it is obviously better to have a normal complement of teeth in the maxillary incisor region. Hence, a partial denture should be provided to maintain the space, particularly if it is felt that the patient's oral hygiene and dental awareness are good enough to cope with this.

An acrylic partial denture can be retained on the maxillary first permanent molars and should have short metal stops placed mesial to the incisors, immediately adjacent to the one that has been lost (Fig. 4.4). This precaution will ensure that the space is maintained should the denture tooth break off. It is essential that the partial denture is provided *as soon as possible* after the accident because space closure can be very rapid. A more robust partial denture or some form of adhesive bridgework can be provided when the patient is older.

If orthodontic treatment is required for these patients later on, then they should be referred for advice at the appropriate time so that a decision can be made on whether the space should be maintained throughout treatment or closed down.

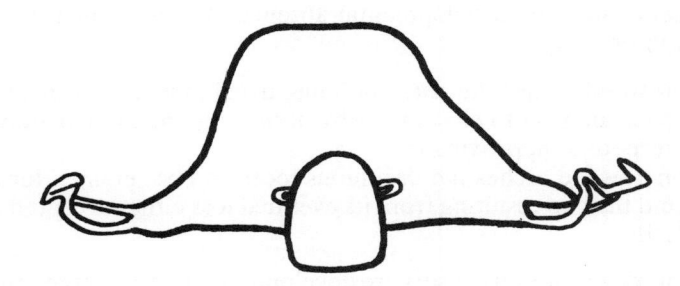

Fig. 4.4 *A single-tooth denture used as a space maintainer. Short metal spurs should be included to contact the teeth on either side in order to ensure that there would be no space loss if the denture tooth breaks off.*

(D) The effects of digit sucking

Digit sucking is common amongst young children. Its effect on the developing dentition will depend on its duration and intensity. Typically, some degree of anterior open bite and increase in overjet is produced. The malformation caused is local in extent and restricted to the dento-alveolar structures. Once the habit stops the incisors show a strong tendency to erupt and align spontaneously. The younger the patient the more rapid and complete is this self-correction.

Should any measures be taken to dissuade thumb suckers in the mixed dentition? Two factors need to be considered.

1. Children will not give up the habit if they don't want to. In fact, some of them obviously derive great psychological comfort from it.
2. Any prolonged orthodontic treatment in the mixed dentition to deter digit sucking is almost certain to encroach upon the 2 years or so of orthodontic goodwill that most patients are prepared to give and which may well be required in the permanent dentition proper — for example, to reduce an overjet.

There is no point in fitting an appliance to break the habit in the early mixed dentition. A possible exception to this advice would be those children having unilateral posterior crossbite with lateral displacement on closure — a commonly associated finding with digit suckers — and who are keen to break the habit. An appliance provided to correct the crossbite at this stage will also work to deter the digit.

If the habit continues until the eruption of the first premolars and maxillary canines, and if orthodontic treatment is to be carried out to reduce an overjet, then the habit will often cease when the appliance is fitted. The open bite usually resolves spontaneously as the overjet is reduced.

Open bites maintained by digit sucking until the teenage years often do not fully resolve if the habit ceases then. In cases such as these fixed appliances would be required to extrude the affected upper incisors to the required level.

(E) Developmental absence of maxillary lateral incisors

As a general rule, the developmental absence of a permanent tooth can be managed in two ways:

1. In crowded arches the corresponding deciduous tooth can be extracted and the space allowed to close, thereby permitting the immediately adjacent permanent teeth to approximate.
2. In uncrowded arches the deciduous tooth can be retained for as long as possible and the gap resulting from its eventual loss either accepted or treated prosthetically.

When maxillary lateral incisors are developmentally absent the canines often develop more mesially. Interceptive treatment should aim to encourage eruption of the canines immediately adjacent to the central incisors.

In crowded cases the extraction of all four deciduous canines and maxillary deciduous lateral incisors should be considered. Crowding in the maxillary arch will be treated, in effect, by the absence of the lateral incisors. In the mandibular arch, crowding will become concentrated in the canine region and can be resolved later by the extraction of first premolars. Prospective cases should be referred for confirmatory advice in the early mixed dentition, unless the practitioner is experienced.

Those cases having unilateral absence of a maxillary lateral incisor are often best treated by including the extraction of the contralateral tooth in order to be able to produce a symmetrical appearance eventually. This recommendation particularly applies to those cases where the lateral incisor to form is microdont.

Cases having spacing in the maxillary incisor region may well have enough room for the permanent canines to erupt mesial to the deciduous canines. In such cases the extraction of the maxillary deciduous lateral incisors should be done so as to encourage the eruption of the canines into more mesial positions. If further space is required at a later date—to reduce an overjet, for example—extraction of the deciduous canines can be carried out then.

Cases having developmental absence of maxillary lateral incisors show an increased likelihood of canines becoming palatally displaced.[4] The timely extraction of deciduous teeth, as mentioned above, has additional use in encouraging the eruption of maxillary canines into the line of the arch.

(F) Supplemental maxillary lateral incisors

These teeth are erupted supernumeraries and are produced by splitting of the lateral incisor tooth germ. The patient will thus present with two lateral incisors in the quadrant concerned.

A supplemental maxillary lateral incisor will increase crowding locally and, if not removed, would make later orthodontic treatment more difficult, as the excess of tooth widths in this region would hinder the satisfactory alignment of the maxillary arch around the mandibular.

Very rarely, a supplemental lateral incisor may be found in a well-aligned arch. Presumably the arch would have been spaced without it! In these cases the supplemental tooth can be left in place. With most cases, however, there will be a local increase in crowding. In these situations the 'extra' tooth should be removed in the early mixed dentition so as to encourage satisfactory approximation of the adjacent permanent teeth.

When confronted with two maxillary right lateral incisors, for example, the clinician would generally want to retain the more mesial of the two, particularly if its size, position and shape are acceptable. If the mesial tooth, however, is chosen for removal because the distal tooth is of better size and shape, there will still be a tendency for the latter to come to the mesial spontaneously. If this improvement is incomplete then appliance therapy would need to be considered later, usually in the permanent dentition proper.

Before extracting a supplemental tooth it is important to check with intraoral radiographs and digital pressure that the roots are not in fact fused! If this is found to be so, then the patient is better referred for specialist advice so that the possible loss of the fused teeth can be considered as part of an overall treatment plan.

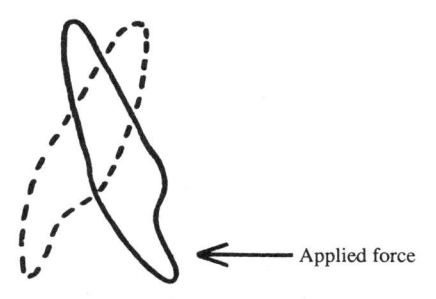

Fig. 4.5 *When the crown of an instanding maxillary incisor is pushed labially then the apex will move palatally. There should be no obstruction to this movement.*

(G) One or more incisors in crossbite

If at least one incisor has a positive overbite and overjet then it would seem reasonable to suppose that those incisors in crossbite would be stable if moved labially to similar positions. Treatment for these cases can be carried out during the mixed dentition. Check first of all, though:

1. *Is the case crowded?* Space can be created in crowded cases by the extraction of the four deciduous canines. This action will transfer crowding to the canine region where it can be treated later, following the eruption of first premolars.

2. *What about the position of the unerupted maxillary canines?* Crossbite correction on maxillary lateral incisors will be hindered and may relapse if the crowns of unerupted canines are more mesially placed than normal and overlie the coronal portion of the lateral incisor roots. Such canine crowns will be palpable labially. Crossbite correction for these cases should be delayed until the permanent dentition proper, when treatment can be started to retract the canines first of all.

Crossbite correction on maxillary incisors will be hindered if the apices of these teeth cannot move palatally as their crowns are tipped labially (Fig. 4.5). Palatally placed canines can provide such an obstruction, as can some unerupted supernumerary teeth. It is essential to take a periapical or nasal occlusal radiograph, if not done previously as a screening procedure, in order to make sure that neither of these obstructions is present. Offending supernumeraries would need to be removed before the crossbite is corrected. The management of palatally placed canines will be considered in a later section.

3. *Are the apices of any maxillary lateral incisors in crossbite palatally placed?* If this is so then ideally these lateral incisors would need to be moved labially in a bodily fashion, so that their apices finish treatment within the line of the arch. If removable appliances are used in such cases, then the crowns of the lateral incisors would be tipped labially with the result that they will be excessively proclined at the end of treatment and may, in fact, have little or no overbite (Fig. 4.6). If there is no overbite, then relapse is likely.

Cases such as these are therefore better treated with fixed appliances in the permanent dentition proper rather than with removable appliances in the mixed dentition.

4. *Is there a forward displacement on closure?* This will occur when the patient occludes as a premature contact in centric relation against the tip of an instanding incisor and then displaces the mandible forward to obtain the intercuspal position.

As to whether these cases can be treated orthodontically it doesn't matter if there is a forward displacement or not. As has been mentioned previously, as long as at least one maxillary incisor has a positive overbite and overjet, then the other incisors will be stable if aligned in similar positions. Treatment is easier, however, in those cases where there is a forward displacement as the incisors to be aligned start off in edge-to-edge occlusion and hence do not need much labial movement.

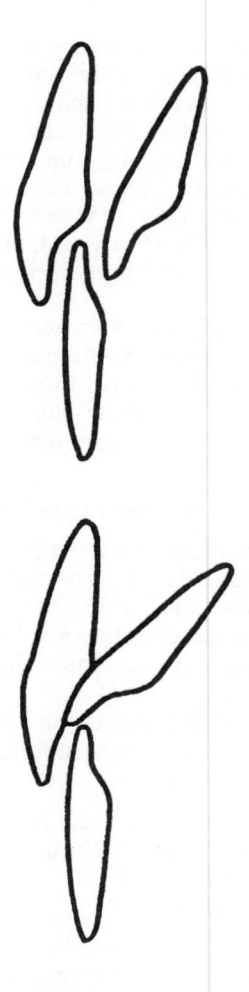

Fig. 4.6 *Top: An instanding maxillary lateral incisor in which the apex is palatally placed. Bottom: If tipping movements are used, then the lateral incisor would be excessively proclined after treatment and there would also be marked reduction of the overbite.*

It should be noted that those cases in which there is a forward displacement on closure will show a greater overjet at the end of treatment on those teeth that had a positive overjet at the start. This is because there is no need for the mandible to displace forwards after the crossbite has been corrected. Any increase in overjet will be proportional to the amount of forward displacement originally present and is usually small.

Those cases having all incisors in crossbite are not always orthodontically treatable and, even if they are, are often better treated in the permanent dentition proper. This aspect is covered more fully in Chapter 5.

(H) Mesiodens

A mesiodens is a conical supernumerary tooth which develops close to the midline between the maxillary central incisors. They can occur singly or in pairs and may, in some cases, be inverted, such that they will remain unerupted and only be discovered during routine radiographic screening. Those that develop pointing towards the mouth usually erupt during childhood and produce a median diastema between the central incisors and/or their mesiolabial rotation. It isn't usual for a mesiodens to prevent the eruption of a central incisor.

Erupted mesiodens should be removed. Unfortunately self-correction of the displaced central incisors is often disappointing and appliance therapy becomes necessary.

An inverted mesiodens may cause no occlusal problems and for this reason could be left alone. The situation would need to be reviewed, however, if its continued presence would hinder any future orthodontic treatment — overjet reduction, for example. In these situations advice should be obtained before starting treatment to align the maxillary incisors.

(I) Abnormally large fraenum of the upper lip

A thick fleshy fraenum extending between the maxillary central incisors to the incisive papilla can reasonably be expected to be the cause of a median maxillary diastema in those cases where there is no spacing elsewhere in this arch. In other words, the fraenum acts as an obstruction in the absence of which there would have been mesial movement of the buccal segments to produce an unspaced arch.

Parents are often concerned about the large space between the central incisors. However, it is important to note that there are other causes of maxillary incisor spacing, for example:

(a) developmentally absent or conical lateral incisors;
(b) generalized spacing of the dentition because teeth are small;
(c) grossly proclined incisors;
(d) an unerupted mesiodens.

A median maxillary diastema can also be present in the mixed dentition only to close down when maxillary canines erupt. In order to avoid needless surgery, possible candidates for fraenectomy (see Chapter 49) should therefore have permanent canines erupted and no spacing distal to the central incisors.

Some spontaneous closure of the diastema will occur after fraenectomy in cases such as these, but appliance therapy is often required to complete it. Also, partial relapse is likely to occur after appliance removal unless some form of long-term retention is employed.

Other reasons for carrying out a fraenectomy are those cases where the fraenum itself is unsightly or is impeding tooth brushing.

(J) A developmentally absent mandibular central incisor

It often occurs that when permanent teeth are developmentally absent there is a tendency for those that form to be small. As a result of this the arches may well be spaced. In the case of a developmentally absent mandibular central incisor the deciduous predecessor will then persist with spacing between it and the adjacent permanent incisors.

This spacing is present because mesial drift of the buccal segments has not closed it down and would be even greater if the deciduous incisor was removed. There is therefore no point in extracting the retained deciduous tooth at this time in the hope of obtaining spontaneous space closure. Its extraction in the permanent dentition proper may be considered, however, as part of an overall orthodontic treatment plan in which appliance therapy, usually fixed, can be used to obtain tooth movement.

Those cases where there happens to be a developmentally absent permanent incisor in an otherwise crowded mandibular arch will usually take care of themselves. In these situations there will be resorption of all the deciduous incisors with the result that these patients present later with three permanent incisors in reasonable alignment. The absent incisor has therefore resolved the crowding to a greater or lesser extent. This in itself is helpful but should tempt the dental practitioner to refer for advice later if orthodontic treatment is considered, in view of the potential difficulty in aligning the maxillary incisors satisfactorily around the mandibulars when one of the latter is absent.

(K) A supplemental mandibular incisor

A patient may present with an additional erupted mandibular incisor the effect of which is usually to increase crowding locally.

If the mandibular arch happens to be well aligned in spite of the extra incisor, a rare finding, then nothing further need be done at this time. Any future orthodontic treatment to align the teeth in the maxillary arch, however, will require careful planning in view of the extra incisor in the mandibular. Specialist advice is useful at that stage.

In crowded cases the extra incisor can be extracted in the early mixed dentition in order to obtain some spontaneous improvement in the alignment of the remaining incisors. The decision as to which incisor to remove is easy in those cases where the tooth concerned is totally excluded from the line of the arch. Other cases aren't so straightforward. If in doubt, then refer for specialist advice.

(L) Serial extraction

Parents often ask whether any treatment can be done to resolve the crowding of their child's recently erupted permanent incisors. The resolution of crowding usually has to await the eruption of the first premolars. However, in very carefully selected cases, the technique of serial extraction can be commenced at about 8 years of age when the mandibular lateral incisors are erupting. Serial extraction can produce good results where:

1. There is a class 1 occlusion with mild crowding in both arches.
2. None of the permanent incisors is rotated.
3. The first premolars are developmentally ahead of the canines as shown on radiograph.
4. The first permanent molars have a good prognosis.
5. All permanent teeth, with the possible exception of third molars, are present.

The procedure for suitable cases is as follows:

1. The four deciduous canines are extracted when the mandibular lateral incisors are erupting so that incisor crowding can resolve at the expense of space for the permanent canines.
2. One year later the four deciduous first molars are then extracted to ensure that the first premolars erupt in advance of the canines. This stage may be omitted if the deciduous first molars are close to exfoliation.
3. Lastly, the four first premolars are extracted in order to provide space for erupting canines. These extractions are usually done no later than when the mandibular canines start to erupt so as to prevent these teeth from being forced buccally.

This sequence sounds very elegant in theory but in practice it is often found that the desired spontaneous tooth movements do not occur; for example, canines may erupt before first premolars. In some situations mesial movement of the buccal segments may be so rapid that appliances are required to maintain the space for erupting canines. For any particular patient this form of treatment should be chosen with care and, unless the dental practitioner is experienced, referral of the patient for confirmatory advice is essential. The alternative to serial extraction is to delay treatment for the relief of crowding until the permanent dentition proper.

(M) Exfoliation of a deciduous canine by an erupting permanent lateral incisor

If this occurs unilaterally there will be a marked shift of the centre line to the affected side. As symmetrical crowding is so much easier to treat, it would be wise to permit some spontaneous correction of the centre line by removing the contralateral deciduous canine.

(N) Lingually erupting mandibular permanent central incisors

In these situations the deciduous incisors will be retained but may be loosening. If this is the case, then the patient should be encouraged to work the loose incisors out for him- or herself, after which the tongue will then be able to mould the permanent incisors labially into a better position.

In those cases where the retained deciduous incisors are firm, their extraction will need to be considered. As a general anaesthetic is often required at this age, it would be wise to consider whether the patient would also benefit from the removal of other deciduous teeth. Clinicians should ask themselves whether the loss of both deciduous central incisors will provide enough space to accommodate both permanent central incisors. In crowded cases it is often better to extract all four deciduous incisors and, occasionally, both deciduous canines as well. The resulting canine crowding can always be treated in the permanent dentition proper.

2. Canine region

Canine teeth are developmentally absent only very rarely. Their main problem is that they can erupt ectopically, particularly in the maxillary arch.

Maxillary permanent canines usually erupt at 11–12 years of age and, if developing normally, should be palpable buccally a year or two beforehand. Maxillary deciduous canines should therefore be loosening and permanent canines be palpable buccally when first premolars are erupting. The clinician should be particularly wary of asymmetry: for example, if a maxillary left deciduous canine is retained and firm at 12 years of age, say, and yet the maxillary right permanent canine is erupted.

With the use of digital palpation and intraoral parallax radiographs it will be possible to determine whether the crown of the ectopic permanent canine is palatally placed or situated high and labial to the lateral incisor root. The angulation of the lateral incisor can also provide useful information as its root may be displaced somewhat by the unerupted canine.

(A) The treatment of misplaced canines

Generally speaking, there are two ways of dealing with this problem:

1. *Align the permanent canine.* The deciduous canine will need to be removed and the permanent canine surgically uncovered. After this the permanent canine can be aligned by orthodontic means. In many cases, however, additional space will need to be created orthodontically in order to accommodate the larger permanent canine.

Treatments such as these often require the use of fixed appliances and may take 2 years or so to complete. A variation would be to reposition the permanent canine surgically and thereby reduce treatment time. Preliminary orthodontic treatment would still be required in most of these cases, however, in order to produce the correct amount of space in the arch for the permanent canine. Also, the prognosis of the transplanted tooth may be less good than if it had been aligned orthodontically.

2. *Retain the deciduous canine.* In these situations consideration should be given to surgically removing the permanent canine rather than leaving it buried.

The advantage of retaining the deciduous canine is that no orthodontic treatment is involved. However, the obvious disadvantage is that the deciduous tooth may not last a great number of years before it exfoliates. Nevertheless, some patients and parents prefer this option because they are not committed to lengthy treatment, and hence will need to be made aware that the space resulting from the later exfoliation of the deciduous canine will either have to be accepted or treated prosthodontically.

Are there situations where it would be safe to leave a misplaced canine in situ? This course of action would be reasonable only if the clinician could be absolutely sure that continued presence of the canine would not result in pathology, such as resorption of upper incisor root apices. Obviously one would be less confident if the crown of the permanent canine was close to incisor apices in a 13-year-old, say, when compared with the chance finding of an identical situation in a 40-year-old and in whom no resorption has occurred.

The author's own view is that misplaced canines in young people still have reasonable eruptive potential and hence are better removed if they happen to be close to incisor root apices. An exception would be where the root apices are not at risk because the canine is more deeply buried. In any case, its removal from situations such as these is often more difficult anyway.

(B) The problem of late referral

The alignment of misplaced canines is better carried out by the orthodontic specialist rather than the dental practitioner, unless he or she is experienced. A major problem, though, is that many ectopic canines are referred too late for the patient to still be willing to accept what is often lengthy treatment to align them. Because of this limitation the treatment of choice for many 14-year-olds and older is often to keep matters as simple as possible by retaining the deciduous canine—particularly if it is firm—and extracting the permanent canine.

(C) The value of interception

Routinely palpating the labial sulcus for maxillary permanent canines at 10 years of age and taking parallax radiographs if in doubt will result in the earlier detection of misplaced teeth. In such cases the extraction of the associated deciduous canine will, at this time, encourage improvement in the path of eruption of the permanent canine. Many then erupt into their proper position. For those that don't then surgical uncovering and orthodontic alignment can be considered at an age when the patient would be more willing to go along with it.

(D) The fate of maxillary deciduous canines when their successors are ectopically placed — a summary

1. *Extraction*. This should be carried out if ectopic permanent canines are detected early, at 10–11 years of age. Parents should still be warned, however, that uncovering and orthodontic alignment will be required if this measure fails.

In older patients spontaneous improvement in the position of the permanent canine is less likely to occur and hence the loss of the deciduous canine should be considered only as part of a course of orthodontic treatment involving appliance therapy to align the permanent tooth.

2. *Retention.* Older patients may be unwilling to wear orthodontic appliances to align a misplaced permanent canine, in which case the deciduous canine should be retained.

3. Premolar region

Commonly found problems in this region of the mouth include developmentally absent second premolars and submerging deciduous molars. Consideration must also be given to the management of those cases in which one or more deciduous molars and/or canines are to be removed because of caries.

(A) Developmentally absent second premolars

Any permanent tooth can fail to form and, after third molars, this condition most frequently affects second premolars. Their absence can complicate orthodontic treatment and, generally speaking, the earlier that this is known of the better. Routine radiographic screening at 8 years of age will enable affected cases to be identified and referred for advice at that time. Subsequent management will depend upon the presence or absence of crowding and on whether the incisor relationship will need treatment in due course.

1. *Uncrowded cases.* If extractions were undertaken in uncrowded arches, then large residual spaces would remain that would be unlikely to close down spontaneously. This would be particularly true if the arches were spaced. Cases such as these with developmentally absent second premolars would therefore be rather worse off if associated second deciduous molars were to be extracted. The latter teeth should therefore be retained particularly if the incisor relationship is class I.

With class II, division 1 or division 2 cases there is the option of extracting second deciduous molars with absent successors at the start of orthodontic treatment to align maxillary incisors. In the case of absent maxillary second premolars then this action will provide space for incisor alignment, although fixed appliances are usually necessary to produce satisfactory contact points between first premolars and first permanent molars. If mandibular second premolars are absent, then the orthodontist at least has the option of considering the loss of the second deciduous molars and of using fixed appliances incorporating intermaxillary traction to align maxillary incisors (Fig. 4.7). A system such as this would have the reciprocal effect of bringing mandibular first permanent molars mesially and thereby closing down residual space.

Similarly, with class III cases the developmental absence of mandibular second premolars need not inconvenience treatment as the extraction of the associated second deciduous molars would provide space for retroclination of mandibular incisors (Fig. 4.8). Also, the space resulting from the extraction of maxillary second deciduous molars when their successors are absent could be closed down by mesial movement of maxillary first permanent molars if intermaxillary traction is used to retrocline the mandibular incisors.

It will be appreciated that the treatments outlined above are complex and are better carried out by specialists using fixed appliances.

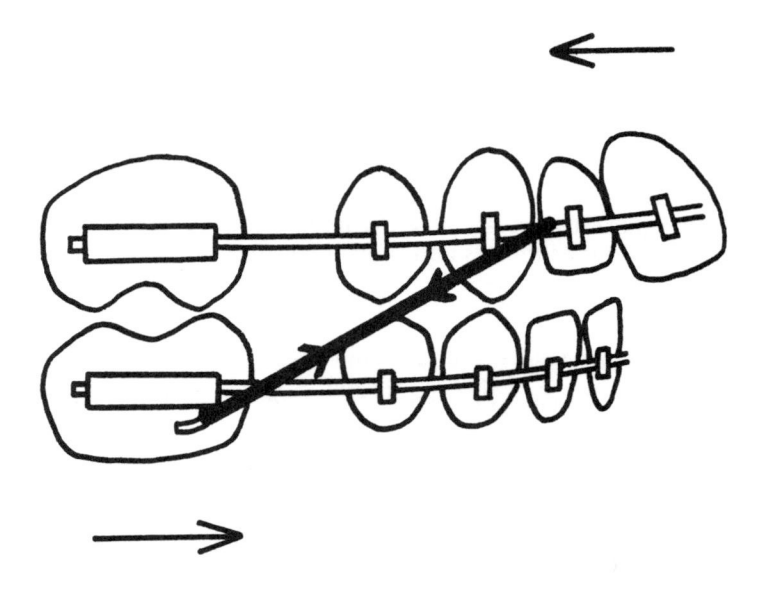

Fig. 4.7 *By using intermaxillary traction it would be possible to bring mandibular first permanent molars mesially whilst reducing an overjet.*

2. *Crowded cases.* The extraction of second deciduous molars having no successors will provide space for alleviation of crowding. If extractions are carried out when first premolars have erupted, then fixed appliances would be required to produce satisfactory contact points between these teeth and the first permanent molars. Their extraction in the early mixed dentition, however, often results in the spontaneous production of a satisfactory contact point. Early referral can therefore considerably simplify treatment for crowded cases. Some cases go better than others, however, and the following points should be borne in mind:

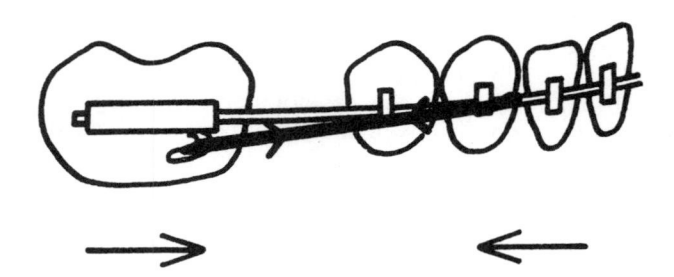

Fig. 4.8 *Mandibular first permanent molars will come mesially if used as anchorage to retrocline mandibular incisors.*

(a) **The degree of crowding** needs to be moderate rather than severe. Suitable cases would be those where not all of the space produced by the extraction of second deciduous molars was required to resolve crowding and hence first permanent molars can be permitted to come mesially to take up the residual space. A typical example would be a class I case with moderate crowding in both arches and having developmental absence of both mandibular second premolars, for example. Following confirmatory advice, all second deciduous molars could be extracted in the early mixed dentition, thereby alleviating crowding and permitting first permanent molars to come mesially. In the maxillary arch, crowding would be transferred to the second premolar region and can be resolved by extracting these teeth when they erupt palatally. Any residual spaces would then be at opposing sites, which improves the chances of further space closure, there being no unopposed teeth to over-erupt.

With severely crowded cases all of the space resulting from extraction of second deciduous molars will be required for the alleviation of crowding. It is therefore important that first permanent molars do not come mesially. In such cases it is better to delay extractions until the eruption of first premolars and canines. Fixed appliances can then be used to align crowded teeth whilst preventing first permanent molars from coming mesially. An alternative method, favoured by some, would be to fit space maintainers before extracting second deciduous molars in the mixed dentition. The appliances used would certainly be simpler but the outcome of treatment would be less certain. Furthermore, appliances would still need to be regularly maintained over what may well be a longer overall treatment time.

(b) **The need for active appliance therapy:** an 'extraction only' treatment will alleviate crowding to a greater or lesser extent but do nothing to align rotated teeth, reduce an overjet or correct a crossbite. As fixed appliances are necessary to treat rotated teeth, it is probably better in these cases to delay the extraction of second deciduous molars until first premolars and canines have erupted. Fixed appliances can then be used to produce satisfactory contact points between first premolars and first permanent molars at the same time as aligning any rotated incisors.

The same reasoning would also apply if fixed appliances were required for other purposes. These would include the application of maxillary incisor root torque to treat deep overbites in class II, division 2 cases. Also, the reduction of an overjet by means of bodily movement of the maxillary incisors rather than tipping in some class II, division 1 cases.

The treatment of cases having one or two incisors in crossbite is usually done in the mixed dentition, and the developmental absence of one or more second premolars need not delay this. Whilst the extraction of deciduous canines is often required to provide space for crossbite correction, the loss of second deciduous molars with absent successors should also be considered to provide space for resolution of crowding. Needless to say, unless the practitioner is experienced, specialist advice should be sought.

3. *The importance of specialist advice.* It must be stressed that in a book such as this it is not possible to give detailed advice on the orthodontic management of patients with developmental absence of one or more second premolars. The subject is complex and the examples mentioned here are included only to

illustrate the various principles involved. As a general rule, cases should be referred for advice earlier rather than later so that timing of extractions and later treatment can be planned. Routine radiographic screening in the early mixed dentition is essential.

(B) Submerging deciduous molars

These teeth 'submerge' because ankylosis of their roots to the surrounding bone prevents further eruption. The earlier that this process starts, then the greater the degree of submergence seen. This is because submergence is dependent upon the amount that adjacent teeth erupt, which in turn is dependent on the amount of growth in height of the jaws.

Submerging deciduous molars are of no functional use and the clinician has to decide whether they can be safely left to exfoliate naturally or whether they should be extracted. It is important to know first of all whether the successional tooth is present or not.

1. *Absence of successional tooth.* Second deciduous molars are most likely to be in this group. The absence of permanent successors means that these teeth will not exfoliate at their normal time and hence are likely to become severely submerged. Generally speaking, they should be removed before they have submerged to the extent that extraction is difficult because the adjacent teeth are beginning to move over their occlusal surfaces. This is particularly true in crowded cases where, of course, it would be advisable anyway to permit first permanent molars to come mesially. Furthermore, the comments on space closure in the earlier section on absent second premolars are applicable here too — i.e. the extraction of an opposing second deciduous molar may also be advisable to permit first permanent molars on that side of the mouth to come mesially together, thereby making it more likely that space will close. Unless experienced, the practitioner should ask for advice.

One situation where retention would be permissible is where submergence starts during the later stages of growth, and therefore will only be limited in extent, and when extraction for orthodontic purposes is not intended.

2. *Presence of successional tooth.* In most cases it appears that the successional tooth erupts normally. If submergence is noted in the late mixed dentition and it can be seen that the successional tooth is close to eruption, then nothing further need be done other than making sure that the affected deciduous tooth is shed normally. Occasionally the erupting premolar becomes deflected, in which case the deciduous tooth should be removed.

If submergence occurs early, before the successional tooth starts to erupt, then there is a risk that submergence will be greater in extent and interfere with eruption of the successor. In these cases the submerging deciduous molar should be removed before its extraction becomes too difficult.

(C) The need for balancing extractions

There are times when conservative measures either fail or are inappropriate and teeth have to be removed. It is important to realize that the extraction of

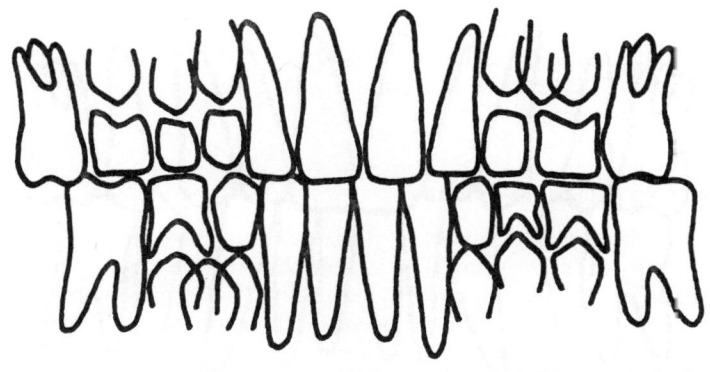

Fig. 4.9 *Diagrammatic representation of the occlusion following early loss of first deciduous molars in the left maxillary and right mandibular quadrants. There has been a shift of centre line in each arch towards the extraction site. The first permanent molars have also come mesially in the quadrants concerned so that the molar occlusions are dissimilar.*

deciduous molars or canines will localize crowding to the extraction sites; first permanent molars will move mesially and crowded incisors will move distally. In the case of a unilateral extraction, the crowding will become concentrated in the quadrant concerned, with the incisors taking on a centre line discrepancy and the molar occlusion becoming dissimilar between the two sides (Fig. 4.9).

The question often asked is whether this resulting asymmetry really matters, particularly as most patients do not notice a shift of the centre line. The answer lies in the complexities that it produces.

Orthodontic treatment of patients with asymmetrical crowding is rendered more difficult. In order to achieve a satisfactory fit of the maxillary arch around the mandibular with the buccal segments properly interdigitated, it would be essential to correct centre line discrepancies and dissimilar molar occlusions during treatment. Fixed appliances are nearly always necessary for the correction of centre line discrepancies.

There is no doubt that orthodontic treatment is simpler if centre lines coincide at the start of treatment, particularly for those cases judged to be suitable for the use of maxillary removable appliances alone and the extraction of all first premolars. With the centre lines coinciding and all the teeth in a class I relationship at the end of treatment, then any remaining spaces at opposing extraction sites will be equal in extent (Fig. 4.10). When the appliance is finally discarded, the buccal segments are then able to come mesially together, thereby closing opposing spaces simultaneously.

Occlusions with asymmetrical crowding, as shown in Fig. 4.9, will still usually require the extraction of all first premolars. However, if fixed appliances are not used to correct the occlusal asymmetries, then an excess of residual space would remain in those quadrants where early loss had not taken place (Fig. 4.11). These excess spaces usually remain after treatment as cuspal locks tend to maintain existing molar relationships.[5] *The price to be paid for not balancing the extraction of deciduous molars or canines is that a case which would otherwise have been considered suitable for treatment with removable*

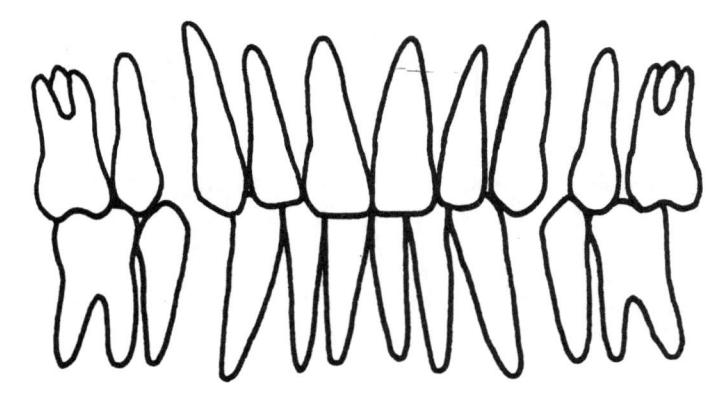

Fig. 4.10 *The desired occlusion at the end of orthodontic treatment if residual extraction spaces are to have a chance of closing spontaneously through mesial drift of the buccal segments. The canine occlusion should match the molar occlusion so that opposing spaces are equal in extent.*

appliances alone may well now have to be treated with fixed appliances in order to correct occlusal asymmetries.

It makes good sense, therefore, to balance the enforced extraction of deciduous molars and canines, if the arches are crowded, in order to prevent displacement of the centre line. The balancing extraction is usually that of the contralateral tooth.

Balancing extractions are *not* required, however, where:

1. The dentition is spaced.
2. The tooth requiring enforced extraction is close to exfoliation.
3. A previous extraction in the same arch was balanced.

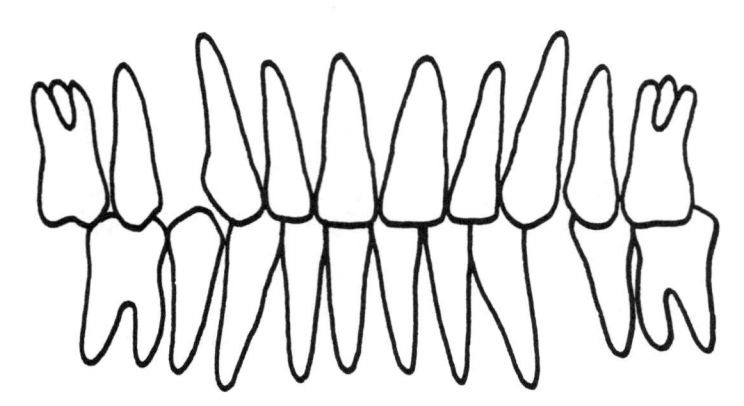

Fig. 4.11 *The occlusion of Fig. 4.9 after orthodontic treatment involving the extraction of all first premolars and where no steps have been taken to correct the centre line discrepancy or dissimilar molar occlusions. Excess residual space therefore remains in the right maxillary and left mandibular quadrants.*

4. Loss of the tooth requiring extraction would actually help to correct an existing centre line discrepancy, provided that the latter is not due to lateral displacement of the mandible on closure.

(D) Compensating extractions

A compensating extraction is when the corresponding tooth in the opposing quadrant is also removed. The effect of these extractions is to maintain the existing molar occlusion so that opposing buccal segments can then move mesially together. If compensating extractions are not done, then the molar relationship may well change and either help or hinder any future orthodontic treatment (Fig. 4.12).

It will be appreciated that when resolving crowding in both arches and producing a class I incisor relationship, one permanent tooth (often a first premolar) is usually extracted from each quadrant. It is obviously helpful in such cases if the buccal occlusion at the start of treatment is class I, for the molar occlusion at the end of treatment would also have to be class I if all residual spaces are to be closed. Thus, in certain situations, compensating extractions of deciduous molars or canines can simplify future orthodontic treatment by preventing the molar occlusion from becoming class II. The following are guiding principles:

1. *Enforced extraction of a mandibular deciduous molar or canine.* Usually there is no need to carry out a compensating extraction when a mandibular deciduous molar or canine has to be lost, as in most cases the molar occlusion merely becomes more class I as a result of mesial movement of the mandibular first permanent molars. Providing the mandibular arch is not spaced, then only a balancing extraction need be considered for these patients.

2. *Enforced extraction of a maxillary deciduous molar or canine.* In addition to balancing, there are reasonable grounds for compensating the enforced extraction of a maxillary deciduous molar or canine where there is crowding in both arches and where the occlusion of the first permanent molars is a half unit class II. The reader will appreciate that the balancing extraction would itself need to be similarly compensated, thus four teeth would be removed. These extractions can be expected to prevent the molar occlusion from becoming more class II. It should be pointed out, however, that this is not too critical, for if compensating extractions are not done, then the correction of the resulting class II molar occlusion would not be a difficult procedure to carry out and can be accomplished with a maxillary removable appliance and extraoral anchorage. The relatively straightforward nature of such an appliance system should be contrasted with the fixed appliances that are often necessary to restore arch symmetry if balancing extractions are omitted. The critical point to note is that it is much more important to balance the extraction of deciduous molars and canines than to compensate.

Finally, there is certainly no need to compensate the enforced extraction of maxillary deciduous molars or canines in those cases where the lower arch is either spaced or well aligned. In these cases it wouldn't matter if the molars did, in fact, become more class II. One possible option of future orthodontic treatment would be to accept the class II molar occlusion and provide the space for producing a class I incisor relationship by extracting maxillary first premolars.

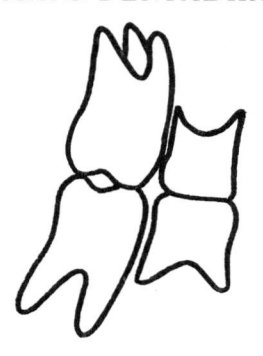

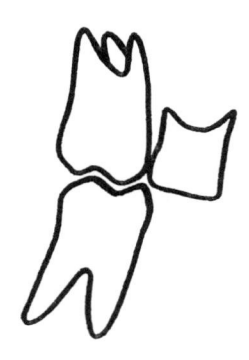

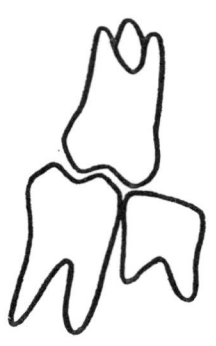

Fig. 4.12 *Top: In the intact mixed dentition the molar relationship is often a half unit class II. Centre: Following the uncompensated extraction of a mandibular second deciduous molar, for example, then the first permanent molar in the quadrant concerned will tend to move mesially into a class I relationship. Bottom: Following the uncompensated extraction of a maxillary second deciduous molar there will be a tendency for the molar occlusion to become more class II.*

4. Molar region

First permanent molars occasionally become impacted, and, more rarely, may become submerged. However, the most frequent problem affecting this region of the mouth, even though caries has decreased markedly in recent years, is the presence of one or more first permanent molars of poor prognosis.

(A) Impacted first permanent molars

These are more commonly found in the maxilla and, depending on the severity of the impaction, will encourage the retention of food debris. The second deciduous molar should be removed to permit eruption of the first permanent molar, which will almost certainly come mesially. The resulting premolar crowding can be resolved in the permanent dentition.

(B) Submerging first permanent molars

These are rare and, like submerging deciduous molars, are ankylosed and fail to keep pace with the eruption of neighbouring teeth.

It is impossible to move orthodontically an ankylosed tooth. Their extraction in the early mixed dentition should therefore be considered to encourage mesial movement of second permanent molars. As will be seen in the next section, removal of the opposing first permanent molar may also be advisable to encourage space closure. It should also be pointed out that ankylosis of their roots often makes removal of submerging first permanent molars extremely difficult and that referral for surgical removal should always be considered. This is particularly true for submerging maxillary teeth where there would be a risk of producing an oro-antral fistula.

(C) First permanent molars of poor prognosis

The long-term prognosis of first permanent molars ideally needs to be considered at 8–9 years of age, before root formation has got underway on second permanent molars. The extraction of poor-quality first permanent molars at this time from crowded arches provides the best chance for the spontaneous resolution of crowding and satisfactory eruption of second permanent molars in contact with second premolars, without excessive tipping (Fig. 4.13). The outcome after extraction at a later age depends on whether crowding has become concentrated in the premolar regions following the previous loss of deciduous molars.

Where there has been no previous loss of deciduous molars and extraction of first permanent molars is carried out when root formation of second permanent molars is well established, then residual space closure is likely to be less complete and second permanent molars more mesially tipped than if the extractions had been carried out earlier (Fig. 4.14).

However, when early loss of deciduous molars has concentrated crowding in the premolar regions, then most of the extraction spaces resulting from removal of first permanent molars would be occupied by erupting premolars. A better result is obtained, therefore, because the second permanent molars have very little residual space into which to tip mesially (Fig. 4.15).

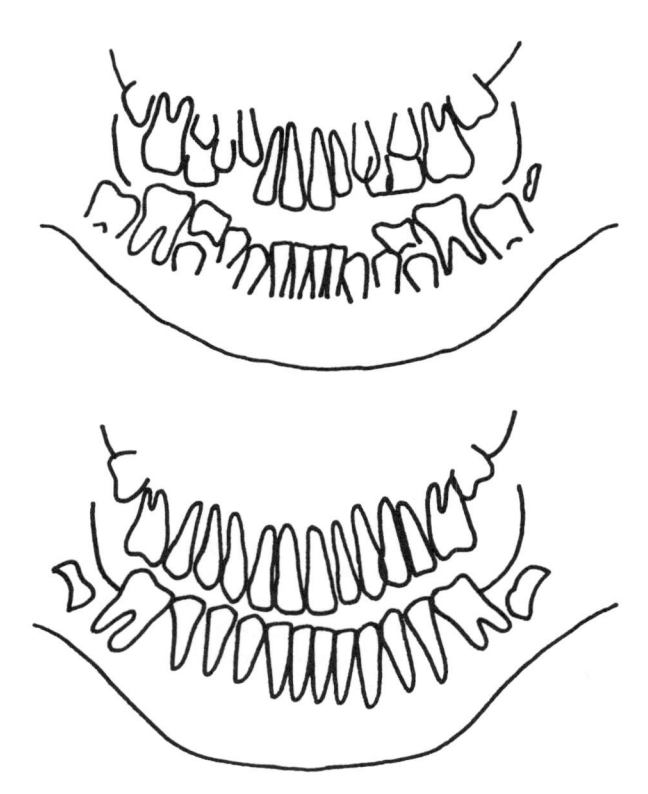

Fig. 4.13 *Top: Diagrammatic representation of an orthopantomograph (OPG) taken at 9 years of age, prior to the extraction of first permanent molars. Note that root formation of second permanent molars has not passed the bifurcation stage. Bottom: OPG tracing showing that satisfactory space closure has occurred at the extraction sites.*

The decision to extract all four first permanent molars from crowded arches is easier if all of these teeth are of poor prognosis. What does the clinician do, however, when this is not the case? The following are guiding principles:

1. *A maxillary first permanent molar with a poor prognosis and the opposing first permanent molar with a good prognosis.* Generally speaking, if a maxillary first permanent molar is to be extracted and the maxillary second molar is unerupted, then only the first molar need be removed. Unerupted maxillary second permanent molars are particularly good at moving mesially and erupting adjacent to second premolars.

If the maxillary second permanent molar is in occlusion at the time the maxillary first molar is extracted, then the second molar would be hindered in its mesial migration on account of intercuspation with the opposing teeth unless the mandibular first permanent molar also is removed. It appears that buccal segments are better at coming mesially if opposing teeth can move forward together.[5] Mesial movement would certainly be helpful if maxillary third molars are present on radiograph.

INTERCEPTIVE ORTHODONTICS 69

2. *A mandibular first permanent molar with a poor prognosis and the opposing first permanent molar with a good prognosis.* Where a mandibular first permanent molar has a poor prognosis, then it is wise to remove also the opposing maxillary first molar. This recommendation would apply whether or not the mandibular second molar had erupted because this latter tooth is not particularly good at moving mesially and such movement can readily be prevented by an unopposed and over-erupted maxillary first permanent molar.

3. *Unilateral opposing first permanent molars with a poor prognosis.* Where opposing first permanent molars on one side have a poor prognosis (or whenever both are to be extracted for the reasons mentioned above) and where those on the other side are to be retained, then it is wise to balance these extractions by removing also the second deciduous molars on this other side. This assumes that no extractions have already taken place in these contralateral

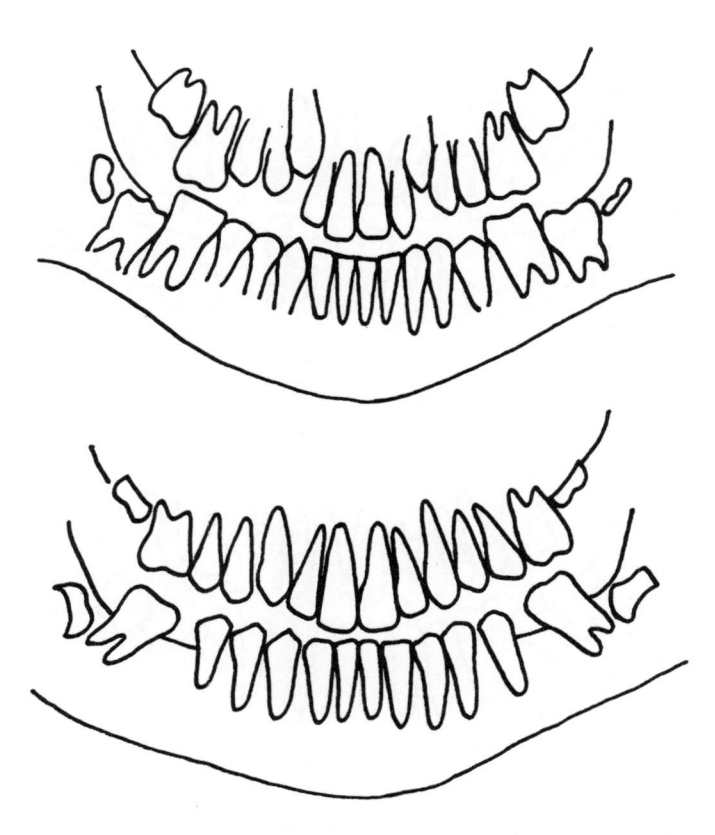

Fig 4.14 *Tracing of an OPG taken at 10 years, 6 months of age when root formation of the second permanent molars was well advanced in a patient with little or no premolar crowding. Bottom: Two years after extraction of first permanent molars. Excessive mesial tipping of mandibular second permanent molars has taken place and incomplete space closure will remain. This is a typical outcome under these circumstances.*

quadrants and that there is labial segment crowding. Crowding will then resolve on the side where the permanent molars were removed and be transferred to the premolar region on the other side. The resulting premolar crowding can be treated by the extraction of first premolars on that side in due course.

4. *What if third molars are absent?* In patients with crowding, the absence of third molars should not affect the decision to extract poor-quality first permanent molars. In any case, many third molars have yet to start forming at the age when the extraction of first permanent molars is usually considered.

These recommendations apply to class I cases with crowding. What if the incisor relationship is not class I?

1. *Class II, division 1 malocclusions*. Present-day thinking on the management of class II, division 1 malocclusions, where the prognosis of the first

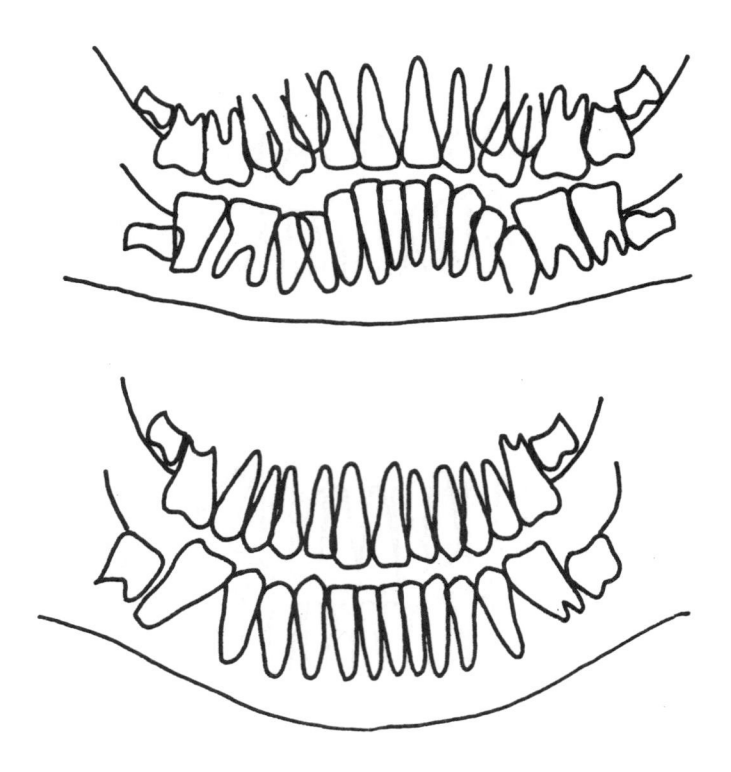

Fig. 4.15 *Tracing of an OPG taken at 11 years, 2 months of age when root formation of the second permanent molars was very nearly complete. Many deciduous teeth had been extracted previously and the patient presented initially with considerable crowding in the premolar regions. Bottom: OPG tracing showing that satisfactory space closure has occurred after extraction of all four first permanent molars.*

permanent molars is poor and where there is crowding in both arches, is that extractions should be carried out at 8–9 years of age as for class I cases. These patients should then be reviewed when second permanent molars, premolars and canines have erupted fully and a decision made at that time on treatment to reduce the overjet.[6]

2. *Class II, division 2 malocclusions*. If fixed appliances are to be used eventually to correct maxillary incisor retroclination in class II, division 2 patients, it is not essential to remove poor-prognosis first permanent molars in the mixed dentition unless symptoms make this a necessity. These extractions can be delayed until the second permanent molars have erupted fully. The production of good alignment between the second molars and second premolars can then be accomplished satisfactorily with fixed appliances at the same time as aligning the incisors.

Furthermore, where a deep overbite is seen to be causing actual trauma to the periodontal tissues in the mixed dentition stage, the extraction of first permanent molars should be delayed, as a maxillary removable appliance will need to be worn to produce some overbite reduction. Such an appliance is best retained on first permanent molars and should be worn until sufficient numbers of permanent teeth have erupted to permit orthodontic treatment to correct the incisor relationship.

Those cases in which the position of the maxillary central incisors is acceptable, and hence can be treated eventually by retracting the lateral incisors with removable appliances, can have poor-prognosis first permanent molars extracted in the mixed dentition, as with class I cases. Orthodontic treatment to align the lateral incisors can then be considered in the permanent dentition proper.

3. *Class III malocclusions*. Where incisor crossbites are to be extracted in the mixed dentition, the extraction of first permanent molars should be delayed until after the incisors have been aligned and the appliance discarded. This is because the maxillary first permanent molars will be required to retain the orthodontic appliance while the mandibulars are needed for the molar capping (posterior bite planes) to occlude against.

As will be mentioned in Chapter 5, those class III patients in which all the maxillary permanent incisors are in crossbite should be carefully assessed in the mixed dentition as regards the timing of orthodontic treatment. If treatment is to be deferred until the permanent dentition proper, and fixed appliances are to be used at that time, then it may be appropriate to postpone the extraction of first molars until then.

Finally it should be appreciated that there are situations when it would be better to retain first permanent molars even though their prognosis is dubious. Where there is spacing in the arches, retention of all the permanent teeth is the only realistic way of maintaining the arches intact, so there is no gain in electively extracting restorable first permanent molars. Clearly, it is also inappropriate to extract a first permanent molar in an arch with crowding if the adjacent second premolar is found to be developmentally absent unless, of course, the first permanent molar is totally unsavable.

THE PERMANENT DENTITION

After the shedding of the last deciduous tooth, the permanent dentition will not be complete until second and third molars have erupted. In many cases, however, third molars will not have enough space to erupt fully and will eventually impact.

Patients frequently ask whether erupting third molars are responsible for the worsening of crowding in their hitherto reasonably aligned dental arches. Unfortunately, the relationship between increasing crowding and the presence of third molars is not a clear one. In fact, crowding can be expected to worsen during the teenage years whether third molars are present or not. The decision on whether potentially impacted third molars should be removed early or late should therefore be made on the basis of wishing to minimize surgical and periodontal difficulties rather than hoping that an increase in crowding will be prevented.

1. Early treatment

There is a choice between either removing second permanent molars to permit eruption of third molars or of removing the third molars themselves.

(A) Removal of second permanent molars

For this procedure to succeed, the third molars must be well placed to erupt. Potential cases must be chosen with great care and, unless the practitioner is experienced, confirmatory advice sought. The problem is that even though maxillary third molars usually erupt satisfactorily after the loss of second molars, the outcome in the mandibular arch is often not so favourable. Extra-oral radiographs are required for assessment and, in the case of the mandibular arch, all of the following signs should be apparent:

 1. The angle between the long axes of first and third molars is in the range of 15°–30°.
 2. Root formation of third molars has yet to start. For most people this would be in the age range 12–14 years.
 3. The crypts of the third molars overlie the distal roots of the second molars somewhat.

(B) Removal of third molars by lateral trepanation

The third molar is surgically removed when the crown is fully formed but before root formation has got underway. The advantage of the procedure is that good periodontal support is ensured on the distal of the mandibular second molar. The disadvantage is that an inpatient general anaesthetic is usually necessary. Also, in the case of the maxillary arch, there is a risk that deeply placed third molars may become dislodged into the antrum.

Probably the only justification for this procedure would be if it was felt that the mandibular third molars were in hopeless positions and would be better removed at this stage rather than as very difficult 'surgicals' later on. Incidentally, if maxillary third molars are felt to be too deeply positioned for easy removal, then the loss of mandibular third molars by lateral trepanation can be combined instead with the extraction of maxillary second molars. Alternatively, the maxillary third molars can be removed on their eruption.

2. Later treatment

Most cases will fall into this category and involves the removal of third molars if impaction makes this necessary. Indeed, if the clinician has doubts concerning the advisability of early treatment, then it is better to do nothing at that time but review the fate of third molars later on.

REFERENCES

1 Todd J. E. (1975). *Children's dental health in England and Wales, 1973*. London: HMSO, pp. 70–3.
2 Dickson G. C. (1974). Long term effects of malocclusion. *Br. J. Orthodont.*, **1**, 63–8.
3 Egermark-Eriksson I., Ingervall B., Carlsson G. E. (1983). The dependence of mandibular dysfunction in children on functional and morphologic malocclusion. *Am. J. Orthodont.*, **83**, 187–94.
4 Bass T. P. (1967). Observations on the misplaced upper canine tooth. *Dent. Practit.*, **18**, 25–33.
5 Stephens C. D., Lloyd T. G. (1980). Changes in molar occlusion after extraction of all first premolars: A follow-up study of class II division 1 cases treated with removable appliances. *Br. J. Orthodont.*, **7**, 139–44.
6 Houston W. J. B. (1976). *Walther's orthodontic notes*, 3rd edn. Bristol: John Wright, p. 83.

Chapter 5

Orthodontic cases to refer, treat yourself or leave alone

In one chapter it is impossible to give detailed instructions regarding the treatment of malocclusion. What can be done, however, is to distinguish those situations which can be satisfactorily treated by dental practitioners using removable appliances from those that are either better left alone or else treated by specialists using more complex techniques.

General dental practitioners wishing to undertake orthodontic treatment for their patients must be selective about what they attempt to do. Generally speaking, they need to know whether it is possible to treat any particular malocclusion with removable appliances alone and, if permanent teeth have to be removed, whether residual extraction spaces will close down satisfactorily of their own accord when appliances are finally discarded.

LIMITATIONS OF REMOVABLE APPLIANCES

Removable appliances can only move teeth by tipping, and for a single-rooted tooth the tipping axis will be in the middle third of the root.

If the maxillary canines are to be moved distally with a removable appliance after extraction of first premolars, for example, then it would obviously be desirable for these teeth to finish upright and parallel to the second premolars. The maxillary canines therefore need to be mesially inclined at the start of treatment if it is intended to retract them distally with removable appliances (Fig. 5.1). Furthermore, for any given case, the canines would ideally need to be mesially inclined by the correct amount so as to be upright when retracted. Such ideals seldom exist in nature.

The reader will readily appreciate, therefore, that many canines which are, at first, mesially inclined will in fact be distally inclined following retraction with removable appliances and, as will be seen in the section on class II, division 1 cases, many maxillary incisors will finish retroclined when overjets have been reduced using these appliances.

Does failure to align teeth in ideal positions really matter? The answer is that minor shortfalls in dental alignment are perfectly compatible with dental health and that if, in such cases the patient is happy with the aesthetic improvement obtained, then treatment with removable appliances was justified. Practitioners must be on their guard, however, for those presenting features which suggest a case would be worse off from either the aesthetic or functional points of view if removable appliances were to be used.

ORTHODONTICS TO REFER, TREAT OR LEAVE ALONE 75

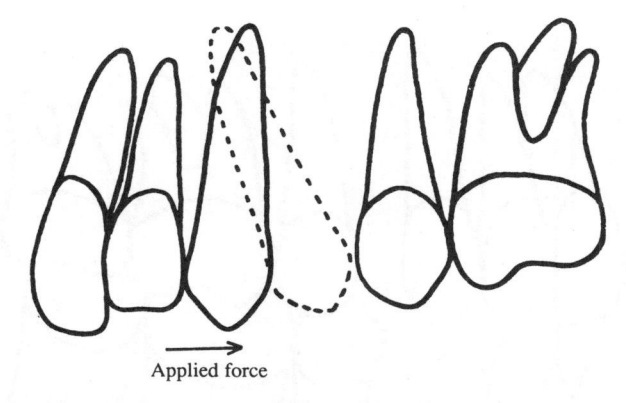

→
Applied force

Fig. 5.1 *Diagram illustrating the tipping distally of a maxillary canine with a removable appliance following extraction of the first premolar.*

Having accepted that removable appliances move teeth by tipping and can produce acceptable results if teeth to be moved are favourably inclined initially, it remains to list those tooth movements which are better carried out using fixed appliances. These are:

(a) apical movements;
(b) bodily movements;
(c) derotation;
(d) intrusion/extrusion.

THE LIKELIHOOD OF SPONTANEOUS SPACE CLOSURE AFTER EXTRACTION OF PERMANENT TEETH

The extraction of teeth will provide space for the alleviation of crowding. In the class II, division 1 case in which all four first premolars are to be extracted and a maxillary removable appliance used, for example, some spontaneous resolution of mandibular incisor and canine crowding can be expected to occur. With such treatments no active steps are taken to close down residual spaces following alignment of the maxillary anterior teeth. Closure of residual space at the extraction sites will be dependent upon mesial drift of the buccal segments when the appliance is discarded. A satisfactory outcome is likely to occur for such treatments when:

1. *The patient's growth potential is good.* The extent to which buccal segments can come mesially appears to be related to growth potential and is likely to be greater in those subjects who still have much of their pubertal growth spurt to come. The mean peak velocity for pubertal growth in girls is 12 years and in boys 14 years. Many girls are therefore well through their growth spurt even when orthodontic treatment is just starting.

If the chances of space closure due to mesial drift are considered small, in view of the patient's more advanced development, then it would be better to

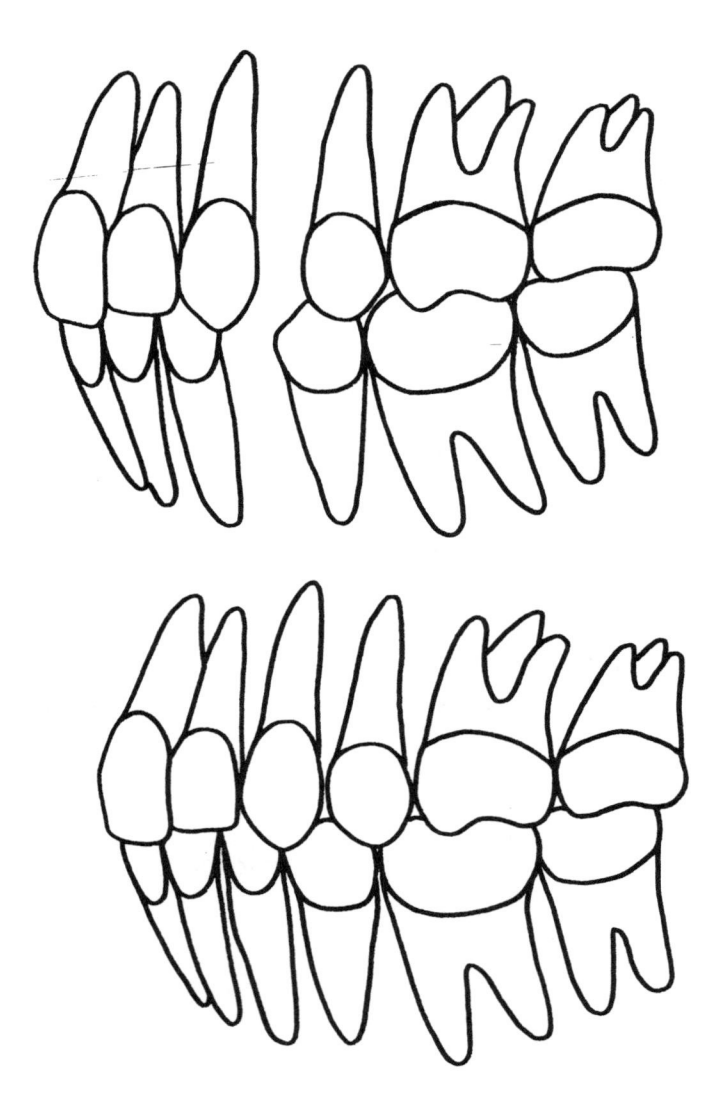

Fig. 5.2 *Top: Equal and opposite residual spaces at the end of treatment in a situation where opposing first premolars were removed. Bottom: Mesial drift of buccal segments resulting in simultaneous space closure at opposing sites.*

treat using fixed appliances so that active steps can be taken to ensure that no spaces remain.

2. *The amount of residual space is small.* Beware of cases with only mild crowding. Much residual space would remain which may well be beyond the capacity of mesial drift to close down. If mildly crowded cases are to be treated, then this is better carried out using fixed appliances so that buccal segments can

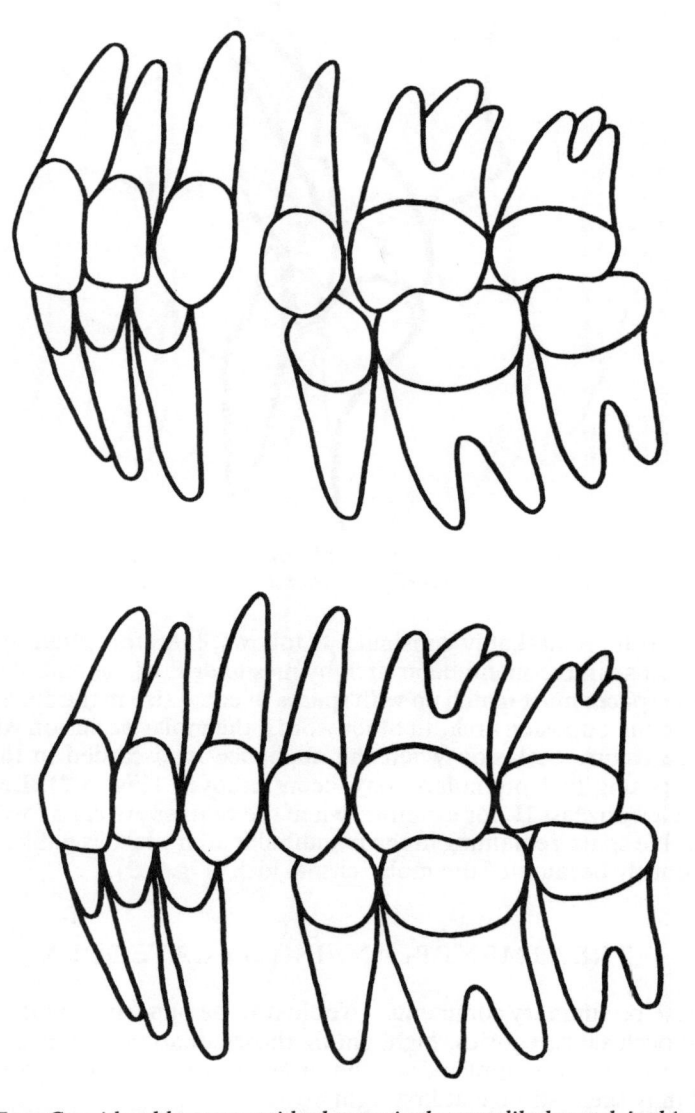

Fig. 5.3 *Top: Considerably more residual space in the mandibular arch in this situation where the molars are one unit class II and the canines class I. Bottom: Mesial drift has closed the maxillary space but the cuspal lock between opposing molars maintains the mandibular space.*

be actively brought mesially. The practitioner should consider, however, the possibility of leaving mild crowding alone; assuming there are no other orthodontic problems. In these days of limited Health Service resources, priority on orthodontic waiting lists should go to those cases with greater treatment need.

3. *The buccal occlusion does not hinder space closure*. The work of Stephens and Lloyd on space closure after orthodontic treatment has shown buccal

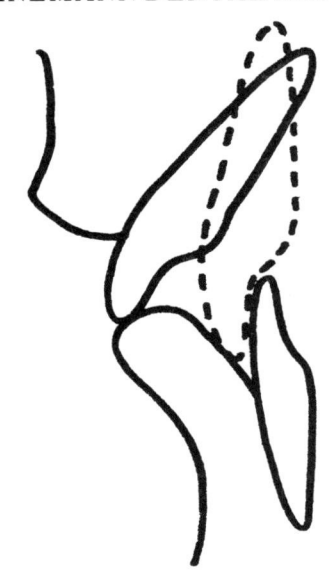

Fig. 5.4 *Crowns of maxillary incisors outside lower lip control at the start of treatment are likely to be retained by the lower lip at the end of treatment.*

occlusion to be remarkably constant.[1] It follows, therefore, that for residual spaces to close in the mandibular arch by mesial drift of the buccal segments, then these spaces must match up with spaces of equal size in the corresponding position in the opposing arch. In other words, the molar occlusion will have to match the canine occlusion when the appliance is discarded in those cases where opposing first premolars have been removed (Fig. 5.2). Leaving the molar occlusion class II, for example, when the canines are class I will result in considerable space remaining in the mandibular arch which is unlikely to close spontaneously because of the molar cuspal lock (Fig. 5.3).

TREATMENT PLANNING BY CATEGORY

After these preliminary comments it would now be opportune to deal with the different occlusal categories, highlighting those situations amenable to treatment with removable appliances. The order in which the categories will be covered may seem strange at first sight:

(a) class II, division 1;
(b) class II, division 2;
(c) class I;
(d) class III.

This sequence is deliberate. A successful understanding of the principles behind the treatment of class II, division 1 cases with removable appliances simplifies treatment planning for class II, division 2 and class I cases.

For all occlusal categories it has been assumed in the clinical situations quoted that all permanent teeth (with the possible exception of third molars)

ORTHODONTICS TO REFER, TREAT OR LEAVE ALONE

are present, are of good prognosis and are developing in their normal positions. If this is not so, then teeth other than first premolars would need to be considered for removal instead. The best advice in these more complex situations is that treatment is better carried out by specialists, unless the practitioner is experienced.

Class II, division 1 malocclusion

With this category the mandibular incisor edges lie posterior to the cingulum plateaux of the maxillary incisors. There is an increase in the overjet and the maxillary central incisors are usually proclined.

Will overjet reduction be stable?

For overjet reduction to be stable the labial surface of the upper incisor crowns must be controlled by the lower lip at the end of treatment. A favourable presenting sign at the start of treatment is to note that the upper incisor crowns are situated outside lower lip control so that the lower lip is 'trapped' between upper and lower incisors (Fig. 5.4).

If the upper incisor crowns lie well inside lower lip control at the start of treatment, then the overjet should be accepted. Overjet reduction in these cases would only take the upper incisors from out of contact with the lower lip and hence would result in relapse when the appliance is discarded (Fig. 5.5). If in doubt, then refer for advice.

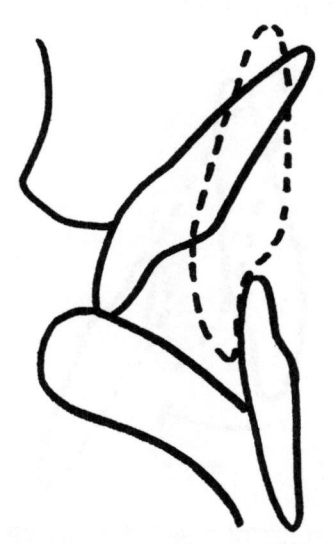

Fig. 5.5 *An everted lower lip resulting in the maxillary incisors being inside lip control is unlikely to be able to retain a fully reduced overjet.*

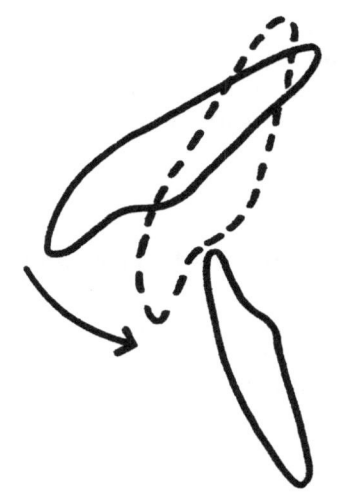

Fig. 5.6 *Maxillary incisors should be sufficiently proclined at the start of treatment for them to have an acceptable inclination after overjet reduction with removable appliances.*

Can the maxillary arch be treated using removable appliances?

1. *Incisor retraction:* maxillary incisors should appear proclined, i.e. tilted labially more than is normal. Assess incisor angulation with respect to the Frankfort plane (superior border of the external auditory meatus to the inferior border of the orbital rim). Patients must be seated upright in the chair so that this plane can be positioned parallel to the ground. In a north-west European population the mean angle between the longitudinal axes of the maxillary central incisors and the Frankfort plane is 107°.

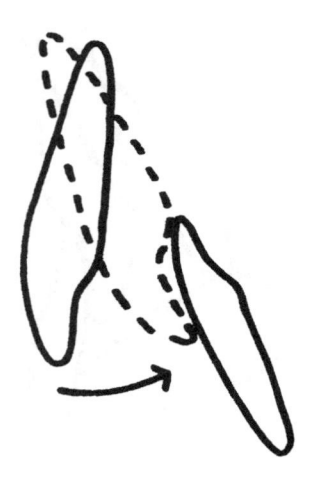

Fig. 5.7 *The likely end result of overjet reduction using removable appliances as the skeletal pattern becomes more class II. The maxillary incisors will become increasingly retroclined.*

Whilst assessing the patient in profile, an assessment should also be made of the skeletal pattern; the anteroposterior relationship of the jaws. Clinicians should be on their guard for skeletal class II cases; those where the mandible is positioned more posteriorly than normal.

The following is a brief outline of the relationship between skeletal pattern and maxillary incisor angulation as it affects the treatment planning of class II, division 1 cases.

If the skeletal pattern is class I then, in the majority of cases, the increased overjet will be due to proclination of the maxillary incisors. In these cases overjet reduction using removable appliances will not over-retrocline the maxillary incisors (Fig. 5.6).

The more class II the skeletal pattern then the more retroclined will the maxillary incisors be if the overjet is reduced using removable appliances (Fig. 5.7). A class II, division 1 malocclusion will have been exchanged for a class II, division 2! Such a change would not matter too much if the resulting class II, division 2 incisor relationship was mild, but the risk of periodontal trauma and breakdown would be present in those with deeper overbites.

Beware— if the maxillary incisors already have a normal angulation as the skeletal pattern is likely to be class II.
Beware— of large overjets, greater than 8 mm, say. The greater the overjet then the more likely that the skeletal pattern is class II, even if the maxillary incisors are proclined.

These more difficult cases are better treated using fixed appliances so that the maxillary incisors can be moved bodily without tipping.

2. *Canine retraction*. Canine retraction must ocur before an overjet can be reduced.

Maxillary canines should be mesially inclined if removable appliances are to be used for their retraction. Initially upright canines will finish distally inclined if moved by this method. If little retraction is required under these circumstances, then it would be quite all right to accept a mild degree of distal tipping at the end of treatment.

Beware— of upright maxillary canines where more than half a premolar unit of distal movement is required.
Beware— of initially distally inclined canines.

Canines in these categories are better retracted using fixed appliances in order to ensure that they finish parallel to second premolars.

Can the mandibular arch be treated without appliances?

If the mandibular arch is well aligned, then the clinician can go on to the next stage of planning which is deciding how space should be provided to enable maxillary canines to be retracted into class I. More about this matter later.

For crowded mandibular arches, clinicians should ask themselves whether crowding will resolve and residual spaces close down spontaneously following extraction of first premolars. Assuming all permanent teeth, with the possible exception of third molars, to be present and of good prognosis, then suitable cases should exhibit:

(a) mesially inclined canines;
(b) incisors and canines not rotated;
(c) around 50% or more of the extraction spaces will be occupied by canines drifting distally as anterior crowding resolves;
(d) a pubertal growth spurt that has yet to finish.

The first two requirements should be present for adequate spontaneous resolution of anterior crowding, the final two to give the best chance of avoiding excessive residual space at the end of treatment that won't close down further.

In the absence of fixed appliances, initially upright canines will become distally inclined after resolution of anterior crowding. Such a change is not ideal but may safely be considered reasonable, as is the acceptance of minor degrees of tooth rotation.

Cases with significantly rotated incisors and/or distally inclined canines should, however, be considered for referral for fixed appliance treatment by specialists.

For how long will crowded mandibular anterior teeth align spontaneously after extractions?

Generally speaking there will be little further improvement in the alignment of crowded mandibular anterior teeth 6 months after extraction of first premolars.[2] Active appliances will therefore be necessary after this time.

Beware of mild crowding

Considerable spare space would remain after extractions which may not fully close, and this may be considered by the patient to be more unsightly than the original crowding. Fixed appliances would be required to ensure space closure.

Beware of very severe crowding

Very rarely the loss of first premolars provides insufficient space for the resolution of crowding. These cases are better referred first of all as additional extractions will need to be considered.

How are space requirements assessed for overjet reduction?

It is important to note the canine and molar occlusions. If using record models for assessment then make sure that their occlusion truly represents that of the patient.

1. *Canine occlusion.* Allowing for relief of mandibular crowding, the amount of space necessary to be able to retract maxillary canines into class I will need to be determined.

2. *Molar occlusion.* If canines finish in class I occlusion then, for all residual spaces to close, the final molar occlusion will have to be one unit class II for those cases where maxillary first premolars only are removed, and class I where all first premolars are removed. This recommendation applies irrespective of the initial molar occlusion.

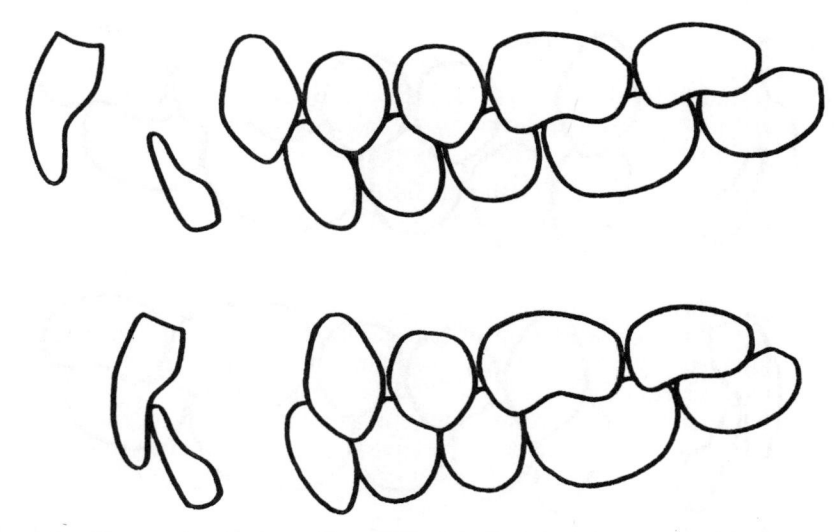

Fig. 5.8 *The extraction of maxillary first premolars provides just enough space in this situation to be able to retract canines into class I and then fully reduce the overjet.*

The decision on whether just the maxillary first premolars or all of these teeth should be removed is taken purely on the basis of space requirements in the two arches. Noting the initial molar occlusion will inform the operator of what steps, if any, need to be taken during treatment in order to ensure that the final molar occlusion is compatible with space closure. The following examples will serve as a guide. In each situation it is assumed that all permanent teeth, with the possible exception of third molars, are present and of good prognosis.

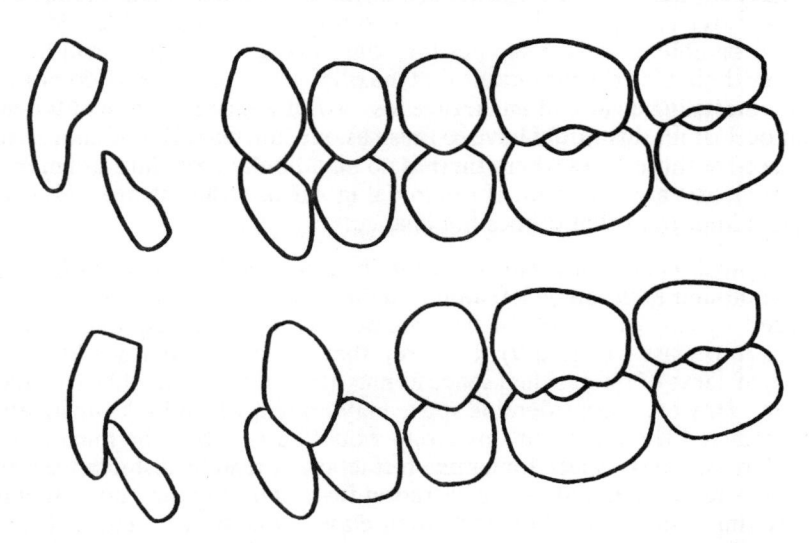

Fig. 5.9 *Half a unit of residual space remains in this situation after the extraction of maxillary first premolars.*

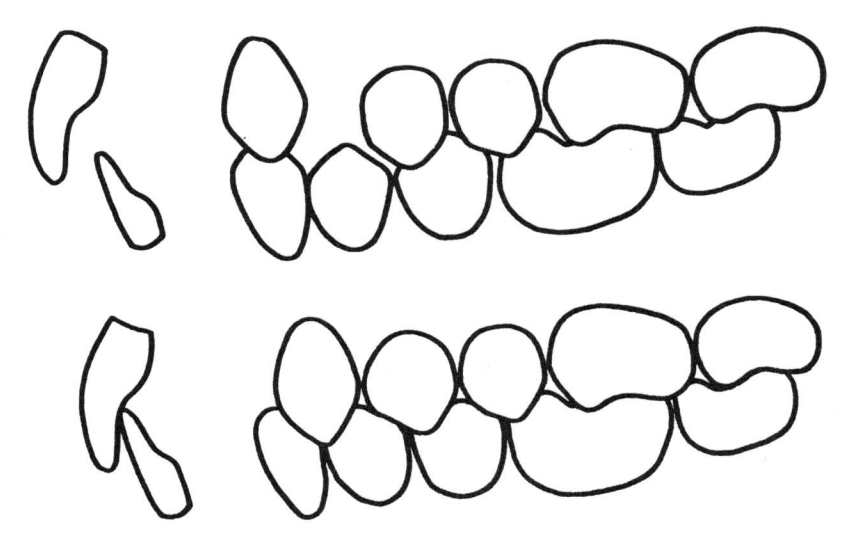

Fig. 5.10 *Often the maxillary buccal segments need to be moved distally until slightly class III to then be able to obtain a class I occlusion on the anterior teeth.*

In addition it is assumed that removable appliances will suffice to retract maxillary incisors and canines, that any mandibular crowding will resolve spontaneously following extractions, and that buccal segments will come mesially sufficiently well to close down extraction spaces of their own accord when appliances are discarded.

Example 1: uncrowded mandibular arch, molars one unit class II. There is obviously no need for any extractions in the mandibular arch. As far as the maxillary arch is concerned, the loss of first premolars will provide just enough space to be able to retract canines into class I (Fig. 5.8). Space will be tight, however, and it is very important that maxillary buccal segments do not come further mesially because of anchorage loss. After all, irrespective of the initial molar occlusion, this would have to finish as one unit class II if all spaces are to be closed for those cases where there is no mandibular crowding and maxillary first premolars are removed. If the initial molar occlusion is one unit class II then it is important that it does not change.

Example 2: uncrowded mandibular arch, molars half a unit class II. Again, the mandibular arch can be left alone. In the maxillary arch only half the space provided by the extraction of first premolars would be required to retract canines into class I (Fig. 5.9). It is true that anchorage loss would result in closure of some of the residual space as maxillary buccal segments are brought mesially. However, considerable space may remain which looks unsightly.

A preferred treatment for this group would be to retain the maxillary first premolars and make space for canine retraction instead by distal movement of maxillary buccal segments using extraoral force. Driving the buccal segments distally until slightly further back than class I will suffice (Fig. 5.10). The extraction of maxillary second permanent molars will need to be considered to provide space for distal movement if third molars are present and of good size.

ORTHODONTICS TO REFER, TREAT OR LEAVE ALONE 85

Example 3: uncrowded mandibular arch, molars class I. As teeth tend to come in matching sets, there should theoretically be enough spacing in the maxillary arch to fully reduce the overjet in those cases where the mandibular arch is well aligned and the molars already are class I. These cases should be judged with care, however, as frequently some distal movement of the maxillary buccal segments until slightly class III is required in order to provide sufficient space to then retract canines into class I.

Example 4: crowded mandibular arch, molars one unit class II. If the extraction of first premolars is considered suitable for the mandibular arch and closure of residual space is to be by means of mesial drift of buccal segments, then the extraction of maxillary first premolars is necessary to ensure that residual spaces are at directly opposing sites. Maxillary buccal segments will therefore need to be moved distally to class I occlusion if opposing spaces are to be equal in extent (Fig. 5.11).

The correction of the buccal segment relationship is also important from another viewpoint. This is because the extraction of maxillary first premolars will not by itself provide sufficient space to be able to retract canines into class I in those malocclusions where the buccal occlusion is a full unit class II and there is mandibular arch crowding. This state of affairs should be contrasted with that where, for the same buccal occlusion, the extraction of maxillary first premolars provides just sufficient space when the mandibular arch is already well aligned. Allowance has to be made of how much space there will then be to retract maxillary canines to class I when crowding has been resolved. This aspect will be covered more fully in the following section.

Cases in this category are difficult and, unless experienced, the practitioner is well advised to refer the patient for specialist treatment.

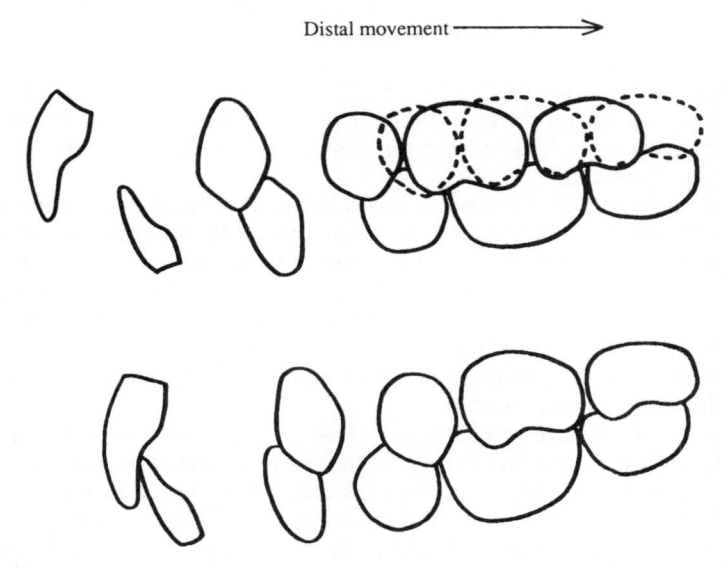

Fig. 5.11 *Distal movement of the maxillary buccal segments is necessary here in order to ensure that the molar occlusion will match the canine occlusion at the end of treatment.*

←——— Mesial drift

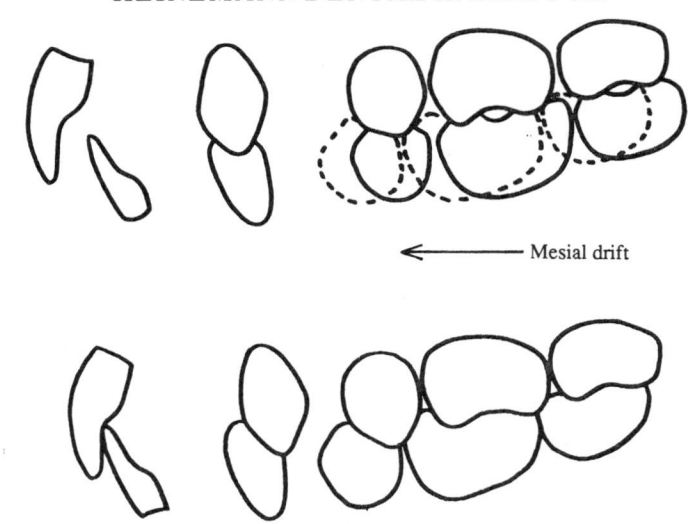

Fig. 5.12 *Provided that maxillary buccal segments do not come mesially because of anchorage loss, then mesial drift of the mandibular buccal segments will correct the buccal occlusion.*

Example 5: crowded mandibular arch, molars half a unit class II. The majority of class II, division 1 cases are of this type and the extraction of all first premolars would normally be considered. As with the previous category, it is important to finish the case with the molars in class I to ensure that any residual spaces are equal in extent at opposing sites. Provided that maxillary buccal segments do not come mesially because of anchorage loss and mandibular buccal segments do come mesially because of natural drift, the molar occlusion should correct spontaneously (Fig. 5.12). In order to ensure that maxillary buccal segments do not move mesially it is wise to use extraoral anchorage to hold their position, at least during the canine retraction stage, after which the need can be reviewed.[3]

When considering those previous cases in which the molar occlusion is a half unit class II but the mandibular arch is uncrowded it was pointed out that the extraction of maxillary first premolars gives more than enough room to retract canines into class I. With the present category, space in the maxillary arch may well be a good deal tighter than it appears to be initially. It is essential to determine how much of the maxillary first premolar space will be required for retraction of maxillary canines until these teeth are in class I with well-aligned mandibular canines and incisors.

If, for a case in the present category, it can be seen that the canine occlusion is a half unit class II and that the mandibular canines need to move distally by half a premolar width, then all of the extraction space would be required in the maxillary arch (Fig. 5.13). Extraoral anchorage would be required throughout treatment in a case such as this, as it is imperative that maxillary buccal segments do not come mesially. It can be appreciated, therefore, that if the molar occlusion is a full unit class II instead of a half unit, then there

ORTHODONTICS TO REFER, TREAT OR LEAVE ALONE

would be insufficient space to obtain a class I canine occlusion once crowding had been resolved, unless the maxillary buccal segments are pushed distally.

When considering the treatment of any crowded case by extractions and the use of maxillary removable appliances alone, the operator should beware of mildly crowded situations as considerable spare space would remain. Even if the position of the maxillary anterior teeth is favourable for alignment using removable appliances, consideration should be given to referring the patient for fixed appliance treatment so that active steps can be taken to ensure space closure.

Example 6: crowded mandibular arch, molars class I. Again, the extraction of all first premolars needs to be considered for this category. The fact that the molars are class I at the start of treatment means that the molar occlusion will not need correction. As with all crowded cases, the comments mentioned previously concerning allowance of how much further distally the mandibular canines will be when aligned also apply here. Space in the maxillary arch may well be a good deal tighter than appeared initially and extraoral anchorage may prove to be necessary.

What about dissimilar molar occlusions?

If centre lines coincide and the left and right molar occlusions are dissimilar, then crowding will be relatively more severe in the maxillary quadrant on the side where the molar occlusion is more class II. As the desired goal of orthodontic treatment is to produce satisfactory alignment of the maxillary arch around the mandibular, treatment will have to include correction of the dissimilar molar occlusions if identical extractions are to be carried out on the two sides of the mouth. In some situations, maxillary removable appliances to produce unilateral distal movement will suffice, in others more complex fixed appliances are necessary. Unless experienced, practitioners should refer for advice.

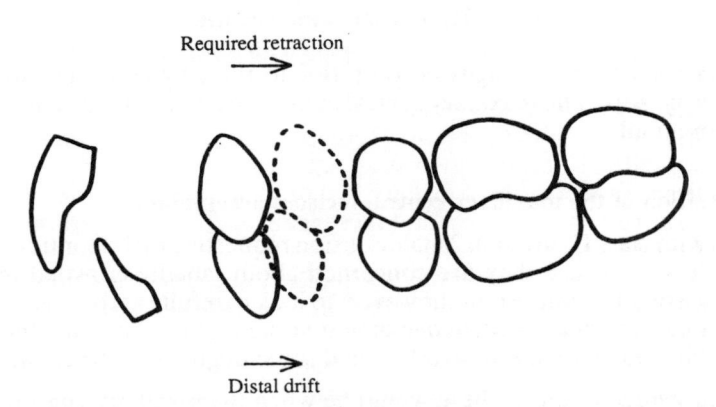

Fig. 5.13 *Maxillary canines must have enough space to be able to be retracted into class I with uncrowded mandibular anterior teeth.*

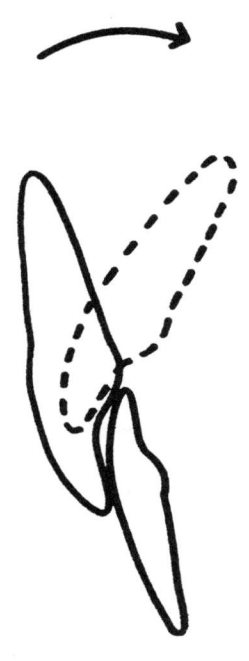

Fig. 5.14 *Palatal root torque to alter the occlusion of the maxillary incisors from class II, division 2 to class I.*

Do centre line discrepancies matter?

The greater a centre line discrepancy then the more difficult it is to satisfactorily align the maxillary arch around the mandibular. Correction of the discrepancy is not straightforward and usually requires fixed appliances.

Class II, division 2 malocclusion

The mandibular incisor edges lie posterior to the cingulum plateaux of the maxillary incisors. The maxillary central incisors are retroclined. The overjet is usually minimal.

Is the position of the maxillary central incisors acceptable?

Patients with class II, division 2 malocclusion requesting orthodontic treatment usually do so because they are concerned about labially crowded maxillary lateral incisors. It is important, however, to look carefully at the position of the maxillary central incisors when deciding treatment aims. Typically these teeth will exhibit some increase in overbite and some degree of retroclination.

1. *Unacceptable cases.* These would be when the maxillary central incisors appear excessively retroclined and/or the overbite is severe enough to place the periodontal tissues at risk.

ORTHODONTICS TO REFER, TREAT OR LEAVE ALONE   89

There is clearly no point in just retracting the maxillary lateral incisors in cases such as these. The aim of treatment should be to produce a class I relationship on all incisors. Referral will be necessary as fixed appliances would be required to produce the required palatal root torque of the maxillary incisor root apices (Fig. 5.14).

2. *Acceptable cases.* The position of the maxillary central incisors can be accepted if they appear only mildly retroclined and the overbite is not deep enough to be traumatic to the periodontal tissues. It would be quite all right in cases such as these to reduce the overjet on labially crowded maxillary lateral incisors so that these teeth are brought into line with the central incisors. Removable appliances would suffice for this procedure as tipping movements are usually all that is required (Fig. 5.15).

For those cases where it is decided that the aim of treatment will be to accept the position of the maxillary central incisors and reduce the overjet on the laterals, a decision should then be taken on whether removable appliances would be suitable to carry out the entire treatment. Much of what was said about class II, division 1 treatment applies here. As before, treatment for the maxillary arch must be planned around that for the mandibular. For simplicity, cases with uncrowded and crowded mandibular arches will be considered separately.

Uncrowded mandibular arches

There is obviously no need to extract teeth from the mandibular arch in these situations. Space will be required in the maxillary arch, however, in order to reduce the overjet on the lateral incisors.

It is important to note that the class I canine rule does not apply to these cases. If space was in fact provided to retract maxillary canines into class I, then excess space would remain mesial to these teeth at the end of treatment as the

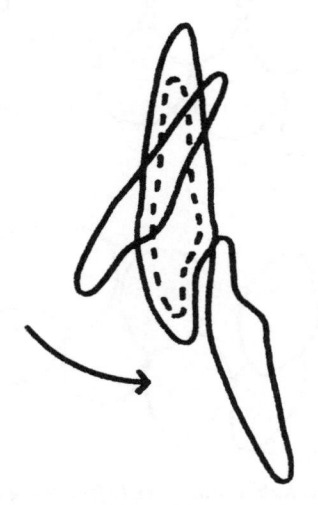

Fig. 5.15 *Overjet reduction on labially crowded maxillary lateral incisors to bring these teeth into line with the central incisors.*

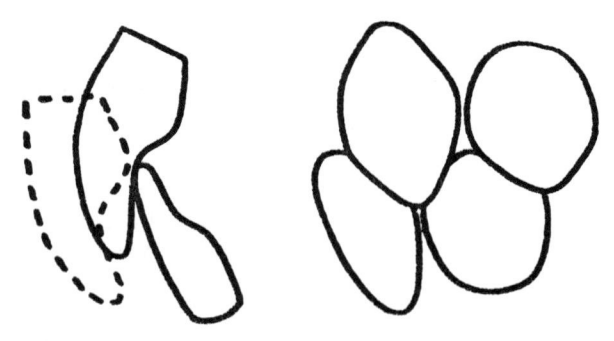

Fig. 5.16 *The deeper the overbite then the more labially placed the maxillary incisors will be.*

incisors would not be class I but still be class II, division 2, albeit uncrowded. The reason for the excess space is that as the overbite increases from class I, then the maxillary incisors would have to be more labially placed (Fig. 5.16).

Maxillary canines therefore need to be retracted until just short of class I — how short will depend upon the depth of the incisor overbite. Judgements such as these are relatively easy if the maxillary central incisors are very nearly class I but will become progressively more difficult as the overbite increases. In fact, as the overbite deepens the question should be asked whether the occlusion would be better treated with fixed appliances anyway, so as to produce a class I result.

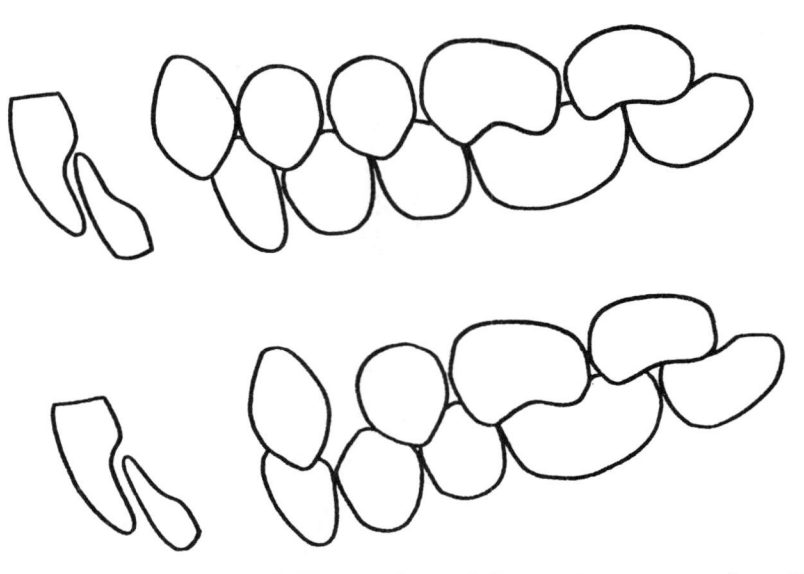

Fig. 5.17 *Canines retracted to half a unit class II following the extraction of maxillary first premolars. Half a unit of residual space remains, which is unlikely to close further because of the cuspal lock between opposing molars.*

Typical cases with uncrowded mandibular arches exhibit buccal occlusions varying from some degree of a half unit class II to a full unit class II. Maxillary first premolars should not be removed to provide space for canine retraction as residual space would remain which is unlikely to close further (Fig. 5.17). A better treatment would be to retain these teeth and provide space instead by pushing upper buccal segments distally using extraoral traction. If third molars are present and of good size, then consideration will need to be given to the extraction of maxillary second permanent molars.

The final buccal occlusion should be just short of class I, so as to match the intended canine occlusion. After correction of the buccal segments, then a second appliance, incorporating extraoral anchorage, would be used to retract the canines before reducing the overjet on the lateral incisors.

Crowded mandibular arches

As with class II, division 1 cases, practitioners should ask themselves whether crowding will resolve spontaneously after the extraction of first premolars, and whether the residual space is likely to close down by mesial drift of the buccal segments.

If the extraction of mandibular first premolars is considered to be suitable, then the maxillary first premolars will also need to be removed so as to ensure that residual spaces are at directly opposing sites. Maxillary canines will need to be retracted until just short of class I and the molar occlusion at the conclusion of treatment will have to match the canine occlusion.

Those cases where crowding is mild and in whom considerable residual space would remain after first premolar extractions are better treated with fixed appliances in order to ensure space closure.

Class I malocclusion

The mandibular incisor edges occlude with or lie immediately below the cingulum plateaux of the maxillary central incisors.

The inter-incisor relationship of these cases obviously does not require alteration unless some of these teeth happen to be crowded from the line of the arch.

Treatment objectives

Treatment will be considered for the correction of the following problems:

(a) crowding;
(b) spacing;
(c) rotations;
(d) crossbites.

The reader will appreciate that these features are not peculiar to class I malocclusion as they can also be found in the other occlusal categories.

Crowding

As has been mentioned previously, alleviation of crowding will require the extraction of permanent teeth. Provided that all permanent teeth, with the possible exception of third molars, are present, are of normal form and of good prognosis, then the most suitable choice for alleviation of crowding will often be the first premolars.

If there has been no previous extraction of deciduous molars and/or canines, then any crowding will be present in the incisor region and the unerupted molar region. When early loss has occurred, then crowding in these regions will resolve at the expense of space at the site of loss; overcrowding will have been transferred to the premolar and/or canine region depending on which deciduous teeth were removed.

1. *Incisor crowding.* Crowded mandibular incisors often resolve spontaneously after the extraction of first premolars. In the maxillary arch, however, appliances are usually necessary and such treatments have much in common with those undertaken for class II, division 1 and division 2 cases because, after all, all that is being done is reduction of overjet on any labially crowded incisors.

Cases judged to be suitable for the extraction of all first premolars and the use of upper removable appliances alone would therefore exhibit:

(a) canines mesially inclined;
(b) no rotations;
(c) no centre line discrepancy;
(d) not too much residual space after extraction of first premolars and resolution of crowding.

Maxillary canines would need to be retracted into class I occlusion. The molar occlusion at the end of treatment would also have to be class I for residual spaces at opposing sites to be equal in extent and hence have a chance of complete closure.

2. *Premolar/canine crowding.* After early loss of deciduous molars and/or canines the permanent incisors may well be acceptably aligned. The aim of treatment will be to resolve crowding in the premolar/canine region, which typically manifests itself as palatally or lingually displaced second premolars and/or labially displaced canines.

The extraction of all first premolars is often done for cases such as these. The best situations to treat using removable appliances are those where there will not be too much residual space after extractions and the alignment of displaced teeth. As before, the molar occlusion at the end of treatment should match the canine occlusion so as to ensure equal amounts of opposing space.

Management of these cases is reasonably straightforward if centre lines coincide at the start. If this is not so, then fixed appliances will be needed to correct the discrepancy so as to permit satisfactory alignment of the maxillary arch around the mandibular.

As with previous categories, fixed appliances should also be considered for those cases where it is felt that space closure after extractions may not occur of its own accord and where teeth to be aligned are unfavourably positioned; for example, maxillary canines may have erupted distally inclined.

Spacing

Spacing can exist for a variety of reasons. Excluding those due to obstructions, such as the midline maxillary diastema caused by an unerupted mesiodens or a large fraenum, it would seem reasonable to list these under two main headings:

(a) missing teeth;
(b) small teeth.

1. *Missing teeth*. An obvious example is when maxillary lateral incisors are developmentally absent. Because of this the neighbouring teeth will be spaced.

Spacing such as this could be closed down somewhat if there happened to be an overjet to reduce! When the incisors are class I, however, then treatment should be considered to concentrate the space in the lateral incisor region so that bridge work can eventually be provided. Fixed appliances are often required as frequently maxillary canines and central incisors in these situations need to be moved bodily rather than by tipping.

2. *Small teeth*. This condition may affect all of the teeth, in which case spacing will be generalized. In other situations spacing will be localized to either side of individual teeth which happen to be microdont — maxillary lateral incisors, for example.

In a class I occlusion there is no satisfactory orthodontic treatment for either of these situations. The spacing can be reduced, however, by building up the affected teeth with composite resin.

Rotations

The extent of spontaneous resolution of rotations after the extraction of neighbouring teeth is disappointing. Appliances will be necessary if the correction of rotations is required. Fixed appliances are to be preferred as removable appliances are not precise enough to obtain the over-correction that is an important requirement in the treatment of rotations.

Crossbites

A crossbite is a transverse discrepancy in arch relationships but may also describe a reverse overjet on one or more of the incisors.

Incisor crossbites are covered in the section on class III malocclusion. When dealing with buccal segment crossbites it is convenient to identify two types:

(a) local;
(b) segmental.

1. *Local crossbites*. These are when single teeth are affected and are usually due to crowding. A typical example would be a palatally placed maxillary second premolar.

Treatment of these crossbites can only be considered as an integral part of treatment to resolve crowding. An option in the case of the maxillary second premolar would be to extract this tooth if it was totally excluded from the line of the arch and the contact point between first premolar and first molar was satisfactory. Alternatively, the first premolar could be removed and the second premolar aligned using a removable appliance. It is essential that the quadrant concerned is not viewed only in terms of providing space to treat the crossbite; additional space may well be required to reduce an overjet, for example.

2. *Segmental crossbites.* These are when two or more adjacent teeth are affected. Often an entire buccal segment may be in crossbite, a typical example being when the buccal cusps of the maxillary teeth occlude medial to the buccal cusps of the mandibular teeth. This situation may occur unilaterally or bilaterally. These conditions are usually caused by a discrepancy in the widths of the maxillary and mandibular bases.

Correction of segmental crossbites is not always essential. Treatment should be based upon functional need as these crossbites usually cause no aesthetic concern. Those unilateral segmental crossbites presenting with associated displacement on closure to the side of the crossbite should be treated by maxillary arch expansion. Cases having bilateral crossbite or unilateral crossbite without associated displacement on closure are better left alone, or, if treated, done so by specialists.

Class III malocclusion

The mandibular incisor edges lie anterior to the cingulum plateaux of the maxillary incisors. The overjet is reduced or reversed.

Many of these cases present with one or more of the maxillary incisors in crossbite. The orthodontic assessment of these individuals will be considered under two separate categories, depending on whether or not all of the maxillary incisors are in crossbite.

1. When some of the maxillary incisors are not in crossbite

Mention has been made in Chapter 4 that if at least one maxillary incisor has a positive overbite and overjet, then it would seem reasonable to assume that those incisors in crossbite would be stable if moved labially to similar positions. Orthodontic treatment for these cases is relatively straightforward and can be considered in two stages; an early phase to correct the incisor crossbite and a later phase to resolve crowding.

(a) *Correction of the crossbite.* This is normally undertaken using removable appliances in the mixed dentition; all deciduous canines being extracted in crowded cases to provide space. The features to take note of during initial assessment are covered fully in the section devoted to this topic in Chapter 4.

Having corrected the crossbite, then any crowding will be transferred to the canine region where it can be resolved in the permanent dentition proper.

(b) *Resolution of crowding.* These cases can now be assessed in the same way as one would a class I case with premolar/canine crowding.

If crowding is present in both arches and all permanent teeth are present and of good prognosis, then the loss of all first premolars can be considered. Space maintenance should be used in those situations where these extractions provide just enough space to resolve crowding.

ORTHODONTICS TO REFER, TREAT OR LEAVE ALONE 95

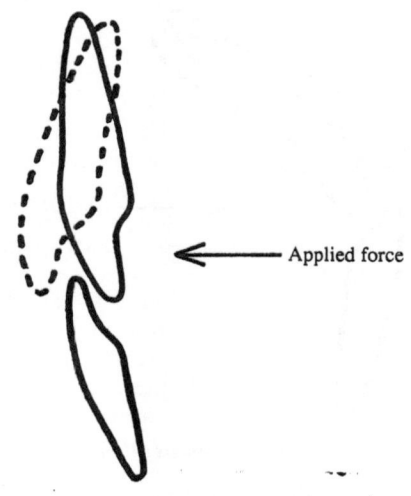

← Applied force

Fig. 5.18 *Little change in the overbite as initially retroclined maxillary incisors are pushed labially.*

If the mandibular arch happens to be well aligned, then consider making space for maxillary canines by moving maxillary buccal segments distally rather than extracting first premolars. Maxillary second permanent molars may need to be removed if third molars are present and of good size.

2. When all maxillary incisors are in crossbite

These cases should be judged with great care as some are orthodontically untreatable.

Generally speaking, if the patient cannot achieve an edge-to-edge contact on the incisors then these cases are too severely skeletal class III for an orthodontic solution on its own, although a combined approach with oral surgery can be considered later when growth has ceased.

If the patient can achieve an edge-to-edge contact on the incisors, then orthodontic treatment can be considered. Rarely the skeletal pattern will be class I or only mild class III, in which case the maxillary incisors will be somewhat retroclined. These cases can be treated using maxillary removable appliances in the mixed dentition. There would be an adequate overbite after crossbite correction to ensure stability (Fig. 5.18).

More commonly the patient will have a definite skeletal class III relationship, in which case the maxillary incisors will have a normal angulation or be somewhat proclined. If treatment is restricted to the maxillary arch, then excessive proclination would be produced with an attendant marked loss of overbite and possible relapse (Fig. 5.19). These cases are better treated by specialists in the permanent dentition proper, as retroclination of the mandibular incisors will be required in addition to proclination of the maxillary incisors.[4]

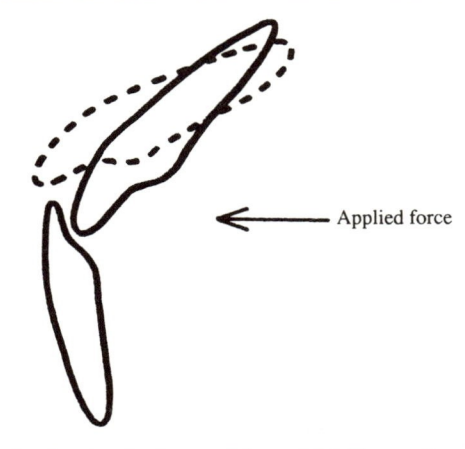

Fig. 5.19 *A marked reduction in the overbite as initially proclined maxillary incisors are pushed labially.*

Unless experienced the practitioner is urged to refer for specialist advice those cases presenting with all maxillary incisors in crossbite. Some of these cases may well be orthodontically treatable in the mixed dentition but some are better treated in the permanent dentition proper and some require surgery.

REFERENCES

1 Stephens C. D., Lloyd T. G. (1980). Changes in molar occlusion after extraction of all first premolars: A follow-up study of Class II Division 1 cases treated with removable appliances. *Br. J. Orthodont.*, **7**, 139–44.
2 Stephens C. D. (1983). The rate of spontaneous closure at the site of extracted mandibular first premolars. *Br. J. Orthodont.*, **10**, 93–7.
3 Lloyd T. G., Stephens C. D. (1979). Spontaneous changes in molar occlusion after extraction of all first premolars: A study of Class II Division 1 cases treated with removable appliances. *Br. J. Orthodont.*, **6**, 91–4.
4 Mills J. R. E. (1966). An assessment of Class III Malocclusion. *Dent. Practit.*, **16**, 452–65.

Chapter 6

The use of fluoride in caries prevention

SYSTEMIC

Water fluoridation

The fluoridation of public water supplies to the level of 1 part per million (p.p.m.) fluoride is the most effective method presently available for preventing dental caries on a community-wide basis.

Over 150 million people in about 30 countries live in areas where water supplies are fluoridated. About 40 million people live in areas where water supplies are naturally rich in fluoride. About 60% of the population in the USA drink fluoridated water, but only about 6% of the UK population.

The safety and effectiveness of water fluoridation have been endorsed by the World Health Organization and other authoritative bodies.

Fluoride drops and tablets

The administration of fluoride supplements to children is an effective method of preventing dental caries in areas served by low-fluoride water supplies. A serious disadvantage of the method is that it is difficult to sustain the interest of even the most highly motivated families for the long-term consumption that is necessary.

Fluoride drops are most convenient for administering to infants. Later, tablets are preferred because, when sucked or chewed, they have a topical as well as systemic effect.

The dosage recommended by the British Dental Association is shown in Table 6.1.

There is no indication for starting fluoride supplementation during pregnancy. Administration may be delayed until the child is about 6 months of age to ensure that kidney function is adequate to excrete excess fluoride.

Fluoride supplementation is most important for children who are classified as 'high risk', who can be described as having one or more of the following characteristics:

(a) a high caries susceptibility, as assessed by previous caries experience and present caries activity;

(b) a medical condition that may be complicated by bacteraemia resulting from infection or from some forms of dental treatment (for example, congenital heart disease);

(c) a medical condition that makes certain forms of dental treatment hazardous (for example, a bleeding disorder);

(d) mental subnormality, which sometimes makes treatment more than usually difficult.

For children who do not fall into a 'high risk' category, fluoride supplementation is less important but may be recommended to highly motivated parents who wish to take every possible precaution to prevent dental caries.

An important period for fluoride supplementation is from birth to the age of 5–6 years, during which time the crowns of all primary molars and of all permanent teeth (other than third molars) are formed. Another important period for fluoride supplementation is from the age of 6 years to the age of 12–14 years; this is the pre-eruptive maturation phase of premolars and second molars, during which time fluoride is taken up from the tissue fluids.

TOPICAL

Varnish, gel or solution

The products used most commonly in the UK for topical fluoride application are:

(i) a varnish containing 5% sodium fluoride;

(ii) an acidulated phosphate-fluoride gel (APF), which contains 2% sodium fluoride and 0.3% hydrofluoric acid in 0.1 M orthophosphoric acid. (An APF solution may be used, but gel is usually preferred.)

Varnish, gel or solution may be applied directly to teeth using any convenient applicator—either a small brush or cotton pledget. Gel may also be applied in a tray.

The main indication for topical fluoride treatment is for children who are classified as 'high risk' for the reasons outlined above. The UK General Dental Service regulations refer to this group as 'children with special needs'.

Since most children in the UK now use a toothpaste containing fluoride, additional topical fluoride in the form of varnish or gel is not strongly justified for children who do not fall into the 'high risk' or 'special needs' category.

APF contains a high concentration of fluoride (12.3 mg/ml)—ingestion of as

Table 6.1
Recommended dosage of fluoride drops and tablets (mgF/day), related to the concentration of fluoride in the drinking water

Age (years)	Water F (p.p.m.)		
	0.3	0.3–0.7	0.7
<2	0.25	0	0
2–4	0.50	0.25	0
>4	1.00	0.5	0

little as 2–3 ml of gel may cause unpleasant gastrointestinal disturbance. The following precautions should be taken when using gel in a tray:

1. Do not use excessive amount of gel in the tray — about 3 ml is sufficient.
2. Use suction apparatus during the 4-min application period.
3. On removing the tray from the mouth, either aspirate or wipe away excess gel from accessible tooth surfaces before allowing the child to expectorate.

Mouthrinse

Mouthrinses are available containing 0.05% sodium fluoride for daily use, or 0.2% sodium fluoride for weekly use. Although it might be expected that the daily regimen would be the more effective, clinical trials have not shown any significant difference in caries prevention.

The main indication for mouthrinsing is the same as for topical application of varnish or gel: for children with 'special needs'. However, since the solution must be kept in the mouth for at least 1 min (preferably 2 min) it is not appropriate for children below the age of 6–7 years.

Mouthrinsing may be recommended in addition to systemic administration and varnish or gel application for 'special needs' children.

Mouthrinsing may also be recommended to highly motivated parents of children who do not fall into the 'special needs' category.

FURTHER READING

Mellberg J. R. and Ripa L. W. (1983). *Fluoride in Preventive Dentistry: Theory and Clinical Applications*. Chicago: Quintessence.

Murray J. J. and Rugg-Gunn A. J. (1982). *Fluorides in Caries Prevention*, 2nd edn. Bristol: Wright.

Naylor M. N. and Murray J. J. (1989). 'Fluorides and Dental Caries.' In *The Prevention of Dental Disease*, 2nd edn. (J. J. Murray ed.). Oxford: Oxford University Press.

Nikiforuk G. (1985). *Understanding Dental Caries. 2 – Prevention: Basic and Clinical Aspects*. Basel: Karger.

Chapter 7

Fissure sealing and sealant restoration

The idea of sealing pits and fissures in teeth before they become carious is not new, but early attempts met with only limited success because adhesion of tested materials to enamel was inadequate. The success of the current sealing technique is based on the discovery by Buonocore[1] that adhesion of an acrylic resin to enamel was greatly increased if the enamel was first etched with acid.

Phosphoric acid, in the concentration range 30–50%, is normally used to etch enamel. Silverstone[2] showed that a 1-min application removes about 10 μm of surface enamel and etches the underlying surface to a depth of about 20 μm. Etching produces a surface layer of enamel into which resin can flow; the porosity provides a large surface area for adhesion of resin and also excellent mechanical retention.

MATERIALS

The resins currently used as sealants are based on the 'BIS-GMA' resin developed by Bowen[3]. Two types are available: those that polymerize after mixing two components (autopolymerizing types), and those that polymerize only when exposed to a suitable light source. Ultraviolet light (wavelength 365 nm) was used initially, but this has been superseded by visible (blue) light (wavelength 430–490 nm).

Most of the resins that have been used as fissure sealants are 'unfilled', that is, they do not contain filler particles, but filled resins formulated specifically to be used as sealants have been introduced recently.

Clear, tinted and opaque resins are available; the regulations of the UK General Dental Service require a tinted or opaque resin to be used.

Glass-ionomer cement has also been suggested as a suitable fissure sealing material.

EFFECTIVENESS

A recent review of the many clinical trials that have been conducted with BIS-GMA resins is that of Ripa[4]. The results, in terms of sealant retention and of caries prevention, show considerable differences between trials but, overall, the evidence points clearly to the conclusion that sealants are well retained if applied correctly and that they are highly effective in preventing dental caries. This conclusion has been endorsed by professional bodies such as the British Dental Association[5] and the US National Institutes of Health[6]. Clear and opaque resins are equally effective but resins polymerized by ultraviolet light appear to be less well retained than autopolymerizing resins. The few studies of resins polymerized by visible light suggest that they are as effective as autopolymerizing resins. Similarly, the few studies of filled resins suggest that they are effective.

The use of glass-ionomer cement for fissure sealing has been studied in only a few clinical trials, and the results of Williams and Winter[7] and Boksman et al.[8] do not suggest that it should be used instead of a BIS-GMA resin.

TECHNIQUE

The procedure described for the application of fissure sealant in the first clinical trial by Cueto and Buonocore[9] was used in subsequent trials and became adopted as the standard technique for clinical practice. Two aspects of the technique have recently been investigated, and the results suggest that some modification of the technique may be justified. Stephen et al.[10] and Eldelman et al.[11] showed that etching for only 20 s instead of the usual 1 min does not affect sealant retention, and Donnan and Ball[12] showed that omitting the preliminary cleaning procedure (brushing the enamel surface, using pumice powder) does not reduce sealant retention.

FISSURE SEALANTS — PREVENTIVE OR THERAPEUTIC?

Fissure sealing was introduced, and has become established, as a method for preventing dental caries — that is, as a primary preventive measure. As such, sealant is applied to surfaces that are assessed as being sound. However, it is not uncommon when examining a pit or fissure to remain uncertain about whether it is sound or carious; early lesions are difficult to diagnose visually or with the aid of a probe.

In the past there has been concern about the danger of inadvertently placing a sealant over a carious lesion. This concern has now been allayed by several studies (for example that of Mertz-Fairhurst et al.[13]) that have shown that caries sealed in by an effective sealant does not progress; microorganisms do not survive and the lesion does not increase in size. This observation is further considered in Chapter 11.

These findings have not only provided reassurance that no harm will be done if a diagnostic error is made and sealant is placed over a carious lesion but have also provided evidence to justify therapeutic sealing, that is, sealing of 'questionable' lesions.

SEALANT RESTORATION (PREVENTIVE RESIN RESTORATION)

The alternative treatment for the 'questionable' lesion is to open up, very conservatively with a small bur, the part of the fissure where caries is suspected. If no caries is found the fissure is sealed but, if caries is detected and a cavity is produced, the tooth is restored with a sealant restoration. The technique that has been tested in clinical trials and found to be effective (for example by

Houpt et al.[14]) involves filling the cavity with composite resin restorative material and then sealing the margin of the restoration and the adjacent fissures.

A related sealant restoration technique involves the use of glass-ionomer cement instead of composite resin to fill the cavity; the glass-ionomer and the adjacent fissures are then covered with sealant. This technique does not appear to have been the subject of a clinical trial but may be expected to be as effective as the technique employing composite resin.

Sealant restorations are considered further in Chapter 12.

THE USE OF FISSURE SEALANTS

In the General Dental Service of the UK National Health Service, fissure sealing is approved as primary preventive treatment only for 'children with special needs' (the 'high risk' group outlined on pp. 97–8). As a therapeutic measure, sealing is approved in the treatment of early carious lesions (see also Chapter 11).

Outside the constraints of the General Dental Service regulations, it might be considered that sealing of all caries-susceptible pits and fissures in all young patients would be ideal treatment. On the other hand, this approach might also be considered to be excessive and unjustified. Therefore some guidelines for selecting patients for treatment are helpful in order to justify the time required to perform the treatment and the expense involved for parents. The British Paedodontic Society[15], after emphasizing the priority of the 'high risk' group, suggested the following guidelines:

1. Seal permanent first molars in children who have experienced extensive caries in their primary teeth.
2. If one permanent first molar becomes carious, seal the other three.
3. Seal permanent second molars if one or more first molars had occlusal caries.
4. Seal as soon as the tooth has erupted sufficiently to permit moisture control, and certainly within 2 years of eruption.
5. Teeth to be sealed should have sound approximal surfaces.

To this list may be added the morphology of the teeth. Although the actual depth of fissures cannot be assessed by mirror-and-probe examination, the caries risk may be expected to be greater when the 'valleys' between the cusps are narrow and fissured rather than when they are wide and smooth.

REFERENCES

1 Buonocore M. G. (1955). A simple method of increasing the adhesion of acrylic filling material to enamel. *J. Dent. Res.* **34,** 849–53.
2 Silverstone L. M. (1974). Fissure sealants: laboratory studies. *Caries Research* **8,** 2–26.
3 Bowen R. L. (1963). Properties of a silica-reinforced polymer for dental restorations. *J. Am. Dent. Ass.* **66,** 57–64.
4 Ripa L. W. (1985). The current status of pit and fissure sealants: a review. *J. Can. Dent. Ass.* **51,** 367–80.

5 British Dental Association (1986) Report of the joint BDA/DHSS working party: fissure sealants. *Br. Dent. J.* **161,** 343–4.
6 National Institutes of Health (1984). Consensus development conference statement on dental sealants in the prevention of tooth decay. *J. Am. Dent. Ass.* **108,** 233–6.
7 William B. and Winter G. B. (1981). Fissure sealants: further results at 4 years. *Br. Dent. J.* **150,** 183–6.
8 Boksman L., Gratton D. R, McCutcheon E. and Plotzke O. B. (1987). Clinical evaluation of a glass ionomer cement as a fissure sealant. *Quint. Int.* **18,** 707–9.
9 Cueto E. and Buonocore M. G. (1965). Adhesive sealing of pits and fissures for caries prevention. International Association for Dental Research programme of meeting, page 137, abstract number 400.
10 Stephen K. W., Kirkwood M., Main L., Gillespie F. S. and Campbell D. (1982). Retention of a filled fissure sealant using reduced etch time. *Br. Dent. J.* **153,** 232–3.
11 Eidelman E., Shapira J. and Houpt M. (1988). The retention of fissure sealants using 20-second etching time: 3-year follow-up. *J. Dent. for Child.* **55,** 119–20.
12 Donnan M. and Ball I. A. (1988). A double-blind clinical trial to determine the importance of pumice prophylaxis on fissure sealant retention. *Br. Dent. J.* **165,** 283–6.
13 Mertz-Fairhurst E. J., Schuster G. S. and Fairhurst C. W. (1986). Arresting caries by sealants: results of a clinical study. *J. Am. Dent. Ass.* **112,** 194–7.
14 Houpt M., Eidelman E. and Shey Z. (1985). Occlusal composite restorations: 4-year results. *J. Am. Dent. Ass.* **110,** 351–3.
15 British Paedodontic Society (1987). A policy document on fissure sealants. *J. Paed. Dent.* **3,** 41–3.

FURTHER READING

Gordon P. H. (1989). Fissure sealants. In *The Prevention of Dental Disease*, 2nd edn. (ed. J. J. Murray). Oxford: Oxford University Press.

Murray J. J. and Bennett T. G. (1985). *A Colour Atlas of Acid-etch Technique*. London: Wolfe.

Nikiforuk G. (1985) *Understanding Dental Caries. 2— Prevention: Basic and Clinical Aspects*, ch. 7. Basel: Karger.

Chapter 8

Conservation of primary teeth

During the primary dentition period, the restoration of carious teeth is always desirable because all the teeth serve important functions: healthy anterior teeth are essential for an attractive appearance and for efficient incising of food, and the posterior teeth are necessary for chewing and for ensuring that the primary molars erupt in their correct positions.

After the primary anterior teeth are shed, the principal function of the remaining primary teeth is maintenance of space for the unerupted permanent canines and premolars; the role of primary molars in mastication is diminished because permanent first molars are present. Although dentists generally prefer to conserve rather than extract teeth, and child patients generally find restorative procedures less stressful than extraction, it should be remembered that the principal function of primary molars during the mixed dentition period is space maintenance. Since space maintenance is more important in some dentitions than in others, it follows that the importance of restoring carious primary molars in the mixed dentition varies.

Restoration of carious primary molars (space maintenance) in the mixed dentition is:

1. **IMPORTANT** — in dentitions in which there is no evidence of crowding:

(a) there is no permanent incisor imbrication;
(b) there is no mesial drift of permanent first molars (all primary molars present).

In such dentitions it is clear that normal development is occurring and that there is adequate space in the arch for the eruption of premolars and permanent canines. It is important to maintain this normal state by restoring carious primary molars.

Rarely (at least in the UK), dentitions show appreciable excess space between teeth. In such dentitions, space maintenance is not so important because there would be little tendency for loss of space following extraction of primary molars.

2. **LESS IMPORTANT** — in dentitions in which there is evidence of mild crowding:

(a) mild imbrication of permanent incisors;
(b) inadequate space for lateral incisors to erupt without a degree of rotation;

(c) mild mesial drift of permanent first molars following extraction of one or more primary molars.

In such dentitions it is clear that there is inadequate space for the eruption of the premolars and permanent canines.

The most common treatment for dental arch crowding involves extraction of a permanent tooth unit from each quadrant, usually a first premolar. In cases of mild crowding, extraction of first premolars will make available more than enough space for the alignment of incisors and the eruption of second premolars and permanent canines. Therefore, loss of primary teeth from the mixed dentition, followed by some loss of space, will not adversely affect the developing dentition. Indeed it may help because loss of space will be partly by distal drift of anterior teeth, which may allow spontaneous alignment of incisors, and partly by mesial drift of permanent first molars, which will reduce the amount of space that remains after the eruption of second premolars and permanent canines.

Thus, there is no strong justification for restoring carious primary canines or primary first molars in mildly crowded mixed dentitions. However, because a greater degree of mesial drift of permanent first molars can be expected after extraction of primary second molars, conservation of primary second molars is always desirable.

3. **IMPORTANT**—in dentitions in which there is evidence of severe crowding:

(a) gross imbrication of permanent incisors;
(b) lateral incisors erupting lingually/palatally, or grossly rotated;
(c) gross mesial drift of permanent first molars after extraction of primary molars.

In such dentitions it is clear that there is gross inadequacy of space for the eruption of premolars and permanent canines. Extraction of a first premolar from each quadrant may provide only just enough space for the alignment of incisors and eruption of second premolars and permanent canines. Therefore it is very important to conserve primary molars (especially the second molars) to maintain what space there is until the premolars are extracted because, if further space is lost, the second premolars and permanent canines may still have insufficient space into which to erupt after extraction of first premolars.

MIXED DENTITION ANALYSIS

Assessment of whether there is adequate space for the eruption of premolars and permanent canines is an essential element of diagnosis during the mixed dentition period. Not only is this assessment necessary in order to fulfil the professional responsibility of supervising the developing dentition but it also affects, as outlined above, fundamental treatment planning decisions concerning the restoration or extraction of primary teeth.

Experienced clinicians may be able to predict whether crowding will occur, and the degree of crowding, by observing:

(a) the degree of imbrication of the erupted permanent incisors;

(b) the extent of mesial drift of permanent first molars (if primary molars have been lost);

(c) (on a radiograph) the axial inclination of permanent first molars and of the unerupted permanent molars — in uncrowded arches the teeth are vertical or mesially inclined; in crowded arches the molars are distally inclined (especially in the maxilla).

Less experienced clinicians may need a more objective method of assessing the degree of crowding. A simple mixed dentition analysis (MDA) may be performed, in which predictions of the total mesiodistal dimension of the unerupted premolars and permanent canines (i.e. the space required for their eruption) are based on the total mesiodistal dimensions of the erupted mandibular permanent incisors. The predicted space required for the unerupted teeth is compared with the actual space available in each quadrant between the distal surfaces of the lateral incisors and the mesial surfaces of the permanent first molars. This type of MDA has been fully described by the author elsewhere.

Although MDA cannot be relied upon to be absolutely accurate in predicting crowding, it is more objective than mere clinical observation and is therefore a useful diagnostic aid, especially for the less experienced clinician.

CAVITY PREPARATIONS IN PRIMARY TEETH

The techniques used throughout this century for cavity preparation in permanent as well as in primary teeth have been based on principles laid down by Black in 1908, which involve preparing a standard cavity outline for carious lesions in each tooth surface. During recent years, however, with the introduction of improved restorative materials and the adoption by dentists of a more preventive philosophy towards dental treatment, modifications in cavity preparations have been advocated.

The authors of most modern textbooks recommend that more conservative cavities should be prepared but they still base their cavity designs on Black's principles. In the UK, Elderton[1] (see also Chapter 12) has argued for more radical change: to abandon Black's principles, and to aim simply to remove carious tooth substance and unsupported enamel rather than to produce a standard cavity shape for each type of lesion.

Elderton's arguments for an ultraconservative approach are based on his own research, which showed that the durability of amalgam restorations in permanent teeth (in Scotland) is only 5–10 years, and that each time a restoration is replaced more tooth substance is destroyed. The case for a conservative approach is clear, but only long-term studies will show whether the techniques he proposes produce restorations that are more durable than those placed in Black-type cavities.

With regard to primary teeth, the case for an ultraconservative approach is less strong. Although it is clearly undesirable to destroy more tooth substance than is necessary, replacement of restorations every 5–10 years cannot occur: one restoration properly placed probably suffices for the life of the tooth. Therefore, conservative, scaled down versions of Black-type cavities, which might be considered unnecessarily destructive for permanent teeth, are acceptable for primary teeth.

RESTORATIVE MATERIALS FOR PRIMARY TEETH

Amalgam has long been the material of choice for restoring primary or permanent posterior teeth. In particular, the high-copper amalgams that have been introduced in recent years have proved to be highly satisfactory materials.

Composite resins have also been shown to be satisfactory materials for Class II restorations in primary molars. Composite resin wears more rapidly than amalgam but this is only likely to become a problem after several years, by which time the primary teeth will have exfoliated. However, the clinical technique required to ensure success with composite resin is more demanding than that required for amalgam, and therefore amalgam remains the material of choice.

Modified cavity preparations have been tested[2] for composite resin restorations, involving very conservative removal of tooth substance without necessarily providing mechanical retention, but results were not as satisfactory as when conventional Black-type cavities were prepared.

Since the cavity preparation required for composite resin and for amalgam is similar, the only advantage of composite resin is better aesthetics, but this is not usually considered to be an important factor when restoring posterior teeth.

Glass-ionomer cement has increasingly been suggested as a suitable material for restoring primary teeth. Few clinical studies, however, have been conducted and the evidence remains equivocal: for example, Walls *et al.*[3] recently concluded that KetacFil is a satisfactory material for Class I and II restorations, but Fuks *et al.*[4] found another glass-ionomer cement (Fuji) totally unsatisfactory. Walls *et al.* used modified cavity preparations for the glass-ionomer restorations, removing only enough tooth substance to remove caries, and relying for retention on the adhesive properties of the cement. For Class I restorations in primary molars this approach seems justified as an alternative to restoration with amalgam, but for Class II restorations further clinical studies are required before the material can be confidently recommended.

Stainless steel crowns may be used for restoring primary molars that have extensive carious lesions; they are more durable than large conventional restorations. They are also ideal for restoring teeth that have been treated by pulpotomy; pulpotomy weakens the tooth crown, which is therefore liable to fracture if not protected.

Two types of stainless steel crown are available in the UK, the Unitek crown (Unitek Corp.) and Nichrome crown (3M). These have six sizes for each primary molar and gingival contours that conform to those of the teeth. Nichrome crowns are crimped at their cervical margins, which sometimes makes further crimping to achieve a good gingival fit unnecessary.

PULP TREATMENT OF PRIMARY MOLARS

When the pulp of a primary molar becomes exposed, usually by caries, either pulp treatment or extraction of the tooth is required. In the primary dentition, conservation by pulp treatment is always preferable, but in the mixed dentition it must be assessed whether the tooth would be serving a useful function as a space maintainer (see p. 104). Other factors will also influence the decision:

(a) the child's cooperation;
(b) the parents' attitudes;
(c) the child's medical history —

(i) pulp treatment is contraindicated in cases of congenital heart disease, or in cases of poor resistance to infection (e.g. diabetes, leukaemia);

(ii) pulp treatment is indicated in cases of bleeding disorders (to avoid the need for extraction).

Forms of pulp treatment

Direct pulp capping

Indications. These are:

(a) no history of spontaneous pain;
(b) no clinical or radiographic signs of periradicular infection;
(c) pulp exposure not more than pinpoint diameter, with sound dentine surrounding it;
(d) gentle bleeding from exposed pulp.

Method. Calcium hydroxide placed over pulp exposure.

Pulpotomy for vital tooth

(Either formocresol pulpotomy or devitalization pulpotomy.)
Indications. These are:

(a) no history of spontaneous pain;
(b) no clinical or radiographic signs of periradicular infection;
(c) pulp exposure greater than pinpoint diameter;
(d) profuse bleeding from exposed pulp.

Methods: 1. *Formocresol pulpotomy.* The steps are:

(a) local analgesia;
(b) pulpotomy (removal of all coronal pulp);
(c) formocresol solution on cotton pledget for 4–5 minutes;
(d) antiseptic dressing (equal parts formocresol and eugenol mixed with zinc oxide powder) over pump stumps.

2. *Devitalization pulpotomy* — an alternative to formocresol pulpotomy if local analgesia is impracticable or ineffective:

(a) devitalizing paste (paraformaldehyde) over pulp exposure; cavity sealed with temporary dressing;
(b) after 1–2 weeks, pulpotomy (of devitalized pulp), antiseptic dressing (as above).

Pulpotomy for non-vital tooth

Indications. These are:

(a) history of spontaneous pain;
(b) swelling, redness or soreness of adjacent buccal mucosa;
(c) presence of a sinus;
(d) tooth mobility;
(e) tooth tender to percussion;
(f) radiographic evidence of pathological root resorption;
(g) no bleeding from pulp.

Method. The steps are:

(a) pulpotomy;
(b) disinfectant on cotton pledget (beechwood creosote, or disinfectant normally used in root canal therapy); cavity sealed with temporary dressing material;
(c) after 1–2 weeks, disinfectant removed, antiseptic dressing (as above).

Ideally, a non-vital tooth requires pulpectomy rather than pulpotomy treatment. Although pulpectomy can be achieved by a skilful clinician for a cooperative child, it is not generally considered practicable for primary molars.

Full details of the techniques recommended for primary teeth are described by the author elsewhere.[5]

REFERENCES

1 Elderton R. J. (1987). *Positive Dental Prevention*, chs. 10 and 12. London: Heinemann.
2 Oldenburg T. R., Vann W. F. and Dilley D. C. (1987). Composite restorations for primary molars: results after 4 years. *Pediatric Dent.* **9,** 136–43.
3 Walls A. W. G., Murray J. J. and McCabe J. F. (1988). The use of glass polyalkenoate (ionomer) cements in the deciduous dentition. *Br. Dent. J.* **165,** 13–17.
4 Fuks A. B. (1984). Clinical evaluation of a glass ionomer cement used as a Class II restorative material in primary molars. *J. Pedodontics* **8,** 393–9.
5 Andlaw R. J. and Rock W. P. (1987). *A Manual of Paedodontics*, 2nd edn. Edinburgh: Churchill Livingstone.

Chapter 9

Trauma to children's teeth

ASSESSMENT OF INJURIES

History

Dental history

1. How did the injury occur?
2. Where did the injury occur? If the wound is contaminated with soil a tetanus toxoid injection may be required.
3. When did the injury occur? This affects the prognosis of treatment.
4. Was a tooth fractured? If so, is the fractured piece available? If not, the child should be referred for a chest X-ray.
5. Is the child in pain? If so, from teeth or elsewhere?
6. Was the child concussed? If so, the child should be referred to hospital immediately after emergency dental treatment.

Medical history

Of special significance:

1. *Congenital heart disease*: endodontic treatment or tooth replantation may be contraindicated.
2. *Bleeding disorders:* if soft tissues are cut.
3. *Allergies:* when antibiotic cover is needed (e.g. replantation) an alternative to penicillin must be used.
4. *Tetanus immunization status:* if vaccination was done more than 5 years previously, a tetanus toxoid injection should be arranged if the wound was contaminated with soil.

Examination

Extraoral

1. Facial swelling, bruising, laceration?
2. Limitation of mandibular movement?
3. Wound contaminated?

Intraoral

1. Teeth fractured? Fracture of enamel only or of enamel and dentine, involving pulp?
2. Teeth displaced?
3. Teeth and/or alveolus mobile?
4. Tooth fragment in lips?

Radiographic

1. Periapical views of traumatized teeth: two views at different angles (in vertical plane) to locate possible root fractures.
2. If lip lacerated: occlusal view of lower lip, extraoral lateral view of upper lip, to locate possible fragments in lips.
3. If jaw fracture suspected: extraoral views.

TREATMENT

Types of injury

(a) no crown fracture, or of enamel only;
(b) fracture involving dentine;
(c) fracture involving pulp;
(d) loosened teeth;
(e) root fractures;
(f) avulsion of teeth;
(g) injury to primary teeth.

These are now considered in turn.

No crown fracture, or of enamel only

1. No treatment required, other than smoothing any rough edges.
2. Splint if necessary (see below).
3. Review for pulp testing after about 1 month, then after about 3 months, then at about 6-month intervals for 2 years.

If the pulp dies:

(a) immature tooth (open root apex)—pulpectomy and root fill with a calcium hydroxide paste;
(b) mature tooth (closed root apex)—pulpectomy and root fill with gutta-percha.

Fracture involving dentine

1. Protect the pulp:
(a) cover the dentine with a hard-setting calcium hydroxide lining material;

(b) protect the calcium hydroxide lining with a layer of composite resin bonded to acid-etched labial and palatal enamel (if time allows the fractured tooth may be restored at this stage with composite resin);

(c) if insufficient labial or palatal enamel is available, place a stainless-steel crown or other form of protection.

2. Review for pulp testing (as above)

Restore the fractured tooth as soon as possible (if not already done) if there is danger of opposing teeth over-erupting or of adjacent teeth tilting into the space (i.e. if they are crowded).

Fracture involving pulp

If the pulp exposure is pinpoint in size, and the patient presents within 2 h of injury:

(a) pulp cap with hard-setting calcium hydroxide;
(b) protect the calcium hydroxide with composite (as above).

If the pulp exposure is larger than pinpoint in size, or the patient presents more than 2 h after injury:

(a) *immature tooth* — perform pulpotomy:
   (i) **either** conventional pulpotomy — removal of entire coronal pulp;
   (ii) **or** partial pulpotomy — removal of pulp at exposure site to a depth of about 2 mm, using a diamond bur at high speed irrigated with sterile water or saline.
   (iii) **in either case** cover the pulp with calcium hydroxide and protect the dressing as above;
   (iv) review for pulp testing and for crown restoration.
(b) *mature tooth*: perform root canal treatment.

Pulp capping may be done as an emergency measure before pulpotomy or pulpectomy. If pulpotomy is the appropriate treatment it should be done as soon as possible after the emergency capping.

Loosened teeth

A tooth may be loose because its periodontal attachment has been broken or because its root has been fractured.

Splinting. 1. No root fracture:

(a) splint only to stabilize a very loose tooth — periodontal attachment will occur without splinting;
(b) splinting period 2–3 weeks; 3–4 weeks if there is an alveolar fracture.

2. Root fracture:

(a) splint if the fracture is in the middle-third region of the root (see below);
(b) splinting period: 2–3 months.

Types of splint. 1. If teeth not spaced:

(a) etch enamel of the incisal third of the labial surface of the loose tooth and of at least one tooth on each side of the loose tooth;

(b) flow epimine or acrylic resin over the etched area (composite resin could be used but is much more difficult to remove).

2. If teeth spaced:

(a) bend a piece of orthodontic wire (or a paper clip) to rest over the incisal third of the labial surfaces of the teeth to be splinted;

(b) attach the wire with epimine or acrylic resin bonded to etched labial enamel.

(This method could be used if preferred whether the teeth are spaced or not.)

3. If insufficient number of teeth present to use methods outlined above:

(a) take an alginate impression;

(b) make a removable splint — either a polythene mouthguard type or an acrylic plate with Adams' cribs for permanent first molars.

Root fractures

Splinting is required if repair of the fractured root is necessary to stabilize the tooth.

1. *Fractured apical one-third*. Then:

(a) no splinting is necessary — periodontal attachment of root coronal to fracture line is sufficient for tooth stability;

2. *Fractured middle one-third*. Then:

(a) splinting is required — repair of the root fracture is necessary because the length of the root coronal to the fracture line is inadequate to ensure tooth stability;

3. *Fractured coronal one-third*. Then:

(a) splinting is not usually justified (unless the fracture line is close to the middle-third region);

(b) either extract the coronal portion, perform root canal treatment on the apical portion and restore with a post crown, or extract both portions and make a prosthetic replacement.

INJURIES TO PRIMARY TEETH

The most common results of trauma to primary teeth are loosening (subluxation) with or without displacement, intrusion and avulsion (complete displacement); crown and root fractures are rare.

Loosened primary teeth

Splinting is difficult if not impossible; fortunately it is not essential because periodontal reattachment occurs rapidly.

For a tooth that is not so loose as to require extraction:

(a) reposition it by finger pressure if it is displaced;
(b) advise the parents to give the child a soft diet and to discourage the child from disturbing the tooth.

Intruded primary teeth

Intruded primary teeth usually re-erupt within 6 months.

(a) reassure the parents;
(b) advise the parents to keep the area clean by swabbing with antiseptic solution;
(c) inform the parents of the possibility of pulp death;
(d) arrange review appointments at about monthly intervals to assess re-eruption and pulp vitality;
(e) inform the parents of the possibility of damage to the underlying permanent teeth and of the need for radiographic examination when the child is about 7 years of age.

Avulsed primary teeth

Replantation of an avulsed primary tooth is feasible but rarely carried out because of the difficulty of splinting adequately in young children.

Crown and root fractures

Fracture of the crown or root of a primary tooth is rare. The principles of treatment are the same as for similar injuries of permanent teeth, but inadequate patient cooperation may make it necessary:

(a) to leave untreated a tooth that has sustained a crown fracture involving dentine (regular review is necessary for signs of pulp death);
(b) to extract a tooth that has sustained a crown fracture involving pulp.

Complications of injuries to primary teeth

Possible complications following trauma to primary teeth are pulp death of the traumatized primary tooth and damage to the underlying permanent successor.

Assessment of pulp death:

(a) symptoms of spontaneous pain;
(b) blue-grey discoloration of the crown—this suggests but does not definitely indicate pulp death. (A yellowish discoloration indicates pulp calcification, not pulp death.);
(c) a sinus in the region of the root apex—this clearly indicates pulp death;
(d) pulp vitality tests are unreliable with young children and therefore of little or no value;
(e) radiographs are often unhelpful because of superimposition of the crypt of the permanent tooth over the periapical area of the primary tooth.

Assessment of damage to underlying permanent tooth:

(a) damage to developing permanent teeth occurs most commonly when the trauma to the primary teeth resulted in intrusion or avulsion;

(b) the most common form of damage to permanent teeth is enamel hypoplasia or hypomineralization — this becomes apparent as the tooth erupts;

(c) less common forms of damage to permanent teeth are dilaceration, odontome-like malformations, and arrest of root formation — these conditions may be detected by radiography when the child is about 7 years of age (there is no advantage in obtaining this information earlier).

Treatment of non-vital primary anterior teeth

Periapical infection associated with a non-vital primary tooth may cause enamel hypomineralization or hypoplasia of the developing permanent tooth. Treatment must involve either pulpectomy and root canal filling, or extraction.

For pulpectomy and root canal filling to be practicable with such young patients, some compromise of ideal endodontic technique may be necessary and justifiable:

(a) having made an adequate access cavity on the palatal surface, a straight small-headed excavator may be used instead of files and reamers to rapidly remove pulp from the pulp chamber and root canal;

(b) the length of the root canal may have to be estimated roughly from a preoperative radiograph — it may not be practicable to take another radiograph with an instrument in place to exactly determine root canal length;

(c) having sealed a small cotton wool pledget soaked in disinfectant solution (e.g. beechwood creosote or camphorated parachlorophenol) in the pulp chamber for 1–2 weeks, a resorbable material (e.g. calcium hydroxide) should be used to fill the root canal.

FURTHER READING

Andlaw R. J. and Rock W. P. (1987). *A Manual of Paedodontics*, 2nd edn. Edinburgh: Churchill Livingstone.

Andreasen J. O. (1981). *Traumatic Injuries of the Teeth*, 2nd edn. Copenhagen: Munksgaard.

Hargreaves J. A., Craig J. W. and Needleman H. L. (1981). *The Management of Traumatised Anterior Teeth of Children*, 2nd edn. Edinburgh: Churchill Livingstone.

Part Three
Restorative Dentistry

Chapter 10

The dental caries process

Dental caries is a bacterial disease of enamel, dentine and/or cementum. Gradual mineral loss takes place as a result of a series of physicochemical events at or near the surface of the tooth following the fermentation of dietary carbohydrates by bacteria in dental plaque. New lesions are referred to as primary caries, whereas lesions commencing in cavity walls or deep to restorations are described as secondary or recurrent caries. Special characteristics of dental caries are that:

1. It occurs at specific (though variable) sites on the tooth surfaces.
2. It is characterized by intermittent periods of demineralization and remineralization.
3. When the net effect over time is demineralization, the organic components of the tissues also disintegrate, leading to cavitation.
4. If the net effect over time changes to one of remineralization, the lesion arrests and becomes static so that cavitation does not increase; rather, the previously softened tissues harden somewhat.

ACTIVITY OF THE DISEASE

The level of activity of the disease varies according to the level of activity of the bacteria involved and the susceptibility of the teeth to the disease process. Dental caries is very much a disease of lifestyle, and it is therefore markedly influenced by social and family characteristics. These are themselves related to economic status and knowledge about dental diseases.

For caries to occur, essential factors are

(a) a susceptible tooth surface;
(b) living dental plaque attached to the tooth surface;
(c) dietary carbohydrate in a readily accessible form to feed the plaque microorganisms;
(d) sufficient time for the above three to interact.

The disease is multifactorial and factors which influence each of the above include the following (pp. 120–1).

Susceptible tooth surface

This is influenced by:

1. The age of the tooth: recently erupted teeth are more prone to enamel caries (see also root caries below).
2. The location of the tooth surface in relation to plaque accumulation. Especially prone sites (in general order of risk) in younger people are:

    (a) pit and fissure surfaces;
    (b) posterior approximal surfaces;
    (c) cervical regions;
    (d) upper anterior approximal surfaces;
    (e) lower anterior approximal surfaces.

In older people (e.g. over age 45 years) where there has been gingival recession, caries may readily commence in the exposed cementum/dentine, especially on the buccal aspects of the teeth. Such root caries may also commence in or spread to the approximal or lingual surfaces.

3. The shape of fissures: deep crack-like fissures are more susceptible (such fissures may relate to a lack of fluoride at the time the teeth were forming).
4. The quality of the tooth tissues, especially the enamel:

    (a) genetically determined factors that cannot readily be assessed, e.g. the precise chemical composition;
    (b) fluoride content: the higher the content, the less likely caries is to become initiated or to progress.

Nature of the dental plaque

1. The age and thickness of the plaque: mature plaque is more likely to be cariogenic than young, thin plaque.
2. The exposure of the plaque to fluoride: if fluoride is available in the mouth, some becomes incorporated into the plaque which acts as a fluoride reservoir. This fluoride inhibits plaque metabolism and therefore acid production.

Dietary carbohydrate

This is a complex matter, but of particular significance is:

    (a) the frequency of intake of even small amounts of dietary carbohydrate, especially if refined;
    (b) the pattern of dietary intake, e.g. refined carbohydrate followed immediately by cheese appears to be less cariogenic than the refined carbohydrate alone.

THE DENTAL CARIES PROCESS

Time

This may be affected by a variety of diverse characteristics including:

(a) the time periods during which the above plaque and dietary characteristics may interact unfavourably.

(b) The medical status of the patient:
    (i) physical or mental handicap may reduce self-cleansing actions of the tongue etc., thereby increasing the time exposure to adverse dietary onslaught;
    (ii) xerostomia (which may be induced by drug therapy);
    (iii) other characteristics of the saliva and salivation, e.g. flow rate and buffering capacity, which may affect the time that is available for mineral loss to take place from the teeth.

THE CARIES PROCESS

The demineralization that characterizes caries results from acids, principally lactic acid, produced in the plaque and within carious lesions. The acids are end-products or intermediaries of:

(a) the Embden–Myerhof glycolytic pathway;
(b) the Krebs tricarboxylic acid cycle;
(c) other chemical pathways used by bacteria in the catabolism of carbohydrates.

When the pH near the surface of the tooth drops to a critical level, calcium and phosphate ions are lost from the enamel crystals. It is not possible to state a precise value for the critical pH because it varies, though 5.2–5.5 may be taken as a guide. A graph showing the change of pH in the plaque over time after a dietary challenge with refined carbohydrate is referred to as a Stephan curve. This shows a rapid fall in pH followed by a gradual rise to normality over a substantial period of time as the saliva clears away food debris and neutralizes acid.

While *Streptococcus mutans* has rarely been found to be numerically dominant in plaque, various strains of this organism have been incriminated as being largely responsible for caries, especially that occurring in smooth coronal tooth surfaces. However, caries can develop in the absence of this organism, and its presence does not necessarily lead to caries. Lactobacilli and other organisms have also been found to be associated with caries progression.

The cariogenicity of streptococci appears to relate to their ability to produce large amounts of extracellular polysaccharides (e.g. dextran) from ingested sugars. These provide a sticky mass which enhances the adherence of plaque to the tooth surface. In addition, the plaque gel hinders the neutralizing, by salivary buffers, of acid produced in the plaque.

CLINICAL APPEARANCE OF EARLY CARIES LESIONS

The earliest clinical evidence of enamel caries is the 'white spot' lesion. Such spots are, of course, areas (which may cover a substantial region of the tooth

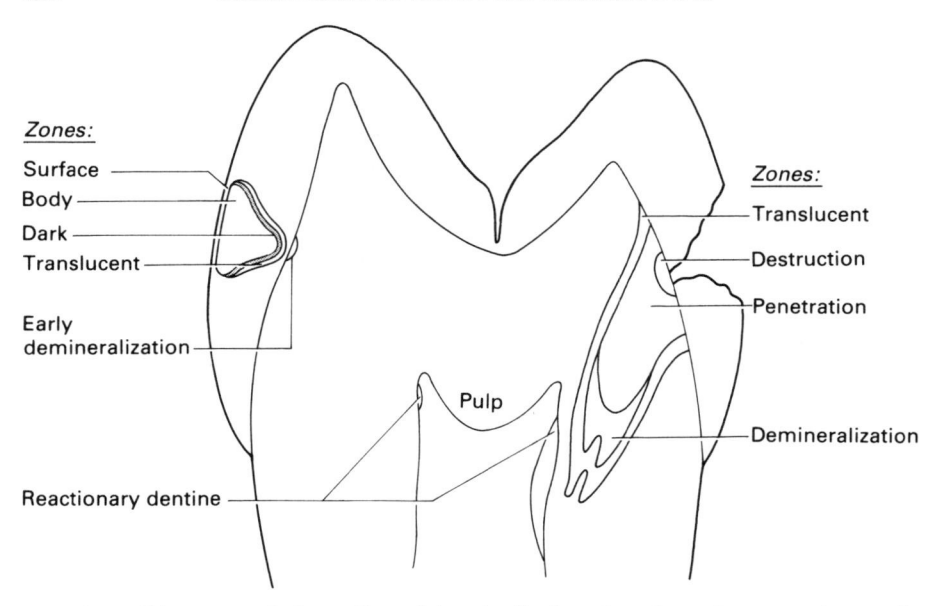

Fig. 10.1 *Diagrammatic buccolingual longitudinal section through a posterior tooth showing: on the left, the zones that are present in a small enamel carious lesion; and on the right, the zones that are present in the dentine deep to a carious cavity in the overlying enamel. Reactionary dentine in the pulp region is also shown.*

surface). In fissures, a small pair of such areas can usually be seen in the cleaned and dried tooth, one in each face of the fissure. Active white spot lesions have a milky appearance, whereas the surface is shiny if the lesion has been arrested.

With the tooth surface often still intact, white spot lesions may progress to a brown colour, whereupon they are described as 'brown spot' lesions. When these arrest they may become dark brown or almost black. With progressing lesions, pitting takes place, followed by increased tissue loss, further staining and cavity formation.

To enhance the accurate diagnosis of caries, the teeth need to be clean, dry and well illuminated. The eye is then the best detection tool for both early and advanced lesions, be they at smooth surfaces or at pit or fissure sites. Probing may damage the tooth and compromise remineralization. It is also important to appreciate that if a fissure is probed, it can seem 'sticky', though there may be no active caries; and the tooth can have active caries but not be sticky.

Radiography

Bitewing radiography may be useful for diagnosing and monitoring approximal carious lesions both in deciduous and in permanent teeth, but it is an insensitive method for assessing the full extent of a lesion. Carious lesions always appear on a radiograph to be less advanced than their histological extent.

The earliest radiographic sign of approximal caries occurs while the surface enamel is still intact (i.e. before any cavitation) and while the lesion is still

THE DENTAL CARIES PROCESS

sterile. There is a small darkened triangular area in the outer part of the enamel. Histologically, however, the lesion will already have penetrated into the underlying dentine.

HISTOPATHOLOGY OF ENAMEL CARIES

Prior to cavitation, an enamel caries lesion typically consists of four zones (Fig. 10.1). From the surface of the tooth inwards, these are:

(a) the surface zone;
(b) the body of the lesion;
(c) the dark zone (present in about 95% of lesions in permanent enamel and 85% of lesions in deciduous enamel);
(d) the translucent zone (present in about 50% of lesions).

The surface zone

This is a thin (approximately 30 μm) but relatively intact and therefore hard layer of enamel which is relatively unaffected by the disease process. Even when demineralization in the body of the lesion has led to mineral loss amounting to 25%, the extent of demineralization (pore volume) in the surface layer will be less than 5%. This is explained by the fact that remineralization takes place in the zone — calcium and phosphate ions from the plaque, or those released by subsurface dissolution, are taken up by the surface enamel.

The body of the lesion

This is the main part of the lesion, and the extent of the demineralization varies widely. The pores are relatively large (pore volume typically = 25%).

The dark zone

The average pore volume is only 2–4% and comprises both relatively large and relatively small pores. Like the surface zone, it is a region of remineralization. It appears that the dark zone sometimes overlaps and obliterates the translucent zone, for it is especially broad and well marked whenever the translucent zone is absent.

The translucent zone

This zone may be restricted to just the lateral aspects of the lesion, near the enamel surface. Adjacent to sound enamel at the advancing front of the lesion, the translucent zone contains about 1% of relatively large pore (compared with spaces amounting to about 0.1% in the sound enamel).

The dynamic nature of enamel caries

The changing distribution of pore sizes throughout the lesion (remember that the small pores of the dark zone occupy positions that, at an earlier stage, contained the larger pores of the then translucent zone) lends considerable support to the understanding that enamel caries is not just a simple process of continuing dissolution, but that it is a dynamic process with phases of demineralization alternating with phases of remineralization. When a lesion regresses, the small pore characteristics of the dark zone come to occupy part of what was once the body of the lesion (which, at that time, only had large pores). Thus, remineralization appears to cause some of the relatively large pores in the body of the lesion to reduce markedly in size.

Enamel crystals

Crystal diameters in sound enamel are some 35–40 nm. However, in a carious lesion they vary in size across the different zones, the ranges of diameters being relatively large in the surface and dark zones (40–100 nm) and relatively small in the body of the lesion (10–30 nm) and the translucent zone (25–30 nm). In addition, some large crystals with diameters of 120–150 nm have been found at the edges of enamel prisms. This knowledge of crystal size provides yet more evidence of the remineralization phases (the large crystals could only have got there by growing) that take place in enamel caries.

As the crystals grow during remineralization, to become about twice the size, on average, of those in sound enamel, so their surface area-to-volume ratio becomes more favourable, resulting in a reduced potential subsequent dissolution rate should circumstances change and the lesion again tend to become active. Certainly, remineralized lesions (with wider dark zones and therefore large crystals) have been found to be more resistant to lesion progression in laboratory studies, in comparison with control lesions.

CARIES IN DENTINE

Once the translucent zone in the enamel has penetrated to the enamel–dentine junction, the caries spreads sideways along this plane of least resistance, so that the enamel–dentine junction becomes the region where the lesion is widest. Overlying enamel tends to become undermined by the process. At a deeper level, the lesion largely follows the dentine tubules, and therefore conforms somewhat to the shape of a cone pointing towards the pulp (Fig. 10.1). Because

THE DENTAL CARIES PROCESS

of the curved arrangement of the dentine tubules in the lateral parts of a tooth crown, it follows that lesions in these regions approach the pulp at a level cervical to that at which the lesion commenced at the surface of the tooth.

Histopathology of early dentine caries

In its relatively early stages, a carious lesion in dentine has two zones (not to be confused with those in enamel):
- (a) the body of the lesion (near the enamel);
- (b) the translucent zone (deeper).

The body of the lesion

Both the peritubular and the intertubular dentine are partially demineralized in this region. Until the stage when cavitation occurs, the lesion is, of course, sterile since bacteria cannot gain access.

The translucent zone

By comparison with the body of the lesion, the translucent zone is a hypermineralized vital response to the lesion and it serves to 'wall off' the lesion from the surrounding dentine. Apatite laid down in the dentine tubules inhibits (for a while) the diffusion, in a pulpal direction, of:
- (a) bacteria;
- (b) proteolytic enzymes;
- (c) acids.

The deep edge of the translucent zone is positioned about half-way through the dentine even when the lesion is quite small.

Reactionary dentine and pulpal response

Deep to the translucent zone there is usually a region of normal dentine, but deeper still a layer of reactionary dentine usually occurs in response to the stimulus brought about by the caries. This is a defence mechanism and it encroaches upon the pulp chamber (Fig. 10.1). At this stage there is a mild degree of inflammation in the pulp. If the stimulus is very severe, then large numbers of odontoblasts die and this reactionary response does not develop.

Histopathology of dentine caries after cavitation of the enamel

Bacteria now start to penetrate the dentine tubules. The acid they produce diffuses ahead of them, causing demineralization as far as the translucent zone. Near the enamel–dentine junction the bacterial population appears to be mixed, producing both proteolytic and hydrolytic enzymes in addition to producing acid, thereby also breaking down the organic collagen matrix of the tissue.

A translucent zone continues to wall off the body of the lesion, but as the lesion progresses and acid succeeds in penetrating it, so a new translucent zone forms in advance of the lesion as the odontoblasts are further stimulated. The body of the lesion comes to occupy the region which was earlier described as the translucent zone. But, by this stage, the body of the lesion has itself become more complex, comprising three sub-zones. From the outside inwards these are (Fig. 10.1) the:

(a) zone of destruction;
(b) zone of penetration (by bacteria);
(c) zone of demineralization.

Zone of destruction

This region at the enamel–dentine junction comes to be fragmented, with little of the normal dentine structure remaining. Clumps of bacteria and necrotic tissue form liquefaction foci by coalescing in the softened matrix. Transverse clefts are also formed (parallel with the incremental lines in the tissue), explaining why large sheets of carious dentine can often be excavated off the floor of a cavity with hand instruments.

Zone of penetration

The bacteria in this zone of bacterial penetration are mainly confined to the dentine tubules. They are sometimes clumped together, showing varying degrees of degeneration as they outrun their nutritional requirements as they multiply. Typical banding is still present in the collagen fibres, which suggests that this organic component is still relatively intact.

Zone of demineralization

This deep part of the lesion, which is usually sterile, marks the advancing 'front' of the demineralization process.

Progress of the lesion

Lateral spread of the carious process along the enamel–dentine junction may undermine considerable amounts of sound enamel. Especially under the direct forces of mastication on the occlusal surface, much of this enamel may break off to give rise to a sizeable cavity in the tooth.

As the carious process continues, so the destruction overcomes the tooth's defence reactions, and increasing amounts of breakdown and disorder are found. Inflammation in the pulp increases progressively, the organisms finally invading the pulp once they have managed to invade the reactionary dentine. In the advanced lesion, this reactionary dentine may be extremely dysplastic; certainly, dentinogenesis is eventually brought to a halt and the tissue is overwhelmed.

PULPAL RESPONSE

Diffusion of bacterial products in advance of the organisms stimulates inflammation in the pulp. Longstanding, slowly progressing caries provides a mild stimulus most of the time, and the inflammation is therefore chronic. Acute pulpitis, a much rarer phenomenon, is a response to the severe stimulus provided by a rapidly progressing lesion, or to the organisms actually reaching the pulp in the later stages of the disease process.

In chronic inflammation, the cellular response predominates over the vascular changes, with aggregations of:

(a) lymphocytes;
(b) plasma cells;
(c) monocytes;
(d) macrophages;
(e) fibroblasts (producing collagen and leading to fibrosis in response to longstanding infection).

With acute inflammation, hyperaemia leads to an exudate of fluid and cells, primarily polymorphonuclear leucocytes. Suppuration and necrosis leading to localized abscess is a likely outcome. Necrosis is brought about by the direct action of the bacterial products and the lytic enzymes which are produced by the disintegrating inflammatory cells. This response is unlikely to resolve. In most other parts of the body, an inflammatory exudate of this type would be manifest as a swelling, but clearly swelling cannot take place inside the rigid pulp chamber. The inflammatory cells increase the oxygen demands on the system, and irreversible degradation is the usual outcome, certainly in teeth with fully formed roots.

In a young tooth where the root apex is still wide open and there is a rich blood supply, the pulpal inflammation will be less severe and may resolve to leave a localized abscess or revert to a chronic inflammatory state. The same may occur if the pulp is open to the mouth as a result of the overlying carious tissue breaking away.

FURTHER READING

Bille J., Thylstrup A. (1982). Radiographic diagnosis and clinical tissue changes in relation to treatment of approximal carious lesions *Caries Res.*, **16,** 1–6.

Silverstone L. M. (1983). Remineralization and enamel caries: new concepts. *Dent. Update*, **10,** 261–73.

Silverstone L. M., Johnson N. W., Hardie J. H., Williams R. A. D. (1981). *Dental Caries: Aetiology, Pathology and Prevention*. London: Macmillan.

Chapter 11

Caries in society and its preventive management

LEVELS OF DENTAL CARIES

The distribution of caries in a population is skewed so that, over a lifetime, some people experience more of the disease than others. In the UK and other parts of the Western world, the disease affected most people during the first two-thirds of this century and an adult who had never experienced caries was a very rare exception. But over the last 20 years or so, the incidence of caries has fallen dramatically and the present young generation contains many individuals who have never had the disease and who are unlikely ever to experience it.

Caries surveys using proper sampling methods and criteria have themselves only been in widespread use for a few decades. The first British national survey of adult dental health took place in 1968 and the first such children's survey was in 1973. The proportion of 5-year-old children in England and Wales with no evidence of caries or of ever having had caries was 29% in 1973. This had risen to 52% by 1983. The mean number of teeth with known decay experience in 12-year-olds dropped over the same period from 4.8 to 2.6 in London and the South East of England, and from 5.0 to 3.2 in the South West. By contrast, in most parts of the developing world, caries levels are rising, indeed they are beginning to overtake present levels in the industrialized countries.

Variation in caries levels in individuals

As every dentist knows well, considerable differences are found in the caries status of any local group of individuals, be they from the same town, school or family.

Pits and fissures are generally the tooth sites that are first affected in an individual, so that it tends to be at these sites that caries or restorations are found in people who have only experienced small amounts of the disease. It should be appreciated, however, that the presence of a restoration reflects a previous diagnosis of caries, yet such diagnoses will not necessarily have been reliable; some will have been frankly incorrect (see p. 137).

Risk factors associated with caries

The reason why some people are more prone than others to caries is explained by the multifactorial nature of the disease. Factors (risk factors) which are thought to affect the level of the disease include the following.

1. Cultural, social and economic status.
2. Age:

   (a) primary caries is more likely to affect a tooth in the first few years after eruption;
   (b) secondary caries adjacent to a restoration may occur at any age;
   (c) root caries commencing in exposed cementum only occurs after gingival recession and therefore in older people.

3. Systemic fluoride intake while the teeth are forming and maturing:

   (a) fluoridation of water supply (or naturally occurring);
   (b) fluoridized salt or other dietary items (e.g. tea, fish);
   (c) fluoride tablets or drops;
   (d) fluoride toothpaste (some will inevitably be swallowed).

4. Topical fluoride usage throughout life:

   (a) topical effect of (a)–(d) above;
   (b) toothpaste;
   (c) fluoride rinses and home-applied gels;
   (d) professional fluoride applications.

5. Frequency of dietary intake, especially of refined carbohydrate.
6. Oral hygiene.
7. General and dental health knowledge (dentists and their families are highly successful at avoiding caries and restorative dentistry).
8. Interaction with dentists and dental personnel (motivating and counselling influence).
9. Medical conditions which affect lifestyle or oral physiology:

   (a) mental or physical handicap (responsible for e.g. dietary or hygiene factors);
   (b) xerostomia;
   (c) long-term use of sugary medicines;
   (d) drugs which reduce saliva flow.

10. Occupation which involves frequent contact with cariogenic food or drink, e.g. food industry, tennis coach (soft drinks on tap at the courts, etc.).
11. Saliva characteristics:

    (a) acid-forming capacity;
    (b) sugar clearance rate;
    (c) buffering capacity;
    (d) flow rate.

12. Plaque levels.
13. Bacterial flora (quantitative and qualitative).

As many of the above characteristics vary from day to day or from year to year, it follows that carious lesions will progress at varying rates and that they may arrest.

Changing status of carious lesions over time

Descriptive status

The status of a carious lesion may be described as one of three types as follows.

1. *Rampant*

    (a) It may take as little as a few weeks for the lesion to spread through the full thickness of the enamel, especially in deciduous incisors.

    (b) Pulpal exposure may take place in just several months from the time the lesion commences. When this occurs, one or more very specific causative factors can usually be identified, e.g. prolonged exposure to a syrupy liquid in a baby's dummy or bottle.

    (c) The condition may also occur in older patients, e.g. in response to a stream of sweets being sucked in an individual who is trying to give up smoking.

2. *Within normal limits.* It will take perhaps 1–5 years to progress through the enamel and as long again to have a major effect upon the dentine.

3. *Arrested*

    (a) This may occur at any stage in the life history of a carious lesion.

    (b) The term applies to lesions in which there is no longer a net loss of mineral over time.

    (c) The lesion tends to darken in colour.

    (d) There is some hardening of the tissues, the mineral for remineralization being derived from the saliva in the outer parts of the lesion, and in the deeper parts through deposition of secondary dentine by the odontoblasts. Some mineral gain in these deeper parts is also thought to come from the saliva.

Progression of caries

The research literature contains a rather heterogeneous array of reports concerning the changing status of carious lesions over time. Most such studies have involved observations on bitewing radiographs and have thus concerned approximal lesions in posterior teeth. Overall conclusions that may be drawn are that:

1. Caries progression is variable.
2. For the majority of people carious lesions progress slowly.
3. Many lesions remain static over periods of years.
4. The mean time taken for lesions to penetrate the enamel is some 3–4 years.
5. There is evidence of some early lesions reversing to a non-carious state.
6. In Western cultures where caries levels are falling:

    (a) the proportion of established lesions that progress appears to be less now than formerly;

    (b) where lesions *do* progress, the rate of progression appears to have become slower.

The reader will appreciate that use of the 'mean' in relation to rates of caries progression is unsatisfactory with respect to the prediction of the future caries activity at individual tooth sites for individual patients, because it concerns pooled information (which inevitably includes that from both arrested lesions and from rapidly progressing or rampant caries).

Carious lesions in pits and fissures also exhibit variable rates of progression, and significant numbers of reversals to a non-carious state have been reported when teeth have been re-examined after several years. It should be appreciated that most 'clinically sound' posterior teeth that have functioned in the mouth for a few years, and have then had occasion to be extracted and examined histologically, reveal the presence of very early arrested caries. Indeed there is some suggestion that the initiation and arresting of small carious lesions in pits and fissures may be considered quite normal in populations with fairly low levels of caries prevalence.

PREVENTIVE MANAGEMENT OF CARIES

In days gone by, the (unstated) maxim in managing carious lesions was undoubtedly 'if in doubt, fill', in accord with the naive and erroneous belief that the restoration would cure the disease. Now, the questions that need to be asked are: *'Is it an active lesion?'*, and if so: *'Can it be arrested?'*

If in doubt as to the state of activity of a lesion, the worst should be assumed and preventive measures instituted in the same way as if the lesion were *known* to be active. Thus, the revised maxim becomes: *'if in doubt, prevent, wait and reassess'*. Clearly, preventive measures cannot work if they are not given time to do so.

Being a disease of lifestyle, management of the disease should concern lifestyle. It will be appreciated that there are certain characteristics of lifestyle that cannot be changed, there and then, for a patient who presents with caries:

(a) general living conditions;
(b) social class;
(c) age;
(d) saliva characteristics (though help can be given to those suffering from xerostomia).

But it should be possible to influence:

(a) dental awareness, e.g. knowledge about the disease including its causes and the realistic possibility of its arrest through self-control;
(b) motivation to attend a dentist frequently enough to allow adequate reinforcement of preventive measures and monitoring of lesions where an attempt is being made to bring about arrest;
(c) oral hygiene;
(d) fluoride usage;
(e) the dietary pattern.

Restorations do none of these things, so it is important to appreciate very clearly the fact that when there is doubt as to whether or not to restore, the higher the caries-risk status, the greater is the chance that a restoration would not serve adequately in the long term, and thus the greater is the need for preventive rather than, or in addition to, restorative management. In other words, the higher the caries activity status is judged to be, the greater is the need to adopt a preventive attitude and shift the patient to a low caries-risk category.

Preventive management of smooth surface lesions

Every dentist has seen early and extensive carious lesions that have arrested because the local environment has changed and a balance has become established between the calcium and phosphate ions in the tooth tissue and those in the saliva. Whilst fastidious application of a battery of preventive measures would be expected to cause any and every carious lesion to arrest, a compromise situation normally prevails, for only a limited uptake of preventive measures usually occurs. Nevertheless, a concerted attempt to motivate the patient to effect sufficient change in habits is very realistic because, often, only minor adjustments may be enough to tip the balance towards arrest and remineralization — and, of course, the lesion *might* be arrested already; after all, arrested lesions exist in most people's mouths, yet such people are not necessarily 'holier than thou' in their day-to-day dietary and oral hygiene habits, etc.

A realistic method for helping a patient to arrest a smooth surface carious lesion is as follows (the intensity of the advice being dependent upon the severity of the disease).

1. Demonstrate the exact site and presence of the lesion to the patient and explain what is going on. It may be necessary to use two mirrors. The patient should be taught to 'find' the lesion. It is often helpful to discuss its radiographic appearance.

2. Encourage the patient to institute improved general preventive measures:

    (a) *Dietary*: reduce the frequency of exposure to cariogenic items, especially refined carbohydrate; and certainly avoid any such items after the final oral hygiene/fluoride application procedure before bed. It may be appropriate to advise giving up sugar in tea and coffee, etc., and substituting 'diet' drinks or water for sugar-containing squashes and sparkling beverages. 'All-in-one-go' chocolate bars are better than 'frequent exposure' sweets that come in packets or bags.

    (b) *Oral hygiene*: raise the quality of overall plaque control. Since plaque takes over 24 h to grow into a pathogenic mass (but can form a definite layer in this time), at least one really good cleaning should take place each day.

    (c) *Fluoride*:

        (i) Ensure at least two applications of fluoride toothpaste each day, one being last thing at night. A third one, or a fluoride rinse, may be appropriate in the middle of the waking part of the day.

        (ii) While there is no scientific evidence to support it, the practice of spitting but not rinsing after using fluoride toothpaste makes a lot of sense on theoretical grounds and should therefore

be encouraged (but children should not normally, at the same time, also be taking systemic fluoride supplements).
(iii) Systemic fluoride supplements (tablets or drops) should be considered for children during the period when the crowns of the teeth are unerupted and the objective is primarily to enhance fluoride uptake into the developing tooth structure as it forms, or to aid subsequent maturation via the tissue fluid.

3. Encourage the patient to adopt specific measures relevant to the particular lesion:

(a) a minute amount of fluoride toothpaste can be wiped (with a finger) directly on to the lesion every night for, say, the initial 6 weeks;
(b) with approximal lesions, interdental flossing every day or two would seem sensible.

4. Say to the patient and/or parent: 'I can't prevent this cavity from progressing, it is largely up to you, for it is *you* who will apply the preventive measures.'

5. Record the site of the lesion and arrange to reassess the patient and the lesion at recall intervals so as to reinforce preventive measures as necessary (or, rarely, if it seems appropriate at that time, restore).

Preventive management of pit and fissure lesions

The presence and activity of caries at pit and fissure sites is sometimes very difficult to determine with accuracy. It follows that any form of 'wait and reassess' method of management is fraught with danger. This is because both the original and the subsequent assessments may be inaccurate, and in the meantime caries may be advancing unnoticed. The accusation of 'supervised neglect' could then be applied justifiably.

If there is any question of active caries being present at a pit or fissure site, it should be assumed that a small active lesion is present and be managed in the same way as pits and fissures with *known* small active lesions; something positive should be done:

(a) either the application of fissure sealant (see Chapter 7);
(b) or an invasive restoration;
(c) or a combination of the two.

Of these options, only the first ensures no over-treatment, for it is non-invasive and reversible.

As correctly applied fissure sealant can be expected to cause arrest of the lesion, this is the method of choice for managing early caries in fissures when the appropriate criteria apply (see below).

There is, indeed, a mass of research evidence to support the efficacy of applying fissure sealant therapeutically to pit and fissure lesions that have been shown by radiographs to extend through up to half of the thickness of the dentine. Providing the sealant remains intact, the caries appears to arrest. Such an outcome would also be expected on theoretical grounds, for by placing a barrier to the nutritional substances required by the bacteria, their demise would be expected. Indeed, over the last 20 years, many millions of carious lesions in pits and fissures must have been sealed over in good faith by dentists who, at the time, considered the teeth to be sound. And the sealants appear to have worked. Providing the sealant remains intact, it:

(a) dramatically reduces the viable bacterial flora to a level which is too low to enable the caries to progress;
(b) leads to a situation whereby the lesion may become sterile;
(c) allows some remineralization of the carious dentine to occur.

Fissure sealants clearly have a significant role to play in the management of relatively early caries at pit and fissure sites.

Criteria for the therapeutic use of fissure sealant

(Compare with the criteria for restorative treatment of pit and fissure lesions — p. 143 et seq, Chapter 12; guidelines for sealant usage are also given in Chapter 7.)

Fissure sealants should normally serve as a preventive/therapeutic treatment when the following criteria apply:

1. A tooth is judged to have *active* or *possibly active* early pit or fissure caries (sometimes white or brown spot lesions can be seen in the sides of the fissure).
2. 'Don't know' situations in which there is doubt as to whether or not a lesion is present, i.e., *if in doubt, seal*.
3. There is a need for temporary management of extensive pit or fissure caries, especially in a patient who will not cooperate with restorative treatment (this is speculative).

The above three criteria apply to all pitted or fissured tooth surfaces, i.e. including:

(a) wisdom teeth;
(b) palatal pits in upper lateral incisors;
(c) buccal and palatal pits and fissures in molars;
(d) deciduous teeth.

Circumstances which contraindicate the use of fissure sealant for the treatment of pit and fissure lesions (and where an invasive restoration is required) are listed in Chapter 12.

Sealant materials. These have been described in detail in Chapter 7. Resin-based materials are in more widespread use than glass-ionomer materials for fissure sealing, and they have been subjected to more clinical trials. But glass-ionomer appears to have a special place as a sealant for deciduous teeth on account of the chemical nature of the bonding system. With glass-ionomer, some clinicians advise that the fissure should first be widened with a very fine bur to permit proper compression of the rather viscous cement into the region. When a resin-based sealant is used, it should be white or coloured (rather than transparent) so as to enhance ease of checking its integrity at subsequent visits.

CARIES AND ITS PREVENTIVE MANAGEMENT

Criteria for the use of fissure sealant for primary prevention

It is appropriate here to consider the criteria for applying sealants for the primary prevention of caries in sound, untreated, pits and fissures in order to put their therapeutic role (above) into perspective.

The prophylactic sealing of all pits and fissures for the whole population of children as the teeth erupt cannot be justified on economic and logistical grounds; indeed such a regimen could be considered to amount to overtreatment. Further, a proportion of the sealants would fail and some of the jagged and cantilevered edges of fractured and partially detached sealants might be partly responsible for predisposing to caries in some of these teeth. The credibility of dentists and sealants would suffer in the eyes of the public.

Sealants as a primary preventive measure are, however, recommended (as part of an overall preventive package) for:

1. Teeth considered to be at special risk of becoming carious, e.g. for:

    (a) caries-prone individuals;
    (b) teeth contralateral to those that have already become carious;
    (c) teeth that have habitually plaque-covered fissured surfaces.

2. Teeth in patients from families in which older siblings have experienced medium or high levels of caries.

3. Teeth in patients whose dental and/or medical history is compromised by circumstances which render them at special risk if they are subjected to:

    (a) dental caries;
    (b) restorative treatment;
    (c) extractions.

4. Teeth in patients for whom restorative treatment would present special problems:

    (a) mentally retarded individuals;
    (b) patients who are especially fearful of restorative treatment;
    (c) those going to, for example, the Antarctic for 2 years.

PREVENTIVE MANAGEMENT OF DEFECTIVE RESTORATIONS

It is noted below (p. 137, Chapter 12) that clinical judgements about secondary caries are remarkably inaccurate. Several studies have also shown very clearly that dentists frequently want to replace restorations, even when caries is thought to be absent — they appear simply 'not to like the look' of them.

In deciding whether or not to replace a morphologically imperfect restoration, it is necessary to weigh the advantages against the disadvantages. The argument that a pulp might be lost if a suspect restoration is not replaced should be seen in proper perspective against the disadvantages of replacing it (weakening of the tooth, etc., and, at the same time, certainly *not* being able to guarantee no loss of the pulp as a result). It would seem that to institute preventive measures and leave the tooth alone, rather than to re-restore, would usually be the correct method of management, unless:

1. Active secondary caries can be demonstrated in the dentine.
2. There are symptoms.
3. There is impairment of function.
4. Aesthetic reasons demand it.

Just as the reduced prevalence of dental caries in most industrialized countries suggests that any carious lesion is less likely to be active today than would have been the case 20 or so years ago, so it may be presumed that caries at the margin of a defective restoration is less likely to be active now than would have been expected in former years. Thus it is likely that fewer restorations should need replacing nowadays. Unfortunately, however, it appears that a diagnosis of secondary caries is often made erroneously (and the restoration then replaced), such as when a probe catches in an innocent crevice at the edge of a restoration.

When active caries is present, preventive measures aimed at improving the environment of the restored teeth should be instituted, whether or not the restoration is replaced. It may then be possible to arrest the caries and thereby eliminate the need to replace the restoration. Where a defective restoration is not to be replaced, it should of course be monitored over time, the option to replace it being taken subsequently if this proves to be necessary.

FURTHER READING

Elderton R. J. (1985). Management of early dental caries in fissures with fissure sealant. *Br. Dent. J.*, **158,** 254–8.

Elderton R. J. (1985). Assessment and clinical management of early caries in young adults: invasive versus non-invasive methods. *Br. Dent. J.*, **158,** 440–4.

Elderton R. J. (1988). Changing scene in restorative dentistry. *Br. Dent. J.*, **164,** 263–4.

Elderton R. J., Mjor I. A. (1988). Treatment planning. In *Modern Concepts in Operative Dentistry* (Horsted-Bindslev P., Mjor I. A. eds.) Copenhagen: Munksgaard, pp. 59–88.

Pitts N. B. (1983). Monitoring of caries progression in permanent and primary posterior approximal enamel by bitewing radiography. *Community Dent. Oral Epidemiol.*, **11,** 228–35.

Todd J. E., Dodd P. (1985). *Children's dental health in the United Kingdom 1983.* London: HMSO.

Chapter 12

Restorative treatment: its problems and criteria for undertaking it

While many carious lesions will arrest spontaneously or can be expected to arrest once appropriate changes have been made to the oral environment, the need for invasive restorative treatment remains. There is no doubt that this can be a very effective cure for pain arising from dental caries, and it has a major role to play in improving function and aesthetics. Indeed, without restorative dentistry, many teeth that are saved would otherwise be lost. But restorative dentistry also suffers from a number of intrinsic failure characteristics which need to be fully understood if criteria for restoring are to be placed within any true-to-life context.

PROBLEMS WITH RESTORATIVE TREATMENT

Problems with caries management

Inaccurate diagnosis of primary caries

Although dentists have been trained to diagnose caries, it should not be assumed that they are infallible in this respect, nor that all dentists even attempt to use the same clinical criteria when trying to do so. Thus, when groups of dentists have been asked to examine the same patients, enormous differences have been found in terms of precisely which teeth, and how many, they consider to have carious lesions. Some of the diagnoses reported must have been incorrect.

Inaccurate diagnosis of secondary caries

When a group of dentists examined extracted restored teeth in a simulated clinical study, there was considerable lack of correspondence between the teeth which the dentists considered had caries, and those which were found, after sectioning, to have caries. And in many instances, the dentists admitted that they did not know whether or not secondary caries was present. As the majority of restorative treatment in the UK concerns replacing existing restorations, the potential consequences of these inaccurate diagnoses are far-reaching.

Idiosyncratic restorative treatment decisions

The above problems with diagnosis are, not surprisingly, reflected in the idiosyncratic nature of many restorative decisions, and considerable variation in this respect has been noted in a number of studies. Thus, in an investigation in which 15 dentists each examined and planned treatment for the same group of 18 young adults, the number of decisions to restore ranged across the dentists from 20 to 153. There is little doubt that many of these decisions must have been wrong; indeed, it is clear that there is considerable confusion among dental practitioners as to precisely what criteria should be used to determine the need to place or replace a restoration.

Problems with replacing restorations

Inability to identify the causes of failure of restorations

Having perceived a restoration as being in need of replacement (i.e. failed), dentists are often unable to state the cause of failure. Thus nine dentists who each examined the same group of 228 restored teeth gave widely differing reasons for breakdown at the edges of the restorations. Whereas four of the dentists most often cited 'excess restorative material' as the main cause of the marginal breakdown, two placed most blame on the quality of the cavity margin, two more said it was because the restorations had not been polished, while the ninth dentist felt that improper manipulation of the restorative material was primarily responsible. Objective studies have shown that most of the reasons given were wrong (or were not the main errors).

Errors are repeated

Replacement restorations frequently contain the same errors as their predecessors.

Thus, as with new restorations, replacement restorations are often doomed to failure from the start because clinicians make mistakes. But worse, clinicians are generally unaware of these faults in their new restorations. Indeed, in a study of occlusal amalgam restorations which were mostly shown, by objective means, to be very poor, the dentists who undertook them nevertheless assessed all of them as satisfactory. This is in spite of the fact that in 23% of instances, these same clinicians reported 'don't know' as the reason for the marginal failure in the restorations they had just replaced. This highlights the somewhat frightening situation whereby a dentist operates to replace a restoration without knowing what has gone wrong before, and therefore without knowing what alterations to make to ensure that the fault does not recur with the new restoration.

Cavities increase in size

This is inevitable as restorations are replaced, but is exacerbated by an apparent desire to 'freshen up the margins'.

Teeth become weaker

This is inevitable as more and more tooth tissue is taken away. Fractured cusps are becoming increasingly common.

Restorations become more complex

This is inevitable as the amount of tooth left to hold the restoration in place diminishes with each replacement.

Restorations become more costly

This is especially the case when crowns or other laboratory-made restorations are used to restore teeth that have had a series of repeat 'simpler' restorations.

Problems relating to dental services

Treatment-orientated approach by dentists

Dentists who adopt an aggressively treatment-orientated approach to caries management may, in addition to doing too many new or replacement restorations, unwittingly fail to allow existing ones to achieve their full potential. Thus, in a 5-year longitudinal study of dental treatment received by a randomly selected group of dentate adults, it was found that 50% of the restorative treatment was directed at just 12% of the people. These individuals were a high-risk group — at particular risk of having their restorations replaced — and it was noted, somewhat inevitably, that the ratio of replacement restorations to first-time restorations increased markedly as the overall amount of restorative treatment rose. It seems that a heavily restored dentition *may* reflect the philosophy of the dentists who have provided treatment, at least as much as the level of caries experienced by the patient.

Inadequate preventive back-up

By placing a restoration, many dentists appear to exonerate themselves from having any responsibility for helping the patient to manage the disease processes, yet modern understanding confirms that restorative treatment for caries should be undertaken in a preventive setting, with attempts being made to help the patient control the disease processes.

Attendance by the patient

Factors relating to the way in which dental services are organized also appear to play a major part in treatment decision-making. Thus, in the above longitudinal study it was noticed that, in general, the more frequently a patient went to a dentist, the more restorations he or she was likely to receive over a fixed period of years; and the more restorations a person had, the more he or she tended to receive in the future — sometimes a vicious circle is created. Frequent attendance should not be seen as providing an opportunity to provide yet more restorations; rather, it should be encouraged to:

(a) enable screening for diseases (including periodontal diseases and cancer);
(b) help effect successful prevention of diseases.

Changing dentist

It was found in the above study that dentate individuals who went to the same dentist approximately annually over 5 years received an average of 7.4 restorations, whereas a similar group of patients who changed their dentist once or more during the 5 years received an average of 13.6 restorations over the same period. It seems that many dentists have a special impulse to want to replace restorations that they did not themselves place.

Remuneration of the dentist

The way in which the dentist is paid and, indeed, its level, *may* have a significant effect upon the pattern of restorative treatment provided, and upon the quality of this treatment.

Problems relating to restorative procedures

Out-dated cavity designs

A very mechanistic approach to cavity design and preparation has typified the treatment of caries for 100 years. Descriptions in text books have tended to relate more to hypothetical situations than to teeth with actual carious lesions. A major problem appears to have arisen from the use of Black's term 'outline form'. This has led to the cutting of cavities (especially for amalgam) with irrational preconceived shapes (Fig. 12.1), especially:

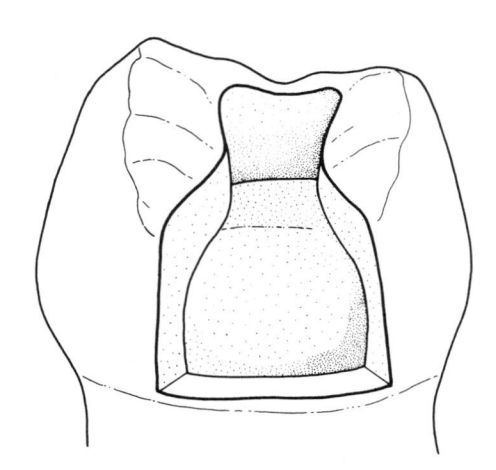

Fig. 12.1 *Diagram showing a molar tooth with an out-dated extended approximo-occlusal cavity preparation for an amalgam restoration. Compare with Fig. 14.1.*

1. Vertical occlusal walls.
2. Flat floors in occlusal cavities.
3. Rectangular approximal 'boxes'.
4. Sharp internal line angles.
5. Occlusal locks in approximo-occlusal cavities.
6. Axio-pulpal line angles in approximo-occlusal cavities.
7. Crazed cervical margins in approximal cavities due to inadequate trimming to remove unsupported enamel prisms that subsequently break away in an uncontrolled manner when, for example, a matrix band is tightened against them. This in turn leads to a poor interface between the tooth and the restorative material in an especially critical area. Marginal leakage is then inevitable.

There is a mistaken, yet widely held, belief that extended preparations with squared-out internal features are essential for allowing a bulk of restorative material and for the prevention of subsequent failure through recurrent caries or material breakdown. It does not require much imagination to realize that maintaining a bulk of sound remaining tooth substance is a more laudable objective.

Incorrectly placed restorations

Some common faults relate directly to the above and include:

1. Weak amalgam margins of occlusal restorations. These occur when the walls of the cavity have been prepared in line with the long axis of the tooth and have high cavosurface angles. The amalgam is then, somewhat inevitably, carved to a 'thin' edge (less than 70° amalgam margin angle) in order to accommodate the opposing occlusion.
2. Poorly adapted restorative material, i.e. the restorative material is left short of the cavity margin or in excess. These are both particularly common with respect to amalgam on the occlusal surface of a tooth, but overhangs and underhangs on all aspects (buccal, lingual, cervical) of the approximal parts of approximo-occlusal restorations are also prevalent.
3. Restored contact points and marginal ridges are often incorrect because the matrix band has been inadequately curved in the occlusocervical plane.

Damage to the adjacent tooth

This often occurs when preparing an approximal cavity. Indeed, sadly, it would be more correct to say that this is the norm rather than the exception — though the damage is often so slight that it may be insignificant.

General lack of attention to detail at all stages

Finesse is often lacking. Widespread use of rubber dam (Chapter 13) and magnifying systems would help.

Moisture contamination

Saliva or blood that are allowed to touch the completed cavity, and during restoration placement, lead to compromises in any chemical treatment that might be applied to the cavity and to the physical properties of the restorative material. The routine use of rubber dam would overcome many of the problems (Chapter 13).

Dentists' often erroneous appraisal of their restorative work

Most dentists erroneously think they carry out technically good-quality restorative dentistry and under the right circumstances; they are not generally prepared to face the fact that they (always the *other* dentist, of course) are responsible for the shortcomings listed above. If it is not dentists who are responsible, who is it?

Problems with restorative materials

Inadequate physical properties

No restorative material has ideal physical properties. Characteristics that are particularly liable to lead to shortcomings in restorations include those relating to:

(a) strength;
(b) wear;
(c) polymerization shrinkage;
(d) dimensional stability over time;
(e) thermal diffusivity;
(f) corrosion;
(g) biocompatibility;
(h) marginal seal;
(i) moisture absorption;
(j) appearance.

Problems relating directly to patients

Inadequate compliance with home care

Many patients appear rather to presume that restorations look after themselves and that they are the dentist's responsibility. Their compliance with home care instructions is therefore often unsatisfactory.

Patients do not 'like' restorative dentistry

Most patients who accept restorative dentistry nevertheless see it as a necessary evil. Other people simply avoid going to a dentist if at all possible, for they do not like what they think they may get if they go. Sociodental research suggests that some of these people might come to accept care in a service with a predominantly preventive image. Certainly, recent data indicate that the present restoratively orientated dental service offers something that many people do not want and that it does not fulfil their needs.

SHORT DURABILITY OF RESTORATIONS

All the above factors appear to work together, with the result that many restorations survive in the mouth for only a short time. While restorations *can* last for many decades, the median survival time of routine restorations in adults has generally been calculated to be only about 5–10 years. Much shorter values have been found in children. The repeat restoration cycle is a very real phenomenon, and helping patients to escape from it is a major challenge for the dental profession. Most dentists have *themselves* succeeded in escaping by virtue of being very careful about who assesses the restorations in their own mouths and makes decisions to replace them. One result of this is that *their* restorations often last a very long time.

CRITERIA FOR RESTORING TEETH

Once the above potential shortcomings of restorations are properly appreciated and understood, the implications of restoring under the wrong circumstances will be very clear.

It stands to reason that a tooth should only be restored if:

1. It has a useful purpose (a buccally placed upper third molar without occlusal function, and not likely to be required for a denture rest, exemplifies a situation where extraction would usually be more appropriate even if the carious lesion were quite small).

2. It is a 'restorable' tooth with a reasonable prognosis (remember that poor-prognosis first permanent molars may be better extracted in children before the second molars have erupted).

3. It has a satisfactory periodontal prognosis.

4. It is not a deciduous tooth about to be exfoliated.

5. It should not be included in a programme of (orthodontic) balancing, compensating or space-gaining extractions.

6. The patient 'wants' the restoration.

7. There are no medical contraindications for it.

Conditions which usually indicate the need for an invasive restoration in a permanent tooth may be considered as general (relating to any carious lesion), or relating specifically to smooth surface or to pit/fissure lesions.

General

A restoration is usually indicated if:

1. There are symptoms believed to be arising from the lesion, e.g. hypersensitivity to various stimuli. A sharp pain of short duration, brought about by hot,

cold or sweetness, etc. (the pain generally lasting only for the duration of the stimulus) usually indicates an excellent prognosis for restorative treatment even though the lesion may extend quite deeply. The pulp must *not* be exposed during cavity preparation (see Chapter 14). If the pulp is irreversibly affected with pulpitis, then endodontic treatment will be necessary before restoring the tooth.

2. The lesion is sufficiently advanced that the pulp is thought to be in jeopardy of becoming 'clinically' involved in the lesion before the next dental examination.

3. Previous attempts to arrest the lesion have failed and there is evidence that the lesion is progressing (an observation of months or years may be needed, and 'risk' factors (see Chapter 11) should be taken into account).

4. Function is impaired or is likely to become impaired if the lesion progresses, e.g.:

(a) drifting of teeth as a result of loss of a contact point;
(b) loss of occlusal stops;
(c) loss of tooth substance for occlusal rests, etc. for fixed or removable prosthetic appliances;
(d) food packing;
(e) presence of a local region of tooth morphology which predisposes towards plaque retention and periodontal ill-health (and which *may* contribute to halitosis);

5. Aesthetic reasons.

6. Secondary caries associated with an existing restoration affecting the dentine and thought to be active.

Smooth surface lesions

Included here are approximal lesions and non-fissural buccal and lingual lesions. A restoration is usually indicated if the lesion is judged to have spread well into the dentine *unless it is known to be arrested* as revealed, for example, after an analysis of previous records or radiographs.

Current understanding in this difficult area suggests that it is definitely *incorrect* to restore when a lesion is judged as being confined, clinically or radiographically, to the enamel. Such lesions *may* already be arrested; and certainly they are amenable to being made to arrest.

The difficult clinical problem is the one that arises when the lesion is judged to spread only into the superficial regions of the dentine (up to half way through its thickness). Dentine involvement per se is definitely *not* a criterion for an invasive restorative procedure. Indeed, in the early stages of dentine involvement, enamel cavitation may not have occurred and the whole lesion will still be sterile. And every dentist has seen cavitated dentine lesions that have clearly been present for decades but which are indisputably arrested (as noted on the approximal surface of a posterior tooth, revealed after removal of the adjacent tooth in an older patient).

When trying to make clinical decisions as to the appropriateness of restoring teeth with lesions extending within the outer half of the dentine, the caries risk factors (see Chapter 11) need to be taken into account.

Pit and fissure lesions

An invasive restoration is required when:

1. There is evidence of direct physical communication between the oral environment and the dentine through an enlarged carious 'hole' in the enamel (unless the lesion is known to be arrested).
2. Caries in the dentine deep to a pit or fissure is visible on a radiograph (unless the lesion is known to be arrested).
3. Fissural caries but where the pit or fissure is sited at a location that is subject to direct occlusion with the opposing tooth (e.g. at or near a ridge on the occlusal surface) and where fissure sealant could not therefore be expected to be retained.
4. Situations where, for whatever reason, the clinician is suspicious that caries may have spread deeply into the dentine, e.g. where there is, perhaps, a greyness shining through the enamel or there are otherwise unexplained symptoms that may be due to caries affecting the pulp–dentine complex.

Sealant restorations

There will be situations when part of a tooth surface fulfils the criteria for invasive caries removal and a restoration (as above), and where another part of the same surface fulfils the criteria for fissure sealant (see Chapter 11). Under these circumstances, both may well be correct and a combined 'sealant restoration' (see also Chapter 7) would be appropriate (Fig. 12.2). A sealant restoration may also serve to conserve sound tooth tissue when a caries-free

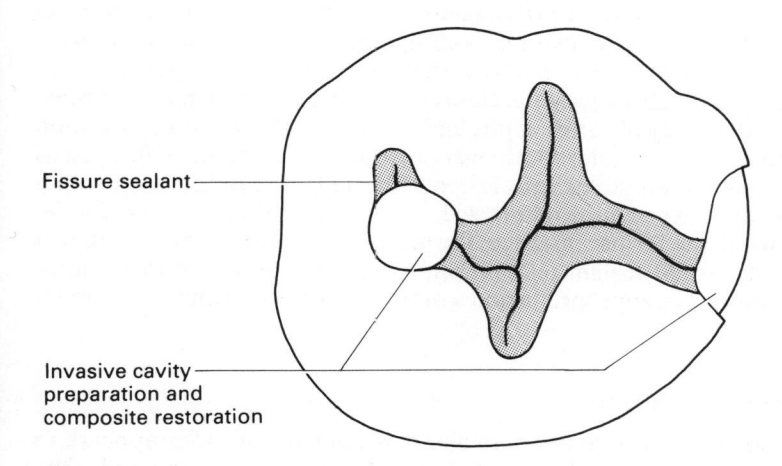

Fig. 12.2 *Diagrammatic occlusal view of a lower molar with a sealant restoration. In this example, there was caries in the mesial (left) part of the occlusal surface and also approximal caries in the distal surface, both lesions fulfilling the criteria for invasive cavity preparation and restoration (cross-hatched). The rest of the fissure system fulfilled the criteria for fissure sealant (stippled). Sealant restorations may involve only the occlusal surface, though extension of the sealant to a buccal fissure (lower molars) or palatal fissure (upper molars) is often appropriate.*

fissured groove radiates outwards from an otherwise completed cavity preparation in which, if amalgam were to be used, it would be necessary to 'extend for prevention' in order to achieve a tenable margin to the cavity and restoration. If amalgam were used in such a situation and the fissured groove *were not* cut away, then flash of amalgam would persist in the fissured region. Most of this would break off in due course to leave a 'ditch' which would be likely to collect plaque, become stained and eventually be a contributory factor to a decision to replace the restoration. A sealant restoration would overcome this problem.

It stands to reason that the materials selected for the 'sealant' and for the 'restoration' components of a sealant restoration should be compatible, and composite resin systems offer this. Amalgam would be contraindicated because it cannot also function as the sealant. A comprehensive sealant restoration might consist of the following materials:

(a) calcium hydroxide lining on the deepest part of the cut dentine;
(b) glass-ionomer cement to make up for the rest of the missing dentine;
(c) composite resin to restore the missing enamel;
(d) resin-based sealant to seal the rest of the fissure system.

If the spread of the caries in the dentine proves to be small, then the cavity preparation in that region will indeed be small; but if the caries proves to be quite extensive, then the cavity preparation will necessarily be extensive (though minimal for that lesion). Large sealant restorations are just as efficacious (perhaps more so) than small ones.

The astute reader will realize that this discussion itself exemplifies one of the benefits of the sealant restoration technique: by having a cavity preparation component, it provides a degree of diagnostic safety with respect to caries in the dentine at the base of the fissure, as compared with the situation where a carious fissure is sealed therapeutically without any attempt at caries removal. It is notoriously difficult to judge accurately, and with confidence, the presence, extent and activity of caries in pits and fissures, so the sealant restoration provides some safeguard against both over- and under-treatment. Thus, just as there will be times when the carious lesion is found (upon penetration with a bur) to be less than expected, so there will also be times when it is found to be more extensive. In the former instance, the procedure is aborted and the defect made good with a small sealant restoration; while in the latter instance, caries removal is continued as appropriate and a more extensive sealant restoration is placed.

Preventive resin restorations

Confusion among dental practitioners about sealant restorations appears to have arisen from some of the descriptions that have been published under the guise of 'preventive resin restorations'. This term, coined in the USA, also embraces a combination sealant and composite resin restoration technique, but it has unfortunately come to be advised sometimes under circumstances that do not warrant it. Indeed illustrations frequently show the cavity preparation part as being restricted to the removal of some enamel (supposedly with active caries) in the region of a fissure, the basal remains of the fissure being in sound enamel. But this is precisely a situation for which fissure sealant alone would be appropriate (see criteria for fissure sealing; Chapter 11) without prior removal of the caries. If cavity preparation is required in order to remove caries, it follows that the lesion must have extended into the dentine (see criteria for restoring pit and fissure lesions; pp. 143–5).

FURTHER READING

Elderton R. J. (1983). Longitudinal study of dental treatment in the General Dental Service in Scotland. *Br. Dent. J.*, **155,** 91–6.

Elderton R. J. (1977). The quality of amalgam restorations. In *Assessment of the Quality of Dental Care* (Allred H., ed.), London: London Hospital Medical College, pp. 45–81.

Elderton R. J. (1984). Treatment variation in restorative dentistry. *Restorative Dent.*, **1,** 3–8.

Elderton R. J., Davies J. A. (1984). Restorative dental treatment in the General Dental Service in Scotland. *Br. Dent. J.*, **11,** 2–8.

Elderton R. J., Nuttall N. M. (1983). Variation among dentists in planning treatment. *Br. Dent. J.*, **154,** 201–6.

Merrett M. C. W., Elderton R. J. (1984). An in vitro study of restorative dental treatment decisions and secondary caries. *Br. Dent. J.*, **157,** 128–33.

Chapter 13

Essentials of rubber dam

Whereas aspiration and absorbent materials are in widespread use for the isolation of the teeth of restorative procedures, the rubber dam is undoubtedly the most effective method. When rubber dam is in place, the patient can still communicate adequately, but excessive chatter is avoided! Particular benefits it brings are:

1. Improved visibility and access to the operating site resulting from retraction of the cheeks, lips, tongue, and gingiva. These advantages allow attention to the finer details of cavity preparation and restorative technique.

2. Control of moisture, allowing complete dryness when required, but also simplifying achievement of this state. Washing away of debris is markedly simplified, especially when chemicals are used, as in endodontic treatment. After removal of a matrix band there can be no onslaught of blood and saliva to obscure the restoration margins and compromise final shaping of the restoration.

3. Control over chemical treatments of enamel and dentine in connection with the use of adhesive systems.

4. Improved detail on elastomeric impressions for laboratory-made restorations.

5. Protection of the oropharynx from instruments and foreign matter like amalgam fragments and mercury.

6. Cross-infection control.

7. Patient comfort—a correctly placed rubber dam leaves the patient to relax and remain free to move his/her tongue, etc.; and it serves to some extent as a mouth prop.

8. Improved quality of life for the dentist—it provides a relaxing working field with reduced stress.

9. Saving of time—this is an undoubted advantage if a high quality of restorative treatment is intended; but mediocre or poor treatment is probably carried out more quickly without the rubber dam.

SUCCESSFUL RUBBER DAM APPLICATION

The overriding prerequisite for successful rubber dam application is for the operator to be mentally attuned to the concept of *wanting* to use it. Several other factors are then of paramount importance, including:

(a) having appropriate equipment;

(b) knowing which teeth to isolate;
(c) knowing a suitable method for applying it;
(d) working with a trained dental surgery assistant (DSA).

RUBBER DAM EQUIPMENT (items marked E are essential)

Rubber dam material[E]

Good quality, thick (tear-resistant) non-white (for enhanced vision) rubber dam in approximately 15 cm ×15 cm squares (12 cm ×12 cm for children) provides the basis for any effective rubber dam application.

Rubber dam stamps and ink pad

The distances between the centres of the holes in the rubber should be similar to the distances between the centres of the teeth and arranged in a similar form. Marking the sheet of rubber with dots to indicate average tooth positions for punching is enormously helpful in this respect.

Punch[E]

In general, the larger the holes, the more easily the rubber dam can be stretched over the teeth and the less is the amount of interseptal rubber to be passed between them. Holes 2.0–2.5 mm in diameter serve for most situations, but a 1.3 mm diameter hole is sometimes desirable for small teeth. The punch *must* be able to make crisp, clean holes in the rubber.

Clamps[E]

One or more of these may be necessary to:

(a) anchor the back of the sheet of rubber dam to the teeth;
(b) enhance gingival retraction.

For most situations (though it is, of course, a matter of personal choice) clamps without wings are preferable to those with wings because they:

(a) are easier to use (less metal to get in the way);
(b) allow better access for dental floss, matrix bands, interdental wedges, etc.;
(c) are more stable on the tooth (less subject to the potential catapulting action of the rubber).

Winged clamps have a special role in single-tooth isolation (see below).

One recently assembled range of clamps (Fig. 13.1) has been labelled A–K according to their most likely usefulness (A=most essential; K=least necessary). In the labelling, a W appended to the clamp's designated letter indicates

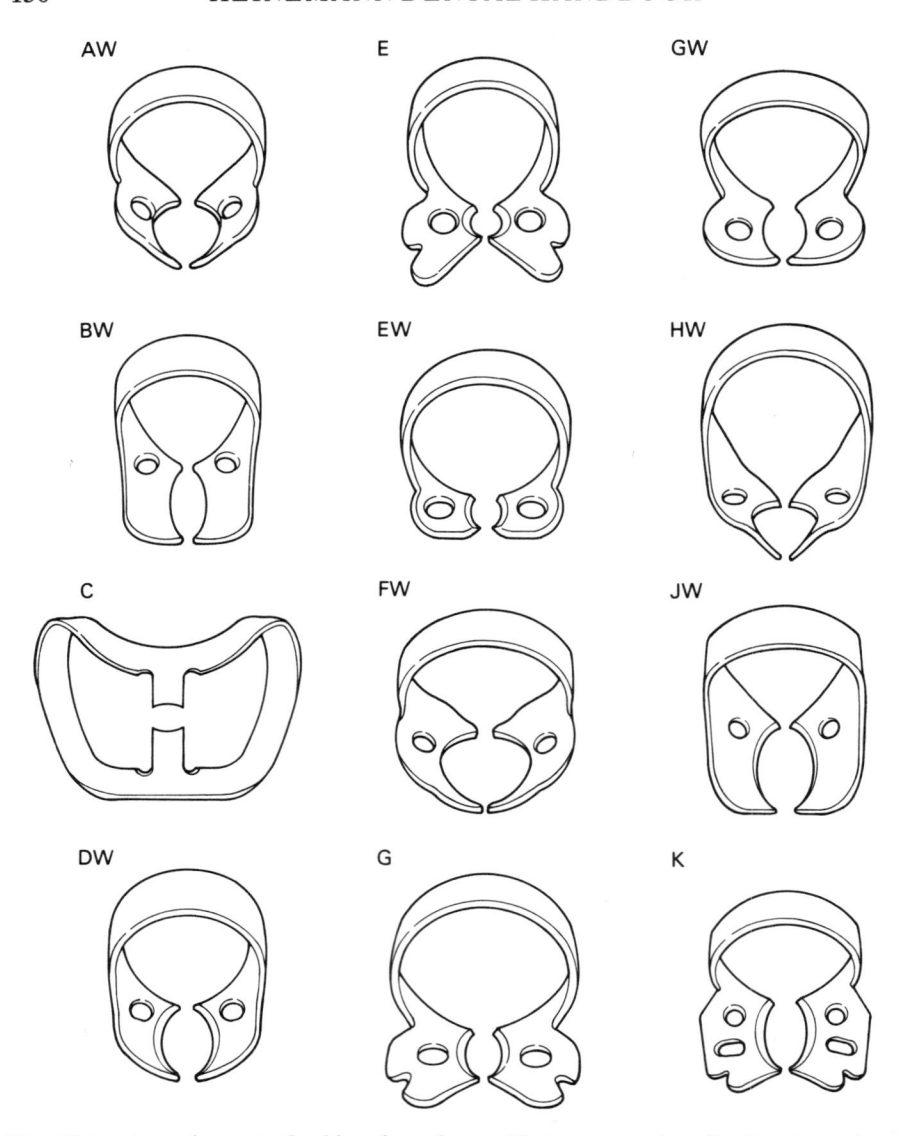

Fig. 13.1 *A modern set of rubber dam clamps (their uses are described in the text).*

that it is wingless (the double-arched C clamp is an exception). The following list describes the uses of the clamps.

1. **AW:** very retentive universal molar anchor clamp (including deciduous second molars), which is especially useful where the tooth is not fully erupted.
2. **BW:** flat-jawed universal anchor clamp for well-erupted molars, also providing better gingival retraction than the AW clamp for cervical cavities and crown preparations.

3. **C:** double-arched (for stability) clamp for definitive gingival retraction around incisors, canines and premolars. There are three versions of this clamp:
   (a) for normal use;
   (b) for situations where extreme buccal retraction is required;
   (c) for situations where extreme lingual retraction is required.

4. **DW:** medium clamp for small molars, first deciduous molars and some premolars. It is useful where the BW clamp is too large.

5. **EW:** universal clamp for incisors, canines and premolars where only limited gingival retraction is required. A winged version (clamp E) is also available.

6. **FW:** very retentive clamp with similar functions to the AW, but it is larger and is usually stable in situations where the AW clamp is unstable.

7. **GW:** general purpose clamp for incisors, canines, premolars and deciduous first molars. It is also useful for upper third molars that are too small to be gripped by the AW clamp. A winged version (clamp G) is also available.

8. **HW:** this is similar to the AW clamp but its arch has been set further back to enhance access to the tooth, e.g. for manipulating matrix bands or taking impressions. However, this clamp is less stable than the AW clamp.

9. **JW:** moderately retentive clamp for large molars, especially where there has been loss of tooth tissue from the cervical regions of the tooth.

10. **K:** winged molar clamp which serves as a compromise between clamps AW, BW, FW and JW in situations where only the occlusal surface of the tooth is involved in the clinical procedure and where the clinician elects to use a winged clamp.

Clamp forceps[E]

These are essential for positioning and removing the clamps from the teeth.

Lubricant[E]

Whenever the rubber dam has to be negotiated past contacting teeth, a wipe of brushless shaving cream over the holes on the tissue side of the rubber just before it is applied to the teeth is mandatory for reducing the friction between the rubber and the teeth.

Dental tape[E]

This is invaluable for carrying the interseptal rubber past tight contact points. Ligatures to hold the dam in place are time-wasting and never necessary.

Petroleum jelly

Applied liberally to the lips and corners of the mouth, this is much appreciated by the patient.

Napkin

Soft absorbent material placed between the patient and the rubber to hold the rubber slightly away from the patient's face further enhances comfort.

Rubber dam holder[E]

This serves to hold the free edges of the sheet of rubber so that they do not obscure vision to the site of operation.

WHICH TEETH TO ISOLATE?

Single tooth isolation

Single tooth isolation can be very effective, quick and simple when the restorative procedure does not involve an approximal surface. If the mesial or distal surface of the tooth is included in the cavity preparation, then at least the contact point of the adjacent tooth will normally need to be exposed through the rubber so that the restoration (permanent or temporary) may be built against it — in which case single tooth isolation is inappropriate. It should also be appreciated that with single tooth isolation of a posterior tooth, the interseptal rubber will usually bunch up in the regions of the occlusal embrasures, thereby obscuring part of the occlusal surface and, at the same time, exerting an elastic and potentially catapulting effect on the clamp.

Multi-tooth isolation

Because most operative procedures involve a mesial or distal tooth surface, it is generally necessary to expose more teeth through the rubber dam than those actually to be operated on. Isolating approximately a quadrant of teeth, or roughly 'four to four', is often simpler and more satisfactory than isolating just two or three teeth. The important thing is to identify two suitable teeth for anchoring the rubber dam at either end of the field:

   (a) a clamp is usually necessary on a molar;
   (b) the contact point between two teeth usually serves to anchor the rubber dam at the front of the mouth or between premolars.

PLACING THE RUBBER DAM

Single tooth isolation

With this method, a winged clamp is engaged in the hole in the sheet of rubber; then the clamp and rubber are placed directly on the tooth. The frame may be attached beforehand or at that stage. The edges of the hole are then freed from the wings of the clamp with a flat plastic instrument. Lubricant is not necessary but local analgesia may be required.

Multi-tooth isolation

This may be more complicated but there need be nothing especially difficult about it. The following steps would, typically, be necessary when placing a rubber dam from the second molar to the midline in order to restore the first molar with a mesio-occluso-distal restoration. The DSA would carry out many of the steps and assist with the others, as follows.

1. Give the local analgesic if required.
2. Test the tooth contacts with floss or tape in order to identify any difficulties (and then, perhaps, avoid them).
3. Decide upon the anchor teeth and select the clamp to be placed on the (probably) second molar.
4. Punch the rubber dam.
5. Lubricate the rubber dam.
6. Open the clamp widely with the clamp forceps.
7. Place the clamp on the second molar (it may, nevertheless, first be appropriate to attach floss around the arch of the clamp and through the forceps holes to safeguard against the unlikely event of the clamp breaking or becoming dislodged.
8. Hold the sheet of rubber so as to stretch widely the most posterior hole; then pass the stretched rubber over the clamp and allow it to hug the tooth.
9. Work the fingers forwards tooth by tooth, trying quickly to pass the interseptal rubber between the tooth contacts. Disregard for the moment any contacts that cannot be negotiated readily.
10. Engage the edge of the anterior hole in the anterior anchor contact point.
11. Apply the petroleum jelly to the lips, etc.
12. Place the napkin.
13. Place the rubber dam holder.
14. Negotiate the interseptal rubber past any contacts that were missed initially. To do this effectively it is essential to use the tape to *pull* the rubber through the contacts. Attempting to push it through is rarely successful. The assistant has an important part to play here in positioning the rubber over the teeth while the dentist passes the tape through the contacts.
15. Evert the edges of the rubber dam where necessary, using tape, an air jet and a pointed instrument as appropriate.
16. Insert wedges to the mesial and the distal of the molar to be treated:
    (a) to aid retraction of the rubber interproximally;
    (b) to protect it from rotary instruments.
17. Wash the field with water spray/air and aspiration.
18. Instruct the patient that he/she can swallow, rather as if the rubber dam were not present.

REMOVAL OF THE RUBBER DAM

Where several teeth have been included in the field, the rubber dam should be stretched out sideways and the interseptal strands cut with scissors. The clamp is then removed with the remains of the rubber and the holder still attached. Where just a single tooth has been isolated, the clamp and dam are simply removed as a unit.

FURTHER READING

Elderton R. J. (1971) A modern approach to the use of rubber dam. *Dent. Pract. Dent. Rec.*, **21,** 187–93; 226–32; 267–73.

Elderton R. J., Marshall K. J. (1988) *Rubber dam*. Dentsview Video 2. University of Bristol.

Chapter 14

Principles of cavity preparation

CAVITY PREPARATION AND RESTORATIONS

A restored tooth represents a compromise when compared with a sound unrestored tooth. Thus, if a tooth needing a restoration is to have the greatest chance of functioning trouble-free in the long term, as much sound tooth substance as possible should be retained, commensurate with satisfying other requirements, so as to:

(a) leave the tooth maximally strong;
(b) place minimal stresses upon the restorative material;
(c) maintain as much occlusal function as possible on enamel;
(d) facilitate correct contouring of the restoration so that it will harmonize properly with the surrounding tooth structure and with the opposing and adjacent teeth;
(e) retain the maximum amount of reactionary dentine;
(f) minimize the extent of cutting (patients do not enjoy the dental drill!);
(g) leave the next dentist the greatest scope for making a replacement restoration in the (likely) event of this subsequently becoming necessary.

Clearly, it behoves the clinician to work to the highest possible standards and to undertake the operative treatment under an umbrella of preventive care so as to maximize its potential.

Before preparing a tooth for a restoration, it is necessary to decide which of the various restorative materials is to be used, for the finer points of cavity preparation vary with the different materials. Characteristics of materials which particularly affect cavity design are:

1. *Physical form:*

    (a) plastic and deformable at the time of placement;
    (b) rigid at the time of placement.

2. *Strength:*
    (a) compressive;
    (b) tensile;
    (c) edge;
    (d) fragility (e.g. with amalgam in thin section, veneers).

3. Biocompatibility.
4. Aesthetic qualities.

5. Method of attachment to the tooth:
    (a) locked into undercuts (including pins);
    (b) cemented into place;
    (c) chemically bonded to the tooth tissue;
    (d) locked mechanically to a roughened enamel surface;
    (e) combination.

PRINCIPLES OF CAVITY DESIGN AND PREPARATION

Cavity preparation should be undertaken in a logical manner. Especially bearing in mind the shortcomings of restorations (Chapter 12), it is important to remove the least amount of sound enamel and dentine commensurate with satisfying certain requirements. But conservative cavities will not necessarily be small; clearly a large carious lesion or large existing failed restoration requires a large cavity preparation, but it should, at the same time, be as small as the lesion or old restoration allows (see Figs. 14.1–14.4).

The principles governing cavity design which are described below are relevant to all tooth preparations, be they for small restorations or for crowns, and whether they are to restore teeth affected by new carious lesions, to replace old restorations or to restore worn, traumatized or aesthetically unacceptable areas.

In considering the principles, it is simplest to think of them in terms of cavity preparation for a new carious lesion. Each principle should be *considered* on every occasion, even though it may not be necessary to take any action.

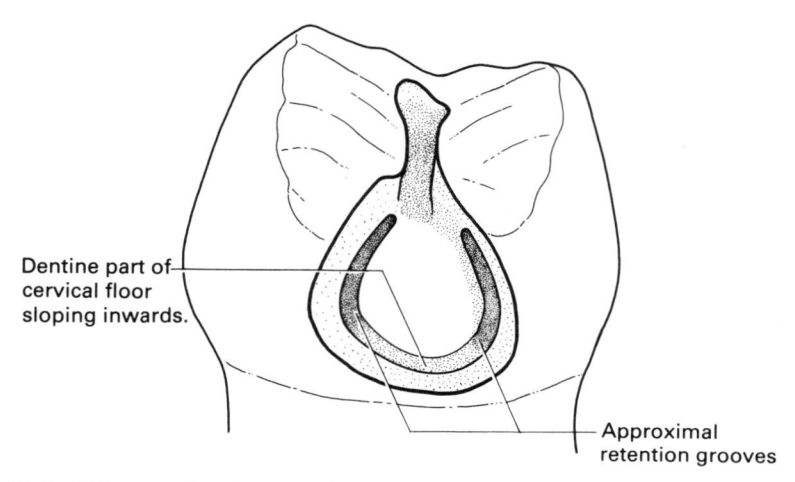

Fig. 14.1 *Diagram showing a molar tooth with a modern approximo-occlusal cavity preparation for an amalgam restoration to restore a tooth with an identical carious lesion to that which resulted in the preparation shown in Fig. 12.1. It is clear that considerably more sound tooth tissue remains.*

PRINCIPLES OF CAVITY PREPARATION

Gaining access to the caries

This is achieved as follows:

1. Penetrate through any overlying enamel so that the lesion in the dentine can be visualized.
2. With Class II lesions, take considerable care to identify the precise buccolingual position of the lesion, whether the marginal ridge is to be sacrificed (conventional preparation) or not (tunnel preparation).
3. Avoid any attempt at cutting a preconceived shape.
4. With Class III lesions, penetrate from the palatal (lingual) side rather than the buccal (labial) if there is a choice, but enter the lesion through the buccal enamel if this is clearly more undermined.
5. Be very careful not to touch and damage the adjacent tooth. Do not use a bur to cut away enamel in contact with the tooth adjacent.
6. When gaining access to secondary caries at the time of removing an existing restoration, take considerable care to cut at the expense of the failed restoration rather than sound tooth tissue.
7. Use a high-speed narrow tapered cylinder (or cylinder) tungsten carbide or diamond bur (or a small round bur in restricted situations). The bur can be used 'end-on' to penetrate the enamel, and 'sideways' with a milling action to open up the cavity. A narrow tapered cylinder bur is a particularly useful, general purpose bur because it is the most realistic for small cavities and perfectly satisfactory for large ones.

Removal of caries at the enamel–dentine junction

This is a very critical step, for it is the primary determinant of the (a) position; (b) size; and (c) shape of the cavity preparation (see Figs. 14.1–14.4).

To remove the caries at the enamel–dentine junction, use a relatively large round bur (e.g. No. 6 for molars and No. 4 for most other teeth). This will leave a caries-free channel at the enamel–dentine junction. Points to note are:

(a) clear the debris frequently to enhance vision;
(b) do not be tempted to work in towards the pulp at this stage.

Removal of actively carious and unsupported enamel

The steps are as follows:

1. Break away any grossly carious or undermined enamel with a hand instrument (e.g. push on it with an excavator or chisel) or use the fine tapered cylinder bur. The latter must be angled correctly to develop the required cavosurface angle (see below). Note that:

(a) a bur is usually more efficient for relatively small cavities on the occlusal, buccal and lingual surfaces;
(b) a hand instrument is usually essential for the mesial and distal surfaces and efficient wherever there is gross undermining in the region of the cusps or incisal edge.

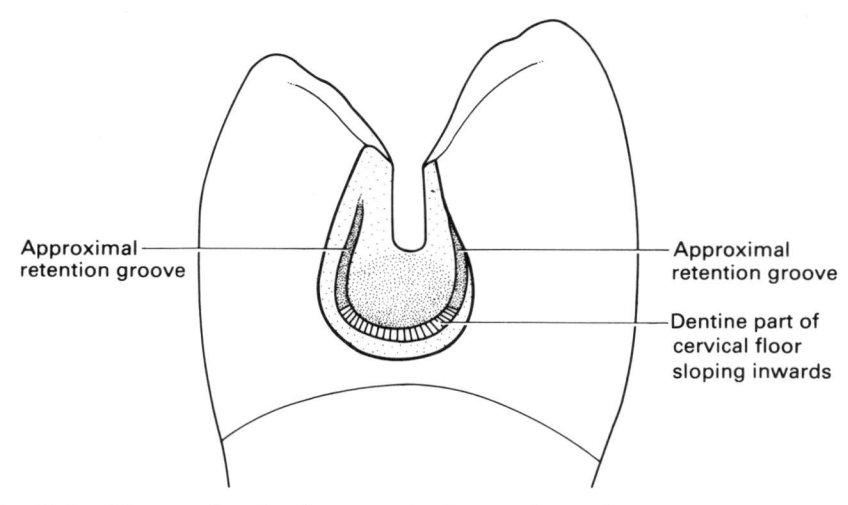

Fig. 14.2 *Diagram showing the approximal view of a modern cavity preparation for amalgam in a premolar in which there had been a moderately sized approximal carious lesion and minimal occlusal caries. As far as possible the cavity has been prepared according to the position, size and shape of the caries at the enamel–dentine junction. The dentine at the cervical floor of the cavity slopes inwards, and there is a retention groove running all around the approximal part of the cavity, just deep to the enamel–dentine junction. Access through the marginal ridge region is as narrow as is commensurate with being able to see the enamel–dentine junction all around. A 'tunnel' preparation (maintaining the marginal ridge) for a lesion of this size would not have been possible because of the extent of the caries. A cavity preparation for composite resin would have been identical, except that the occlusal fissure would have been retained and sealed (to make a two-surface sealant restoration — as at the distal end of the tooth in Fig. 12.2). Likewise, if the occlusal fissure had not been confluent with the approximal cavity, again the fissure would not have been cut away even if amalgam were to have been used: the approximal part of the preparation would, of course, have been identical to that shown here for amalgam (and similar to that shown at the distal in Fig. 12.2).*

2. It is important to develop the final cavosurface angle at this stage. This will be a compromise dictated by the average orientation of the enamel prisms and the physical properties of the restorative material. It should:

(a) never be less than 90° (and if near 90°, the margin should be scraped or planed with a hand instrument to ensure that it is strong);

(b) only be markedly greater than 90° when:

(i) the restorative material can withstand having a 'thin' edge, e.g. gold,
(ii) the restorative material can be bonded firmly to the enamel,
(iii) the enamel prisms tend to run in an apical direction in the cervical regions of teeth, e.g. at the 'bottom' of a Class II cavity;

(c) generally be about 105–110° on the inward facing slopes of cusps where amalgam, composite or glass-ionomer (or cermet) is to be used (Fig. 14.4). The exception is for ultra-narrow extensions to remove fissures in cavities for amalgam, where the cavosurface angle may

PRINCIPLES OF CAVITY PREPARATION

unavoidably be up to about 140°. Fortunately, here the amalgam can be carved flat as in Fig. 14.4c (to give it a high margin angle). Such narrow extensions should never arise in cavity preparations for composite restorations, because such regions should be fissure-sealed directly (see sealant restorations; Chapter 12).

3. Gingival margin trimmers (Fig. 14.5) are a special set of chisels that should be considered essential for removing carious and unsupported enamel from the approximal parts of cavities. Correctly used, they serve especially to:

    (a) split off precisely the unsupported enamel and no more;
    (b) leave the cavosurface angle precisely correct;
    (c) instrument the cavity margins without damaging the adjacent tooth.

4. Where the caries undermines a cusp tip it is necessary to cut away the cuspal enamel and include it in the restoration.

5. It is sometimes appropriate to leave in situ some arrested, or readily arrestable, enamel caries:

> (a) at the edge of a cavity preparation in a smooth tooth surface where there has been no loss of contour and where complete removal would require a much more extensive cavity;
>
> (b) in a fissure where it is to be covered with fissure sealant as part of a sealant restoration.

Extension of the cavity for accessibility and aesthetics

The cavity wall in some regions may have to be cut back slightly to enhance the accessibility of the cavity margin for:

1. The instruments that prepare it (e.g. the orifice of a cavity should not be so narrow that instrumentation is compromised).

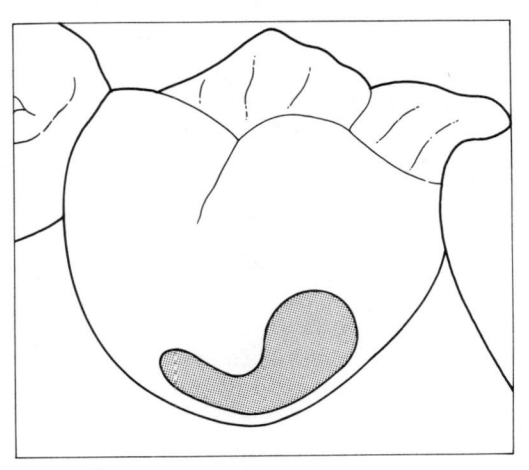

Fig. 14.3 *Diagram of a lower molar showing a modern Class V buccal cavity preparation for amalgam. The preparation is entirely dependent upon the position, size and shape of the carious lesion. This lesion happened to be a rather irregular shape.*

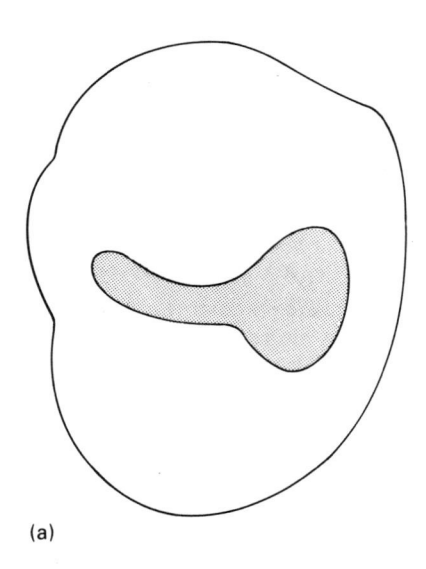

(a)

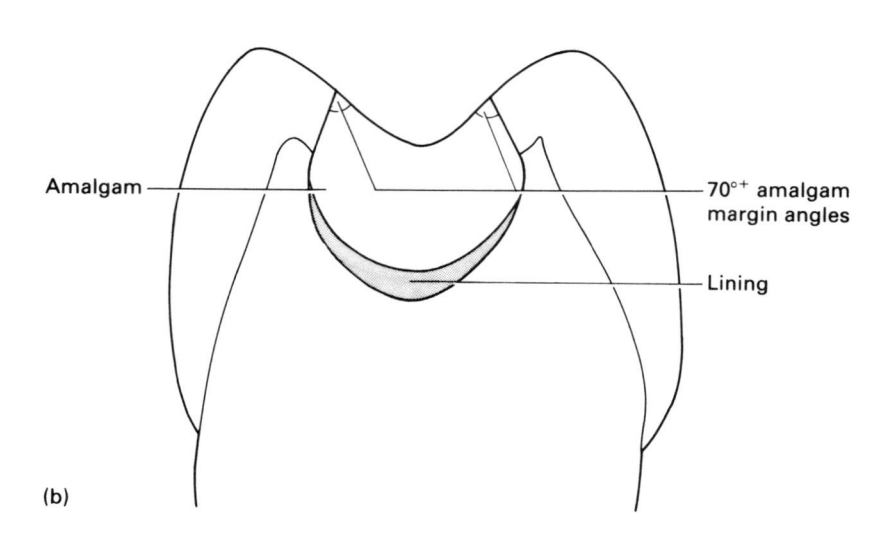

Amalgam — 70°⁺ amalgam margin angles

Lining

(b)

PRINCIPLES OF CAVITY PREPARATION

2. The instruments that will adapt and shape the restorative material. Of special note here is the fact that amalgam cannot be carved to a fissured groove radiating from a cavity; extension of the cavity ('extension for prevention') would usually be correct (see Fig. 14.4a and c) — if amalgam were indeed the right material to be used (rather than changing to a sealant restoration; Chapter 12).

3. The needs of the restoration, e.g. to avoid an undercut in a cavity for a cast restoration or to achieve a broad region in the restoration to contain a precision attachment for a partial denture.

4. Examination and assessment by the dentist at the time of operation and at recall appointments, e.g. paring back an embrasure wall with a gingival margin trimmer so that it lies just clear of a contact point.

5. Cleaning by the patient. In the old days, embrasure walls were cut widely in a vain attempt to place them in so-called 'self-cleansing' regions at the

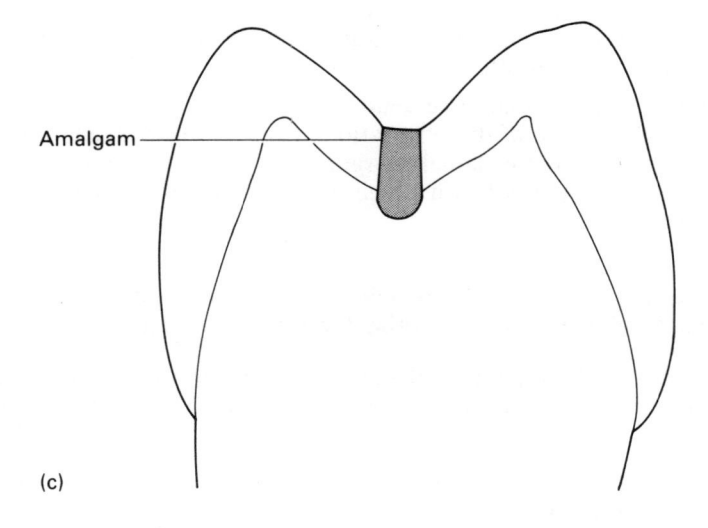

(c)

Fig. 14.4(a) *Diagram showing the occlusal view of an upper premolar with a modern occlusal Class I cavity preparation for an amalgam restoration. The cavity is wide on the right on account of extensive caries in this region, but narrow on the left (cut with a single sweep of a 330 bur) where a fissured groove was confluent with the wide part of the cavity (extension for prevention) or had early caries. If the whole fissure had only had such early caries, fissure sealant would have been the treatment of choice without any cavity preparation. (b) Buccolingual section through the wide region after lining and restoring, showing: that the cavity is widest at the enamel–dentine junction (where the caries would have been most widely spread); the curved shape of the floor which remains after removal of the caries; the correct cavosurface angles of about 105°–110°; and the desirable amalgam margin angles of 70°–75°. The same features would hold if composite resin were to be used as the restorative material. (c) Buccolingual section through the narrow part of the cavity after restoring (there is no room for lining), showing how the amalgam margin angles are optimal at about 90° by virtue of the amalgam being carved flat, even though the cavosurface angles are high. With the preparation as narrow as this (about one-eighth of the intercuspal width) there will be no occlusal interference with the amalgam carved flat in this way.*

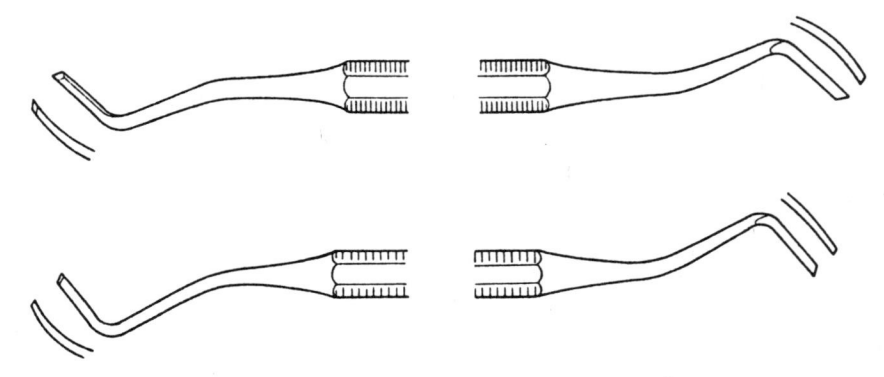

Fig. 14.5 *A pair of double-ended gingival margin trimmers.*

'corners' of the tooth. Such self-cleansing regions do not normally exist. Today, it is sometimes realistic to just free (by a hair's breadth only) any remaining contact with the adjacent tooth.

It will sometimes be necessary to extend a region of the preparation in order to improve the appearance of the restoration. There is rarely a need for this, but cervical extension of the labial margin of a crown preparation into a subgingival region for a patient with a high lip line exemplifies a situation that arises from time to time.

Shaping the cavity so that both the remaining tooth tissue and the restoration will be able to withstand biting forces (resistance form)

It is necessary to consider separately the integrity of the tooth and the integrity of the restorative material so as to be sure that both will tolerate occlusal forces.

The tooth

In respect of tooth integrity:

1. Check for weak cusps where there is little or no dentine remaining and replace them with restorative material — lean on them with a chisel and see if they break away.
2. Check for and remove fragile enamel near the tip of a cusp (gnarled enamel) even where there is good dentine support.
3. Check for, and remove if necessary, thin regions of enamel that remain between two closely approximating cavities in a tooth.
4. Check for and remove *any* unsupported enamel (this should have been accomplished earlier).

The restoration

The tooth preparation may have to be adjusted to prevent:

(a) major fracturing of the restorative material;
(b) minor breakdown at the margins.

PRINCIPLES OF CAVITY PREPARATION

Thus cognizance should be taken of, and adjustments made, where necessary to the tooth preparation, to ensure certain specific things.

1. There needs to be provision for adequate thickness of restorative material:

>   (a) **amalgam:** at least 2–3 mm over cusps and at least the thickness of the enamel elsewhere;
>   (b) **cast gold:** at least 1 mm on the occlusal surface and 0.5 mm elsewhere (though, of course, it inevitably thins to zero thickness at the edge of a bevel).

2. There needs to be provision for an adequate material edge angle. This should rarely be less than 70° except where a bevel (see pp. 168–9) is required; 85–90° is generally appropriate. It should never be less than 70° for amalgam on the occlusal surface of a tooth for fear of markedly increasing the chances of subsequent marginal breakdown.

3. Especially where amalgam is used, the cavity preparation needs to be such that the restorative material will not be subjected to undue tension. Such tension occurs in a multi-surface amalgam restoration, e.g. a mesio-occlusal restoration. Here, the occlusal forces resolve into occlusal and mesial components. The dentine part of the floor of the mesial part of the cavity needs to be cut at a right angle to these forces so that the restoration will resist them. It is even better if it inclines inwards slightly so that the mesial part of the restoration tries to 'dig' itself into the cavity as occlusal forces are applied. If the cervical floor of the cavity were to incline outwards, the amalgam in this region would have a tendency to be forced in a mesial direction, with the result that the cervical part of the restoration would tend to move mesially. This could cause the restoration to be lost or a fracture to occur in the so-called isthmus region between the occlusal and mesial parts (as the mesial part moved and the occlusal part stayed behind). Correct inclination of the cervical floor of such a cavity is clearly of critical importance (see Fig. 14.2). With a single-surface restoration, the flatness or inclination of the cavity floor is of no consequence.

Cavity design to restore cuspal enamel

When restoring cuspal enamel, the following options exist.

1. *Cast gold* in the form of an onlay (or crown if appropriate) which grips the prepared remains of the cusp(s). This:

>   (a)   is the strongest and most durable;
>   (b)   requires a minimum of 1 mm of cusp reduction;
>   (c)   may be unacceptable aesthetically.

2. The use of *cast ceramic* or *laboratory-cured composite resin* may, in due course, be shown to overcome this problem, while, at the same time, being as satisfactory as cast gold with respect to (a) and (b) above.

3. *Amalgam*. It is necessary to cut the cusp back to make room for at least 2–3 mm for strength purposes. This may be unacceptable aesthetically.

4. *Acid etch-retained composite resin* applied directly to the tooth. However, it should be appreciated that:

(a) it is early days with this material, but it may prove to be the most conservative method — in that partial onlaying of cusps may prove to be acceptable;

(b) however, it is doubtful whether composite resin allows enamel to be retained which is not itself supported by dentine;

(c) wear of the material against the opposing teeth may be unacceptable.

5. *Stainless steel.* As pre-made crowns, these are excellent for deciduous molars (Chapter 8).

Shaping the cavity so that the restoration will be retained in the tooth (retention form)

It is essential that the restoration remains firmly in intimate contact with the cavity in the face of:

(a) general wear and tear;
(b) sticky foods;
(c) dimensional instability with temperature change, etc.

Possible movement of each component (surface) of the restoration in each direction must be prevented and, to this end, adjustments may have to be made to the cavity preparation to make it retentive.

Potentially an occlusal restoration could only be lost in an occlusal direction, but a mesio-occlusal restoration could be lost in a mesial or an occlusal direction. Further, such a restoration could fracture and separate into its two component parts and then just one part might not be retentive.

There are three main ways in which cavities may be prepared so that restorations are retained.

1. By undercuts for plastic restorative materials including amalgam — making the cavity wider in its interior than at or near its orifice.

2. By near-parallelism, for laboratory-made solid restorations — enabling a laboratory-made restoration to slide tightly into place.

3. By direct attachment of the restorative material to the dental tissues.

Undercuts

Where this method of retention is to be used, the following points are of particular note.

1. A pair of opposing concavities are required in the cavity with respect to each surface of the restoration.

2. The enamel must not be undermined with respect to its dentine support.

3. The undercut regions must not inadvertently be covered over by lining material.

4. On the occlusal surface an undercut shape to the cavity will result automatically after removal of the caries which is most widely spread at the enamel–dentine junction (Fig. 14.4b).

PRINCIPLES OF CAVITY PREPARATION 165

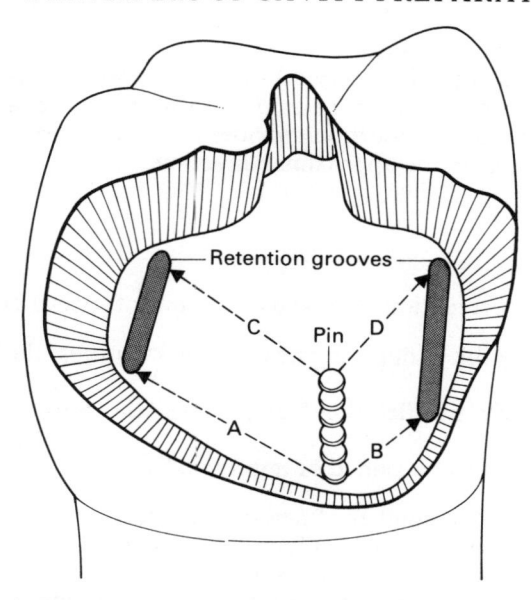

Fig. 14.6 *Diagram showing a wide class II cavity preparation for amalgam with divergent approximal cavity walls. The approximal retention grooves in the dentine only become effective once a pin has been placed, for this has the effect of creating undercuts between itself and the grooves. Thus, dimensions A and B are greater than C and D respectively, thereby preventing dislodgement of the restoration in an occlusal direction. Note that the pin is situated in the mesio-lingual corner of this lower molar, occupying the position that would have been assumed by a lingual approximal retention groove in a smaller mesio-occlusal cavity preparation.*

5. With approximo-occlusal cavities, loss of the approximal part of the restoration in the occlusal direction is prevented by the relatively narrow part of the preparation in the region of the marginal ridge. Loss in the approximal direction is prevented by approximal retention grooves running cervico-occlusally in the dentine of the buccal and lingual embrasure walls of the cavity (usually cut with a fine tapered fissure bur at low speed) (Fig. 14.2).

6. With approximal cavities in anterior teeth, a buccolingual groove in the cervical dentine complements an opposing undercut in the incisal dentine.

7. With buccal and lingual Class V cavities, occlusal and cervical grooves in the dentine are appropriate. Mesial and distal undercuts would tend to undermine the curving mesial and distal enamel unless the tooth were very flat in these regions and in the same plane as that of the cavity.

8. Pins placed in the dentine serve to create undercuts where there is insufficient dentine for the purpose. They should be used in conjunction with conventional undercuts, i.e. maximum use should also be made of conventional undercuts (Fig. 14.6). Pins should only be placed into bulky regions of dentine where there is good access for instrumentation. Places best avoided for fear of exposure into the pulp or perforation into the periodontal membrane include:

(a) the furcation regions;
(b) the mesial and distal cervical regions of posterior teeth.

9. An occlusal dovetail in an approximo-occlusal cavity preparation for an inlay with an occlusal path of insertion provides a useful undercut with respect to retention of the inlay in the approximal direction.

Near-parallelism

Where this method of retention is to be used, points of special note are:

1. The longer the pairs of opposing near-parallel features, the more retentive the restoration.
2. The more nearly parallel the features are, the more retentive the restoration.
3. Near-parallelism can be gained or improved by:

(a) increasing the number of near-parallel features;
(b) 'squaring up' the internal features of the preparation;
(c) adding near-parallel grooves or slots;
(d) adding veneers to cause the restoration to embrace additional parts of the tooth, e.g. by surrounding part of a cusp or additionally veneering the side of a tooth;
(e) adding pin holes for cast pins;
(f) adding a pin-retained or adhesively retained core with near-parallel sides;
(g) converting a rather non-retentive coronal stump or core into a post crown;
(h) combination of the above.

Direct attachment

This method may, of course, be used in combination with undercuts, etc. Direct attachment systems include the following.

1. Composite resin applied to acid-etched enamel.
2. Glass-ionomer cement chemically bonded to the enamel or dentine.
3. Composite resin bonded to the dentine by means of a dentine adhesive system or glass ionomer cement.
4. Metal bonded to enamel or dentine by means of a dentine adhesive system.
5. Combinations of the above (Fig. 14.7).

With all of these methods, cavity preparation should be minimal, the removal of the carious tissue and unsupported enamel being the major essentials.

It is important to appreciate the need for the right direct attachment system for the particular circumstance. Thus, for example, sole reliance upon acid etch-retained composite would be inappropriate for the cervical regions of a tooth where the enamel is very thin or non-existent.

Adjustment of the cavity walls and margins so that they are appropriate for the restorative material

Greatest efficiency is achieved when all the cavity walls and margins are cut to their optimum form at the same time as the cavity wall itself is first prepared. Bevels for gold restorations are clearly an exception and these should now be placed. Indeed, it is appropriate at this late stage to examine systematically all the way along the entire length of the cavity margin, whatever the restorative material to be used, and to make minor adjustments as appropriate.

1. Round off any jagged or sharp corners of enamel which project into the cavity.
2. Consider adding small veneers to regions of preparations for large inlays so as to reduce the overall marginal length of the restoration.
3. Run a gingival margin trimmer or other hand instrument along any lateral or cervical cavity margins where there is a possibility of friable enamel — and remove it. This will mitigate against such things as 'matrix band fractures' whereby minute chipping of the enamel occurs as a matrix band is tightened around the tooth.

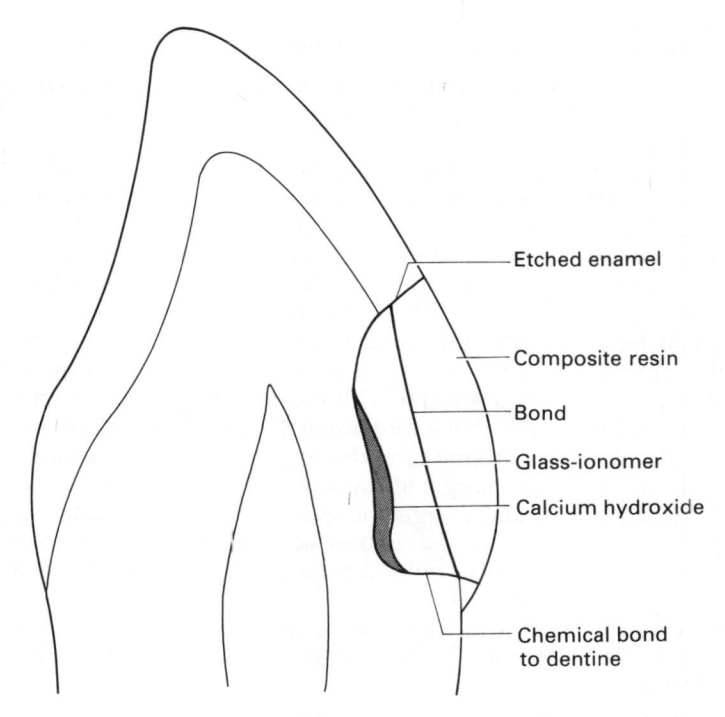

Fig. 14.7 *Diagrammatic vertical section through an upper canine showing the use of a combination of glass-ionomer cement and composite resin to make a restoration. In this class V cavity, the glass-ionomer is bonded to the dentine (and constitutes, in effect, artificial dentine). This is overlaid with composite resin which is acid etch-retained to the enamel and adheres also to the glass-ionomer cement.*

4. It is important to appreciate that tungsten carbide burs running at high speed produce the smoothest and most cleanly cut cavity walls and margins, especially when cutting approximately along the lengths of the enamel prisms and in towards them (bur 'entry' as opposed to bur 'exit' margins). Subsequent use of steel 'finishing' burs will reduce the quality of the margin and should be avoided. Their use would also make the cavity larger. The trick is: hold the first bur (high speed) at the correct angle to start with and cut the cavity wall and margin once, getting it right, first time.

Bevels for cast gold restorations

Bevelling is desirable for some of the margins of preparations for cast gold in order to enhance the chances of a good fit between the gold and the tooth. Note in particular:

1. The effect of a bevel at an otherwise butt joint margin (like a shoulder) is to go some way towards providing a sliding relationship, and hence towards achieving closer adaptation of the gold to the tooth should there be:

(a) any shortness of the casting arising from a dimensional error during its fabrication;
(b) any impediment to the complete seating of the casting.

2. An overwhelming advantage of a bevel is that it allows for a region of thin gold near the margin, which can be pushed or burnished into close adaptation with the enamel.

3. Care must be taken, when placing bevels, not to create undercuts with respect to the path of insertion of the restoration (e.g. at embrasure margins of Class II cavities in regions that are cervical to the 'survey line').

4. Bevels should be of the order of 45° (cavosurface angle, 135°). If they are markedly more severe than this they are difficult to identify and the margins of the intermediate wax pattern will be very thin and friable.

It should be noted that the ultimate theoretical bevel, a 'knife edge', is virtually impossible to manage with routine success and would be better avoided. It will also be appreciated that chamfers are only helpful in overcoming points (a) and (b) above, providing the final cavosurface angle is of the order of 135°. Without extreme care, the edge of a chamfer can easily approach that of a butt (shoulder) margin at the most critical part, the actual margin.

5. Bevelling of occlusal margins is generally contraindicated adjacent to steeply sloping cusps because the cavosurface angle in these regions is generally approximately 135° already, once the necessary slightly divergent occlusal cavity walls have been prepared.

6. Bevels may be cut with burs, fine stones or hand instruments, depending upon access. The important thing is not the instrument, but the obtaining of a clearly defined finishing line.

Bevels for composite resin restorations

Disadvantages. Bevelling is generally contraindicated because:

1. Bevels increase the surface area of the restoration, thereby:

(a) placing more direct function on the composite rather than on the enamel;
(b) possibly increasing the wear of the opposing tooth.

2. It is more difficult to adapt and finish the composite precisely to such a margin because it is less obvious visually.

3. If the restoration ever has to be replaced (a likely event), then its removal may involve the inadvertent removal of sound tooth tissue in the process, as the dentist will not necessarily be aware of the presence and extent of the bevel.

4. Any substantial bevelling of a 'deep' cervical margin reduces the accessibility of that margin, thereby compromising:

(a) visibility at the time of operation and at subsequent examinations;
(b) isolation from moisture;
(c) matrix adaptation;
(d) chemical treatment;
(e) (sometimes) the amount of enamel left for retention purposes; indeed such bevelling may convert an enamel margin into a cementum/dentine margin.

5. At visible margins, the presence of a bevel provides an enhanced opportunity for unsightly staining.

Advantages. In spite of the above, theoretical advantages of bevelling are:

1. It usually results in the enamel prisms being cut more transversely, thereby allowing more satisfactory etching and bonding.

2. It usually produces a larger area of enamel for bonding (but this may not be clinically relevant).

3. At visible margins, an improved aesthetic outcome may result (in the short term only?) on account of the gradual blending from composite to tooth.

Removal of deep caries

Up to this stage in cavity preparation, only caries in the vicinity of the enamel–dentine junction should normally have been removed, together with all the carious enamel. The only exceptions are:

(a) when the removal of arrested or readily arrestable, non-cavitated white or brown spot caries that extends laterally from a cavity (e.g. a Class V cavity) would markedly increase the size and complexity of the cavity (e.g. cause it to extend around to another surface of the tooth);

(b) when caries is left in the region of a fissure and is to have fissure sealant applied over it as part of a sealant restoration (see Chapter 12);

(c) small amounts of arrested secondary caries in cavity walls.

There may or may not be deep caries remaining, but if there is, it should, by this stage in the cavity preparation, be restricted to one or more isolated zones surrounded by sound dentine at the enamel–dentine junction. When removing this diseased tissue, an orderly method is required so as to avoid accidental pulp exposure.

1. Have the cavity well isolated and clean and dry (but not desiccated).
2. Use a large, slowly rotating, round bur or large sharp excavator (a bur is, in effect, a series of excavators and is therefore often more efficient than an excavator).
3. Commence near the enamel–dentine junction and work around the zone of caries, gradually reducing it in size.
4. Carious tissue may be lifted off the centre periodically in order to maintain access to the peripheral parts. The reader will appreciate that by following out and removing caries as described in steps 1–4 the pulpal aspect of a deep cavity will assume a rounded shape, be it the 'floor' of an occlusal cavity or the axial 'wall' of a cavity on the side of a tooth. Any discussion about 'flat' floors (as in many textbooks) can be dismissed as irrelevant (see Fig. 14.4b).
5. Keep washing and lightly drying the tissue to enhance proper vision (but, importantly, avoidance of desiccation must be stressed).
6. Probes should not be used for detecting deep caries or for testing that it has been removed. An excavator is an excellent and safe instrument for this purpose.
7. Do not expose the pulp (unless, of course, there is or has been irreversible pulpitis, in which case endodontic treatment should already have been planned or the tooth extracted). Thus, excavation should be halted if a hint of the redness of the pulp tissue (not a frank exposure) is seen looming through the softened area. Gradual sterilization and remineralization of the residual carious dentine would be expected to take place without action by the dentist, subsequent to covering it with a calcium hydroxide lining material and a restoration.
8. Should the removal of deep caries inadvertently lead straight into the pulp, this will probably be a blessing in disguise, for the pulp will usually have undergone irreversible degenerative change, in which case:

   (a) either the pulp will bleed readily;
   (b) or a bead of pus will be expressed;
   (c) or clear serous fluid will exude;
   (d) or the pulp chamber will appear empty.

In each of these cases, endodontic treatment (subject to no medical contraindication) or removal of the tooth is indicated. A corticosteroid/antibiotic dressing and a temporary restoration will usually provide a satisfactory 'holding' operation if necessary. (Should a 'traumatic' exposure take place in the absence of the above, then pulp capping with a calcium hydroxide material is usually appropriate as a medium term measure.)

9. It should be noted that any pins that are required for retention purposes are best placed after the removal of the deep caries. Once in position, pins are liable to interfere with caries removal.
10. Complete caries removal from the whole tooth, including its root, should always be carried out before commencing endodontic treatment. Indeed, only when all the caries has been removed may it be possible to examine the extent of tissue loss and make a rational decision as to the feasibility of restoring the tooth as opposed to extracting it.

Washing and drying of the preparation

This important step can usually be accomplished with an air/water spray syringe and high-volume aspiration, though a scrubbing action with a small moist pledget of cotton wool may also be required, so as to remove:

(a) enamel and dentine chips, powder and carious tissue;
(b) saliva, blood and crevicular fluid contamination.

The process is markedly simplified when rubber dam is in place, because recontamination cannot then occur. Especially when adhesive systems are to be used, any such contamination (at any stage) would be disastrous. Saliva and blood cannot simply be 'blown' away.

Great care should be taken not to desiccate the dentine.

Chemical treatment of the enamel and/or dentine

Chemical treatment to alter or condition cavity walls and margins in preparation for adhesive or bonded restorative materials should take place at this stage and immediately prior to the placement of the material itself. It is, however, sometimes appropriate first to place a matrix system, for any leakage occurring as the rubber dam is stretched while the matrix is applied would otherwise contaminate the chemically treated tissues.

CAVITY PREPARATION FOR REPLACEMENT RESTORATIONS

Important points to note are:

1. Where an existing restoration has failed and the criteria for operative intervention (Chapter 12) are fulfilled, the options are to:

(a) replace it completely;
(b) repair it by partial replacement;
(c) cover it with a larger restoration, e.g. a crown.

2. With any of the above, all the principles of cavity preparation apply and should be considered, with action being taken to make modifications to the existing cavity as necessary. Questions to be asked and answered include:

(a) what is wrong with the existing restoration?
(b) why did this fault occur?
(c) what steps should be taken to prevent recurrence of the fault or, more precisely, what changes should be made to the cavity preparation and/or choice of restorative material?

3. The repair of a locally defective region of a restoration is usually preferable to total replacement of the restoration because:

(a) it is likely that less sound tooth tissue will be removed (which would weaken the tooth);
(b) total concentration can be placed upon improving the defective region;

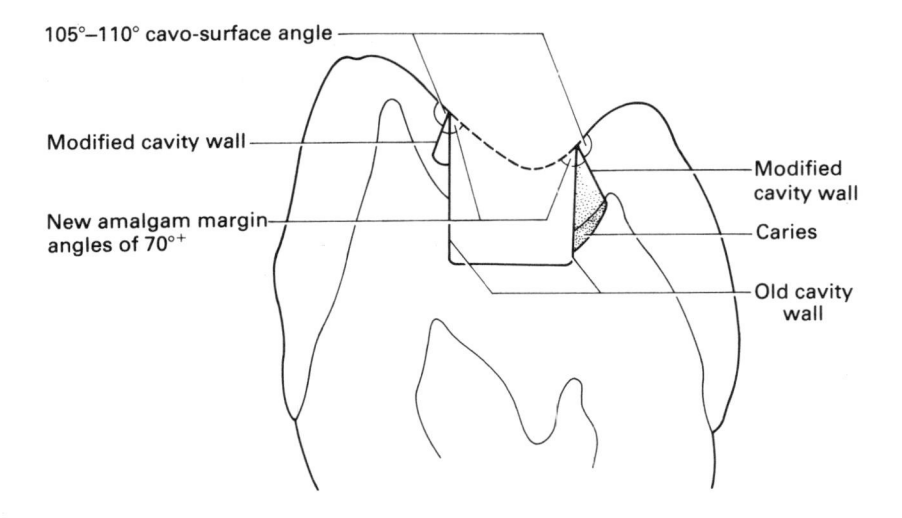

Fig. 14.8 *Diagrammatic buccolingual section through an upper premolar. The box-shaped cavity indicates a commonly found but incorrect cavity preparation for amalgam in which the buccal and lingual cavity walls have been prepared in the long axis of the crown of the tooth (see also Fig. 12.1). Where the restoration is to be replaced and there is secondary caries (stippled), the cavity wall should be cut back as on the right (and as in Fig. 14.4b) so as to allow for a 70° amalgam margin angle. In regions where there is no caries, as on the left, the outer part of the enamel wall of the cavity should be cut back so as to reduce the cavosurface angle and thereby allow a strong amalgam margin angle, again of 70°. No dentine is removed and the cavity is not made wider at the surface of the tooth in this region.*

(c) with complete replacement, regions of the old restoration that were themselves satisfactory may well end up worse after replacement (objective studies have shown this very clearly with respect to the replacement of occlusal amalgam restorations);

(d) the operative procedure is:

    (i)   simplified,
    (ii)   quicker,
    (iii) less likely to require local analgesia,
    (iv) 'kinder' on the pulp,
    (v)   less likely to lead to adverse after-effects,
    (vi) more acceptable to the patient;

(e) postoperative marginal leakage is likely to be less.

4. With respect to marginal leakage:

(a) there is less leakage between new amalgam and old amalgam than between new amalgam and cavity wall (some amalgamation occurs between new and old amalgam, but none occurs whatsoever between amalgam and tooth tissue);

PRINCIPLES OF CAVITY PREPARATION

(b) glass-ionomer cement seals well against freshly cut old amalgam;
(c) composite resin seals well against old composite resin;
(d) cohesive gold seals well against cast gold;
(e) indeed it should be appreciated that most combinations seal better than new amalgam against cavity wall and it is *probably* satisfactory to place new composite resin or glass-ionomer against the remains of any previous material.

5. Access to secondary caries or to the defect should be gained, as far as possible through the defective region and at the expense of the restorative material rather than by cutting sound tooth tissue.

6. The region where failure occurred should, in effect, be treated as if it were a primary carious lesion, while the remaining parts of the restoration should be treated as sound tooth tissue.

7. The enamel–dentine junction and the interface between any existing lining material and dentine should be made completely free of active caries. If in doubt, more or all of the old restoration should be cut away.

8. Removal of parts of the old restoration should be made by cutting *within* the substance of the material and breaking out the weakened fragments with a hand instrument.

9. The walls and margins of the cavity should then be modified selectively as necessary to improve them, e.g. by:

(a) removing caries;
(b) cutting back undermined enamel in such a way as to leave the cavity wall and cavosurface angle optimal (Fig. 14.8) (see also p. 157 and below).

Improving the cavosurface angle

This is necessary where the cavosurface angle is too high or too low. In particular, occlusal margins of cavities that have contained amalgam restoration often have irresponsibly high cavosurface angles where the cavity has been prepared with a fissure bur held approximately in the long axis of the crown of the tooth: the adjacent amalgam then has a ditched margin, but this is rarely associated with active secondary caries. To put right the defect, the outer part of the enamel wall of the cavity should be cut back (Fig. 14.8) so as:

(a) to reduce the cavosurface angle;
(b) to leave the marginal width of the cavity unchanged, thereby
  (i) maintaining occlusal function on the enamel,
  (ii) not adding to the complexity of contouring of the new restoration (because its surface will not be any larger);
(c) to enable a new amalgam margin angle of at least 70° (see p. 163).

Root-treated teeth

When a posterior tooth with a satisfactory occlusal restoration requires endodontic treatment it is often appropriate to remove just the central part of the restoration to gain access to the pulp chamber. Gold crowns opened in this way may be repaired effectively with occlusal cohesive gold, amalgam or composite resin plugs.

Root-treated teeth undoubtedly become more brittle than vital teeth, and restorations which protect them from splitting are more likely to be needed. There are specific situations that may indicate the need for more extensive restorations than existed previously.

1. A posterior tooth with a medium to large approximo-occlusal cavity. An onlay embracing the cusps is generally appropriate. The role of intracoronal bonded composite restorations for this purpose remains to be fully researched.

2. A previously crowned anterior tooth that is subsequently root treated is often best served with a post crown.

FURTHER READING

Elderton R. J. (1984). Cavo-surface angles, amalgam margin angles and occlusal cavity preparations. *Br. Dent. J.*, **156,** 319–24.

Elderton R. J. (1984). New approaches to cavity design with special reference to the Class II lesion. *Br. Dent. J.*, **157,** 421–7.

Elderton R. J. (1986). Restorative denistry: 1. Current thinking on cavity design. *Dent. Update*, **13,** 113–22; 240.

Elderton R. J. (1990). Operative treatment of dental caries. In *The Dentition and Dental Care* (Elderton R. J., ed.). Oxford: Heinemann Medical, pp. 263–305.

Chapter 15

The way forwards with caries management in dental practice

With the UK National Health Service (NHS) having been in operation since 1947, there has been long enough for the population to collect together some opinions as to the effectiveness and relevance of the dental service. Over the years, official reports have been increasingly forthright in their observations and recommendations about dentistry. Thus the Dental Strategy Review Group in 1981 (which was set up in response to recommendations of both the Royal Commission on the National Health Service in 1979 and the Nuffield Inquiry into Dental Education in 1980) noted that a problem area calling for remedial action was:

- 'Wastefulness arising because some dental treatment provided is either unnecessary, inappropriate or ineffective insofar as it has to be regularly repeated'.

The report went on:

- 'The time is right for a change of emphasis within the service from being essentially reparative to preventive' . . .

and indicated that:

- 'Inherent in this will be the need to encourage practitioners to limit clinical intervention to the absolute minimum and give prevention the opportunity to work'.

The Group placed some blame on the dental schools for:

- 'Failure to instil at all levels of undergraduate teaching a preventive as opposed to a reparative philosophy'.

Barmes, Chief of Oral Health at the World Health Organization, had already preempted these statements when in 1979 he stated:

- 'The time is long overdue for the whole dental profession to become much more actively and practically oriented to prevention as the first priority of all its endeavours'.

One outcome of the whole scenario has been the considerable media coverage over the last few years concerning various aspects of dental treatment. National and local television and radio channels have devoted whole programmes to dental treatment, and major and minor newspapers and magazines have produced a stream of articles. And this situation continues.

While some of this publicity has been favourable concerning, for example, the aesthetic benefits of certain types of treatment, other coverage have been extremely adverse, including both forthright and implied accusations that dentists have sometimes been guilty of carrying out treatment for their own gain rather than for their patients.

THE COMMITTEE OF ENQUIRY INTO UNNECESSARY DENTAL TREATMENT

The Government responded in 1984 by setting up the official 'Committee of Enquiry into Unnecessary Dental Treatment' to look at the General Dental Service in England and Wales. Published in 1986, its Report was comprehensive, balanced and forthright.

Forms of unnecessary treatment

In trying to distinguish between the different forms of unnecessary treatment, the following were defined:

- 'a. Treatment which is not necessary at all, e.g. where a dentist fills a non-existent cavity or fills a small cavity where most dentists would wait to see if the caries developed;
    b. Cases where some treatment is necessary but what is proposed is in excess of treatment which is reasonably necessary—e.g. where the great generality of dentists would fill with amalgam but a dentist does a crown to earn a larger fee;
    c. Cases where the treatment is inappropriate. These fall into two separate groups: those cases of elective treatment, where the dentist prescribes treatment which requires the cooperation of the patient which the dentist has no reasonable expectation of receiving; and those where the surrounding tissue has been so damaged that the extensive restoration is bound to be short lived or ineffective'.

Caries management and restorative treatment

Clearly the above categories a–c are not always inseparable, and many of the statements made in the report reflect this situation. Thus, it was noted that:

- 'The possibility of caries being arrested or even enamel lesions being remineralized suggests that premature intervention may be unnecessary and do positive harm to a patient'.

Indeed, the Committee made it clear that:

- 'The treatment philosophy of twenty years ago was one of early intervention and wholesale restoration. The present philosophy is one of prevention . . . and for intervening as little as possible'.

The preventive approach

Times certainly have changed, for the Report went on:

- 'All the evidence we have received has supported the preventive approach. This suggests that we have gone beyond the stage where there are in the profession two respectable alternative approaches, the 'restorative' and the 'preventive'. It is now clear that those who follow the restorative approach and carry out more than the minimum number of restorations necessary are undertaking unnecessary treatment. It follows that those who trained twenty or thirty years ago but who have not kept up with modern methods or approaches will be practising the kind of restorative dentistry which should now be regarded as involving unnecessary treatment'.

The Committee was clearly aware of the way in which things had changed, for they made it clear that:

- 'The preventive philosophy, which has gained increasing acceptance over the past few years, has grown out of an improved understanding of how caries develops. This has led dentists to realize that it is better to leave some lesions untreated in the knowledge that they may develop no further or become remineralized ... It has been gradually realized that doing avoidable restorative treatment is harmful since any fillings undertaken now will involve larger replacements at a later date'.

Overcoming the problems

There was then consideration in the Report as to how to address some of these problems, thus:

- '... more positive steps need to be undertaken by the profession to establish criteria for what is acceptable intervention and what is not'.

Indeed the Report went on:

- '... the time had come for a general reappraisal of the idiosyncratic nature of decisions as to whether fillings should be placed or replaced and that this should be a high priority in clinical dental research'.

The Committee did, however, draw from their evidence an appreciation of the fact that:

- '... there may be a wide and legitimate difference of view between dentists as to the amounts of treatment which many patients need'.

Then, in considering the eventuality of an invasive restoration being appropriate, the Report endorsed modern approaches to cavity design and confirmed their view that:

- '... it was important to ensure minimal tooth destruction when carrying out restorations'.

Out-of-date treatment philosophy

It is evident that in facing up to the realities of unnecessary treatment the Committee was alert to the fact that none of the evidence was conclusive on its own, but that in general it points to there being:

- '... a small but significant and unacceptable amount of *deliberate* unnecessary treatment ... and a larger amount attributable to an out-of-date treatment philosophy'.

The identification of this out-of-date treatment philosophy seems to hit the nail on the head. Indeed, the Report went on:

- 'We have received evidence that leads us to believe that there is a substantial amount of unnecessary dental treatment being carried out by dental practitioners in good faith. Aspects of this are treatment for purely cosmetic purposes; out-of-date dentistry; inappropriate training; or one dentist re-doing work done by another dentist'.

Problems

Statements in the Report from individual dental practitioners seemed to sum up quite well sentiments that might have been widespread among dentists. It would seem to have been a sensible and committed dentist who said:

- '... surely all reasonable practitioners must welcome the first serious attempts to plug the hole which everyone knows but few will admit exists in the General Dental Service'.

But then, there is the practitioner who voiced what he considered to be a problem confronting the average dentist:

- 'You get professional satisfaction from the delight of patients who after years of fillings are told they only need a scale and polish. It, alas, does not pay the bill'.

The Committee appeared to be sympathetic to this view, for it indicated that:

- '... an increasing number of dentists have a motive to undertake unnecessary treatment, for in many areas there are too many dentists to carry out the available work'.

This is in line with the British Dental Association noting in their evidence to the Committee that some dentists have too few patients and declining incomes:

- 'This may carry with it the temptation to provide more expensive treatment than is strictly needed or treatment which may lead to no more than marginal improvement in the dental health of the patient'.

Change of direction

In order to foster the desired change in direction in providing dental care, the Committee believed that:

THE WAY FORWARDS WITH CARIES MANAGEMENT 179

- '... members of the public should be made more aware of the need to seek preventive rather than restorative treatment, and to discuss with their dentist whether the latter is really necessary and, if not satisfied, decline to accept the treatment'.

In overall conclusion the Committee certainly gave the benefit of the doubt when it stated:

- 'Although the evidence has led us to conclude that unnecessary dental treatment is significant, it has not led us to believe that it is so widespread that patients in general should lose confidence in their dentists. In our view the vast majority of dental practitioners in the General Dental Service provide a thoroughly professional service on which the general public can continue to rely'.

THE NEW ROLE OF TODAY'S DENTIST

Clearly we in the profession need to be taking the lead here. We must collectively be debating and agreeing just what is right for patients and what constitutes good dentistry. We need to be very clear how best to help our patients control dental diseases and be very sure how to provide the very highest standards of treatment—and under the right circumstances. To do this, we must be fully aware of the many shortcomings of restorative dentistry (Chapter 12) so that we fully understand the basis for the treatment measures we elect to provide.

The days of mechanical, stereotyped restorative treatment, which is often alien to the patient's needs and which enters the dentist into a repetitive mode of practice, should have gone years ago. But there has been a considerable lethargy by the profession with respect to facing up to the shortcomings of restorative dentistry, and in keeping up-to-date with current concepts of cavity design and high-quality use of materials.

It is abundantly clear that the time has well and truly come for dentists to realize that greater caution is required in treatment planning for caries management than is generally thought necessary. Much more emphasis should be placed upon the assessment of each and every carious lesion with a view to allowing a possible natural arrest of the process to occur, aided by specific preventive measures as appropriate. And restorations should not necessarily be replaced just because there is a moderate degree of marginal breakdown. The universal adoption of a preventive approach to making treatment decisions could be by far the most powerful factor in reducing the restorative burden of dental service and, in so doing, provide a type of dental care which the consumer will more readily accept.

It would seem that the supply and demand forces of the market place will put increasing pressure upon dentists to adopt a more preventive approach to the management of caries and defective restorations, and that the regular attender will become less ready to accept an apparently unending commitment to restorations and re-restorations. The dental visit is likely to become more of a screening exercise, with the dentist providing much more of a diagnostic, advisory, supervisory, monitoring and counselling role than at present.

There is a very real need for dental practitioners to move forwards and manage carious lesions as far as possible by preventive means. Patients should be motivated to accept responsibility to change the environment of their teeth so that the calcium and phosphate balance favours remineralization (Chapters 10 and 11), though with the dentist placing therapeutic fissure sealants (Chapter 11) or modern, high-quality restorations as appropriate.

The case for adopting this preventive approach to the management of caries becomes very strong once the many serious problems with the restorative approach are fully appreciated (Chapter 12). And as long as dentists continue to be powered by an aggressive restorative approach, the repeat restoration cycle seems likely to continue for a while. But with increasing awareness by the public of the possibilities for prevention, consumers can be expected more and more to demand this type of care in preference to the treatment-orientated methods of the past, which they do not like. Indeed such changes are already well underway and there already are many practices in the UK where the psychological switch has been made and health promotion rather than 'restorative' treatment is the main driving force.

FURTHER READING

Carrington H. B., Elderton R. J. (1985). Reflections on Elderton's 'Restoration '85'. *Br. Dent. J.*, **160**, 36–8; 342–3.

DHSS (1986). *Report of the Committee of Enquiry into Unnecessary Dental Treatment*. London: HMSO.

DHSS (1981). *Towards better dental health-guidelines for the future*. The report of the Dental Strategy Review Group. London: Department of Health and Social Security.

Elderton R. J. (1984). The prevention of dental caries in the General Dental Service. *J. Dent.*, **12**, 215–20.

Elderton R. J. (1985). Scope for change in clinical practice. *J. Roy. Soc. Med.*, **78** (suppl. 7), 27–32.

Elderton R. J. (1985). Implications of recent dental health services research on the future of operative dentistry. *J. Publ. Health Dent.*, **45**, 101–5.

Elderton R. J. (1986). Restorative dentistry: 2. Prospects for the future. *Dent. Update*, **13**, 161–8.

Elderton R. J. (1990). *Evolution in Dental Care*. Bristol: Clinical Press Ltd.

Chapter 16

Endodontics

The scope of endodontic treatment ranges from procedures designed to preserve the vitality of compromised pulps to surgical techniques for removing diseased tissue that cannot be dealt with by other, more conservative means. There is still a commonly held misconception that periapical pathology requires a surgical approach for a successful result. In the last 20–30 years, however, research has demonstrated that root canal therapy alone will provide conditions that permit the healing of the periapical region in the majority of cases.

The first requirement is for careful, accurate diagnosis. A wide differential diagnosis must be considered when radiographic examination reveals an area of lucency in association with the apex of a tooth root. Where the tooth in question has a non-vital pulp and there is a satisfactory explanation for the loss of vitality, such as extensive caries, restorations or evidence of trauma, then the likelihood is that the lesion is either a periapical dental granuloma or cyst. It is not possible, on the basis of radiography alone, to distinguish with certainty between these possibilities. In any event the distinction is unnecessary since the first choice of treatment will be the same, namely root canal therapy followed by careful follow-up examination and only if the lesion persists, endodontic surgery.

When properly performed, root canal therapy has a very high success rate of over 90%. However, success can only be expected if the basic principles are understood and put into practice when treatment is undertaken.

If, after careful clinical and radiological assessment, pulp disease is diagnosed and root canal therapy selected as the treatment of choice, the aims of treatment are as follows.

1. To **cleanse** the pulp space, thoroughly, to remove pulpal tissue and breakdown products, microorganisms and debris.

2. To **shape** the pulp space so that an adequate filling can be placed subsequently.

3. To **obliterate** the pulp space, completely, in three dimensions.

In many cases, the achievement of the second objective requires preparation additional to that necessary for the first.

After treatment, careful follow-up examination is required to establish whether the treatment has been successful. In order to be judged successful, the following criteria must be fulfilled.

1. *On clinical examination* there should be:

   (a) no pain;
   (b) no sinus;
   (c) no swelling;
   (d) no tenderness on biting, palpation or percussion;
   (e) the tooth should be a functioning unit of the dentition both aesthetically and from the point of view of the occlusion.

2. On *radiographic examination* there should be:

   (a) maintenance of the normal apical appearance or resolution of pathology.

Once treatment has been completed, periodic radiographic assessment should be performed to ensure that any apical pathology present before treatment has resolved and that if, initially, no pathology was present, any that develops subsequently can be treated promptly. Such periodic assessment must continue for as long as the tooth is retained in the mouth since it has been shown that late failure of root canal therapy can occur after several years of apparent success.

There are many factors which influence the success of root canal therapy but the most important appear to be:

(a) the presence of apical pathology;
(b) the position of the root filling;
(c) periapical disturbance during treatment;
(d) lateral compression of the root filling.

In the presence of apical pathology of pulpal origin, success can only be expected if meticulous attention is paid to the technical details of all phases of treatment. The margin for error is much smaller than when the tooth has a vital pulp before treatment commences.

The ideal point of termination of a root filling is the most constricted portion of the root canal, corresponding with the dentine–cementum junction, since this reduces the residual space within the canal and reduces the area of contact between the root filling and the adjacent connective tissues. This latter is desirable because the materials used for filling canals are not totally inert biologically. Damage to the apical tissues resulting from over-instrumentation, leakage of irritant medicaments or forcing debris, possibly infected, through the apical foramen, is a potent cause of failure. It is preferable for the root filling to be slightly short rather than too long. The function of the filling is two-fold; it should prevent microorganisms from gaining access to the pulp space from the mouth or via the bloodstream and it should prevent diffusion of tissue fluid into the pulp space, where it would act as a culture medium for any microorganisms which may remain after the cleansing process. These functions can only be performed if the root filling obliterates the pulp space completely.

Root canal therapy can be divided into three stages:

(a) access;
(b) canal preparation;
(c) canal filling.

Table 16.1
Average working distances of teeth

	Average (mm)	Range (mm)
Maxilla		
Central incisor	22	17–27
Lateral incisor	21	16–26
Canine	27	19–32
Premolars	21	16–27
Molars	21	16–24
Mandible		
Incisors	21	16–25
Canine	25	20–32
Premolars	21	17–26
Molars	21	17–26

ACCESS

Anatomy of the pulp space

Before attempting to gain access to the pulp space it is essential that the anatomy of the root canal system is understood. Root canals are not simple, straight, round channels but have complex, irregular shapes. The majority have some degree of curvature and are broader in a buccolingual direction. The apical foramen is seldom found at the apex but usually 0.5–1 mm from it. With increasing age, however, increased amounts of secondary cementum are deposited apically and the 'apical' foramen may be 2 mm short of the anatomical apex of the root. The apical foramen is not the narrowest part of the canal. The apical constriction is to be found 0.5–1 mm short of the apical foramen, and it is at this apical constriction that the root filling should terminate. The average working distances for the different teeth are shown in Table 16.1.

Accessory canals are a common occurrence, being present in over 50% of teeth. They are often wider than the apical foramen and may be found at any point along the length of the root. In roots containing more than one canal—for example the mesial root of a lower molar—lateral communications or anastomoses between them are commonly found. The incidence of multiple roots or multiple canals within a single root is higher than is generally thought; the results of a number of surveys are summarized in Table 16.2.

Anatomy of individual teeth

Maxillary central incisors

The overwhelming majority of these teeth have one canal, although two canals have been reported. Radiographically the canal appears to be straight and tapering, and is the one which is most likely to be nearly round in cross-section. There is often a slight curvature towards the labial side in the apical third which cannot be detected from a standard radiographic projection.

Table 16.2
Incidence of multiple root canals (%)

Maxilla	
First premolar	85
Second premolar	40
First and second molars (mesiobuccal root)	50
Mandible	
Central and lateral incisors	40
Canines	18
First premolars	28
Second premolars	6
First molars:	
mesial root	87
distal root	30

Maxillary lateral incisors

Slightly shorter than central incisors with usually one canal, which may have a fairly severe, distally directed curvature in the apical third.

Maxillary canine

The longest of all teeth with a distinctly oval canal, wider buccolingually than mesiodistally. The canal narrows abruptly in the apical third, which is often curved towards the labial side and sometimes distally also.

Maxillary first premolar

Approximately 85% of these teeth have two roots and 5% have three, each with its own pulp space and apical foramen. If three roots are present, two are located buccally. The apical thirds of the roots are fine and delicate and may be curved in any direction. The pulp chamber tends to be very wide buccopalatally.

Maxillary second premolar

Usually single-rooted but approximately 40% have two canals within a single root. Although the canals may join and share a single foramen, two separate foramina are sometimes found. The apical third of the root may curve distally.

Maxillary first molar

Usually has three roots but the majority of mesiobuccal roots have two canals, which should be sought for routinely. The palatal root is the largest and longest, and tends to curve buccally. The distobuccal root is the thinnest and tends to curve distally. The mesiobuccal root is broad buccolingually and the two canals are placed buccally and lingually. On the floor of the pulp chamber, the orifice of the main canal is found well buccally, and that of the second canal is to be found along the groove connecting the orifice of this main canal to that of the palatal canal.

Maxillary second molar

Similar to but smaller than the first molar. The roots may be fused but there are usually still three canals.

Mandibular incisors

The anatomy of the central and lateral incisors is similar although the lateral incisor is slightly longer. About 40% have two canals within a single root but only approximately 1% have separate foramina. Where there is one canal it tends to be very much wider buccolingually than mesiodistally, and if two canals are present they are situated buccally and lingually.

Mandibular canine

Usually single-rooted although two roots may occur. Approximately 18% have two canals even if there is only one root.

Mandibular first premolar

This tooth may cause considerable problems because of its pulpal anatomy. Approximately 28% have two canals, situated buccally and lingually, in the apical third. The opening of the lingual canal can be very difficult to locate.

Mandibular second premolar

Similar to the first premolar but only about 6% have two canals.

Mandibular first molar

Usually has two roots and three canals, two in the mesial root and one in the distal, although approximately 30% have two canals in the distal root also, making a total of four canals. Occasionally, three roots are found. The fine canals in the mesial root are usually curved both buccolingually and mesiodistally, and frequently anastomose. Accessory canals are common in the furcation area.

Mandibular second molar

Similar to the first molar but the roots are closer together. Two canals in the distal root are uncommon.

Third molars

In both jaws these teeth may be similar to the other molars or exceedingly complex. Severe distal curvature of the roots is a common finding.

All available radiographs should be studied carefully before making an access opening and on occasions additional views taken from differing horizontal angulations may help in visualizing the anatomy to be encountered. The radiographs may be expected to provide information relating to:

(a) the length of the tooth;
(b) the size and position of the pulp chamber;
(c) the number of canals present;
(d) the relationship of the canal orifice to the pulp chamber;
(e) the size, direction of curvature and branching of canals;
(f) the presence of calcifications or other solid objects such as old root fillings, fractured instruments, etc.

Preparation of access openings

The recommended designs for access openings can be seen in textbooks of endodontics. Whilst it is desirable to retain useful coronal tooth substance to simplify subsequent restoration of the tooth, this should not be done at the expense of adequate access for the manipulation of instruments within the canal. If the root canal therapy cannot be carried out effectively, the prognosis for the tooth will be poorer. The opening should be extended to provide unimpeded access to the apical third of the canal and should be as near 'straight line' as possible.

Before commencing access cavity preparation, any caries or defective restorations should be removed and the tooth restored in such a way that it may be isolated using rubber dam and that it will remain intact during treatment so contamination of the canal will not occur. This may necessitate the placement of a temporary crown, copper ring or possibly a pinned amalgam core. If a pinned core is placed, care must be exercised when choosing the sites of pin placement to ensure that they will neither impede access to the root canals, nor be destroyed during the preparation of the access opening, thus resulting in a loss of retention for the core.

The outline of the access cavity should be established and the cavity extended deeply into dentine, without entering the pulp space, using an air-rotor handpiece. The rubber dam should then be applied. Rubber dam application is seen by many as a difficult and time-consuming exercise and is all too often omitted. With a small amount of practice and using a suitable technique (see Chapter 13), it can be applied in most situations in well under 1 min. For endodontic purposes, only the tooth being treated needs to be isolated and this makes the application much easier and quicker. The benefits of its use are that it prevents the inhalation or swallowing of instruments; it retracts the tongue and cheek, thereby improving access for vision and manipulation of instruments; it prevents gross salivary contamination of the pulp space; and it permits the use of sodium hypochlorite solution for irrigation, which otherwise is not well tolerated by patients because of the unpleasant taste. The greater ease of treatment and consequent reduction in the time taken with a rubber dam in place fully justifies the small amount of time taken for its application.

Penetration into the pulp chamber should be performed using a round or dome-ended bur in a slow handpiece. The cooling spray from the high-speed handpiece might result in infected debris being forced out of the canal and into the periapical tissues. Compressed air from a triple syringe should not be directed into an opened root canal for the same reason. In the case of posterior teeth the initial penetration should be directed towards the axis of the largest canal, that is the distal canal in lower molars and the palatal canal in upper molars. The pulp space will be greatest in these areas and consequently easier to locate. The entire roof of the pulp chamber should be removed and the walls of the cavity made smooth. The walls should diverge so that the temporary seal will not be dislodged into the pulp chamber since this would result in salivary contamination of the pulp space.

A successful access preparation is one in which:

(a) the floor of the pulp chamber is visible;
(b) the canal orifices are identifiable;
(c) there is no overhanging enamel or dentine;
(d) there is a direct approach to the apical third of the canal.

CANAL PREPARATION

The first step is to explore the pulp space to determine the number of canals present. Then the working length is determined for each canal found. Electronic measuring instruments are useful but do not replace radiography. They are helpful in positioning the instrument before exposing the working distance radiograph. They will also reduce the number of occasions when radiographs are exposed with instruments remote from the apical constriction; such errors necessitate further exposures to determine the working length accurately and thereby unnecessarily increase the exposure of the patient to radiation.

Canal preparation has two objectives. The first is the removal of all organic material that might support the growth of microorganisms, from the root canal system. The second is the development of a preparation whose form simplifies the placement of a dense and permanent filling. This cleansing and shaping process is carried out by the manipulation of instruments within the canal, accompanied by frequent, copious irrigation to flush out organic material and the debris created by instrumentation.

Hand instruments continue to be the most suitable means of preparing the root canal. Used correctly, they will create a preparation having a predictable shape, which can then be filled accurately using relatively simple techniques.

Reamers should not be employed in curved canals. They are designed to cut on rotation around their long axes. In curved canals this results in an eccentrically shaped apical preparation with a constriction short of the working distance. In these circumstances it becomes very difficult to obliterate the space totally. A better approach is to use files with a short 'in-out' action. The dental manufacturers are now producing new designs of files, using improved materials, that are sharper and more flexible than their predecessors. It is now possible to negotiate and prepare tortuous canals and to prepare them effectively.

In the ideal preparation, there should be:

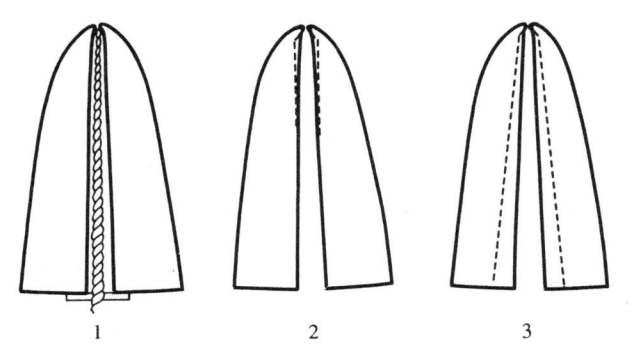

Fig. 16.1 *Sequence of preparation of straight, wide canals. (1) Determination of the working distance. (2) Preparation of the apical stop. (3) Flaring of the coronal portion to produce a smooth, flowing canal shape.*

(a) minimal enlargement at the apical end of the root canal;
(b) an apical 'stop' within the root canal;
(c) a smooth, progressive taper from the apical stop to the pulp chamber, following the natural curvature of the root.

The precise way in which the canal preparation is carried out will depend on the width and degree of curvature encountered. In wide, moderately curved canals, files should be tried sequentially, and the size of the first one to bind at

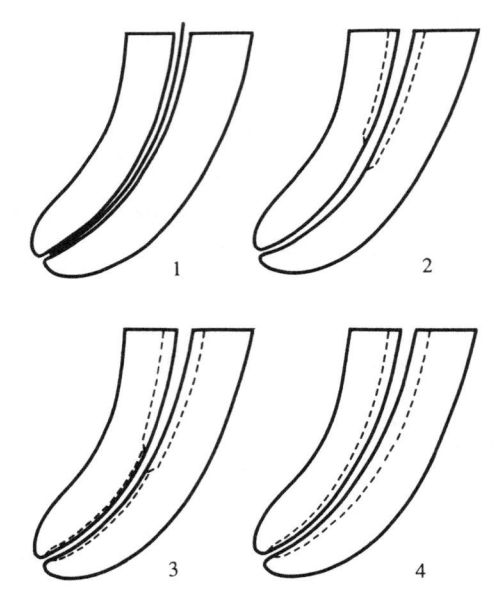

Fig. 16.2 *Sequence of preparation of narrow, curved canals. (1) Determination of the working distance. (2) Enlargement of the canal orifice. (3) Preparation of the apical stop. (4) Flaring of the coronal portion to produce a smooth, flowing canal shape.*

the full working distance noted. The canal is then prepared three full sizes above this and the size of the file which fits the prepared canal at the working distance becomes the 'master apical file'. The remaining coronal portion of the canal is then prepared with hand files alone, using a step-back technique, or in combination with Gates–Glidden drills, so that it is flared sufficiently to allow a spreader to reach to within 1–2 mm of the working distance. During the preparation of the canal, frequent 'recapitulation' with the master apical file should be performed in order to avoid impaction of debris in the apical portion of the canal (Fig. 16.1). In narrow, more severely curved canals a different approach is called for (Fig. 16.2). After exploration of the canal and determination of the working distance, it is advantageous to enlarge the orifice of the canal before preparation of the apical stop. Enlargement is accomplished by using small then large hand files or Gates–Glidden drills, short of the working distance, to widen the coronal portion of the canal. Next, the apical stop is prepared as for wider canals, and finally the canal is flared to produce the required enlargement to allow the spreader to within 1–2 mm of the full working distance. The size of the master apical file will obviously depend on the initial diameter of the canal but, because of the difficulty in handling very fine gutta-percha points, should not be smaller than ISO #25.

When using hand instruments:

(a) maintain control of the working distance;
(b) use copious irrigation;
(c) precurve instruments before use in curved canals;
(d) never force an instrument if it binds;
(e) never rotate instruments in curved canals;
(f) use a short in-out filing action;
(g) clean instruments frequently;
(h) use each file until it fits loosely in the canal;
(i) do not miss or skip an instrument in a series;
(j) discard damaged instruments;
(k) use an anticurvature technique in curved canals;
(l) consider modifying instruments in difficult situations;
(m) clear sudden blockages with copious irrigation together with the use of a small, curved file.

The importance of frequent irrigation cannot be overemphasized. Sodium hypochlorite, in 1–2% concentration, has been found to be most suitable. Its advantages are that it:

(a) dissolves organic material;
(b) is bactericidal;
(c) has a lubricating action for instruments;
(d) flushes out debris;
(e) bleaches the tooth and reduces staining.

Endosonic instruments, as alternatives to hand instrumentation, show considerable promise. They are capable of effective debridement and irrigation but the precise shape of the preparations produced has not been evaluated in all cases and they should be regarded as adjuncts to hand instruments rather than replacements for them. Perhaps their greatest use is to speed up the flaring process once the shape of the apical preparation has been established.

Once the preparation of the canal has been completed, it may be dried with paper points and the access cavity sealed temporarily if it is not to be filled at the same appointment. Antibacterial medication is seldom necessary since the biomechanical preparation described is the most important factor in eliminating microorganisms from the canal. If a medicament is to be used it should not be an irritant to the periapical tissues should it inadvertently escape from the canal. Non-setting calcium hydroxide preparations are suitable for most circumstances.

CANAL FILLING

The root filling is designed to provide a favourable biological environment to enable soft tissue healing to occur, by preventing the percolation of exudate from the periapical tissues into the root canal space and also preventing reinfection of the canal via the bloodstream.

The ideal root filling material should be:

(a) non-irritant;
(b) dimensionally stable;
(c) non-resorbable;
(d) easily introduced into the canal;
(e) plastic on insertion;
(f) rigid on setting;
(g) adherent to dentine;
(h) bacteriostatic;
(i) radiopaque;
(j) non-staining;
(k) easily removed if necessary;
(l) inexpensive;
(m) endowed with a long shelf-life.

A multiplicity of techniques is available for filling the root canal system but the use of laterally condensed gutta-percha combined with a sealer provides a reliable means of obliterating the space created by the canal preparation techniques described above. The function of the sealer is to fill in any *minor* discrepancies between the gutta-percha and the walls of the canal, to act as a lute for the gutta-percha, and to lubricate the canal to facilitate insertion of the solid cones. The advantages of gutta-percha are that it is:

(a) inert;
(b) tolerated by the periapical tissues;
(c) compactable;
(d) dimensionally stable;
(e) radiopaque;
(f) has known solvents.

Its disadvantages are few:
(a) it is not rigid;
(b) it shrinks on solvent evaporation;
(c) it shrinks on cooling;
(d) it is difficult to use in small sizes.

The properties of the ideal root-filling material, listed above, apply equally to the sealer as to the solid core material. In the past there has been a preoccupation with the use of strong antiseptics to compensate for less than adequate canal preparation in attempts to achieve sterility, and many sealers incorporating such drugs have been advocated. The results of modern research show that the cleansing and shaping process is the most important factor in reducing the population of microorganisms in the root canal. Many strong antiseptics, when used in concentrations capable of destroying bacteria, are also irritant to the periapical tissues. It is more important for a sealer to be insoluble and inert than to have a bactericidal effect. Those sealers based on mixtures of zinc oxide and eugenol appear to have most of the desirable criteria, although newer materials incorporating calcium hydroxide show considerable promise.

When the filling stage of treatment has been reached, the first step is to confirm that a finger spreader can be inserted into the empty canal to within 1–2 mm of the working distance and, if not, to carry out further preparation until it is possible. Next a master cone of gutta-percha corresponding in size to the master apical file is tried in the canal and adjusted until it fits snugly to within 0.5 mm of the working distance. When its position and fit have been checked radiographically, it is removed from the canal and sealer is introduced using a file one size smaller than the master apical file. A thin layer only of sealer is applied to the walls of the canal, the master cone is 'buttered' with sealer and then introduced into the canal and seated into position. Immediately, the previously selected finger spreader is inserted alongside the master cone and firm apical pressure is applied for 8–10 s to condense the gutta-percha both apically and laterally. It is unwise to rock the spreader from side to side because of the risk of splitting the root. The spreader is then rotated to free it from the gutta-percha and sealer in the canal, withdrawn, and an accessory cone, either the same size as or smaller than the spreader, is inserted into the space created. This process is repeated until the spreader can no longer be inserted further than 1 mm apical to the labial crestal bone. Using a heated instrument the gutta-percha is removed from the coronal access cavity down to the level of the cementum–enamel junction. In multi-rooted teeth, one canal at a time should be filled, commencing with the one to which access is most difficult. As each canal is filled the gutta-percha is removed to the level of the canal orifice. The excess gutta percha from the last canal should be warmed and condensed firmly onto the floor of the pulp chamber to ensure that any lateral canals in the furcation region are adequately sealed.

A radiograph of the completed root filling should now be taken and retained as a baseline record against which to measure any changes in the periapical region. If this radiograph reveals the filling to be defective in position or adequacy of fill the gutta-percha should be removed, the canal prepared further, and then refilled.

Successful restorative dentistry demands that any restorations or appliances be supported by roots with sound, healthy supporting structures. If the pulps of the teeth are not intact, they should be replaced by materials handled and placed in such a way that the health of the periapical tissues will be maintained. There are no short cuts! Only meticulous attention to detail during every phase of treatment will allow the operator to be confident of the outcome of root canal therapy.

Chapter 17

Elastic and non-elastic impression materials

SECTION ONE   ELASTIC IMPRESSION MATERIALS

Classification

Impression materials are generally classified as being either elastic or non-elastic in nature. All these materials are plastic on insertion but will set to form either a rigid or elastic material. The obvious advantage of the elastic impression materials is that they can be withdrawn from undercuts without fracturing or distorting. A detailed classification is as follows:

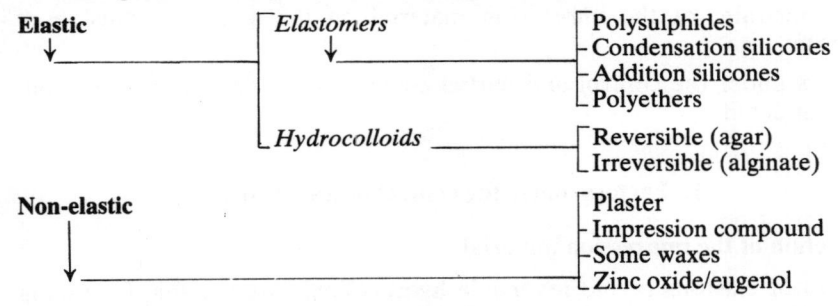

Elastic
- *Elastomers*
  - Polysulphides
  - Condensation silicones
  - Addition silicones
  - Polyethers
- *Hydrocolloids*
  - Reversible (agar)
  - Irreversible (alginate)

Non-elastic
- Plaster
- Impression compound
- Some waxes
- Zinc oxide/eugenol

Properties of an ideal impression material

1. Easy to mix and handle
2. Fluid or plastic on insertion into the mouth
3. Reasonable working time
4. Reasonable setting time
5. Non-toxic and non-irritant
6. Elastic when set, so that undercut areas can be recorded without distortion
7. No dimensional changes on setting or storage
8. Ability to record fine detail accurately
9. Compatible with die and stone materials
10. Acceptable to the patient

The hydrocolloids and the elastomers fulfil all the above criteria except that they all change dimensionally on setting and storage and the polysulphides have a rather unpleasant odour, and therefore questionable patient acceptability.

Factors affecting the accuracy of an impression

1. Factors under the control of the dentist
   (a) selection of the impression material;
   (b) impression technique;
   (c) selection of an appropriate tray and correct adhesive;
   (d) proportioning, mixing and loading the impression material;
   (e) seating and stabilizing the impression in the mouth;
   (f) setting time in the mouth.

2. Factors under the partial control of the dentist
   (a) distortion on removal from the mouth;
   (b) storage conditions of the set material;
   (c) duration of storage.

3. Factors not under the control of the dentist
   (a) dimensional changes during setting process;
   (b) thermal contraction on cooling from mouth to room temperature;
   (c) constraint of the impression material on the setting expansion of gypsum.

Factors under the control and partial control of the dentist are now considered in detail.

1. Factors under the control of the dentist

(a) Selection of the impression material

All types of elastomers and reversible hydrocolloids are suitable for taking impressions for crown and bridgework, whilst alginate is only suitable when study models are required.

Elastomeric impression materials

Polysulphides

These were the first elastomeric materials to be used in dentistry in the mid 1950s. They are sometimes called thiokol, mercaptan or rubber base. They have been produced in all consistencies, usually as two paste materials in their characteristic brown and white colours with their distinctive sulphurous odour.
   Examples: Permlastic and Coeflex.

Their **composition** is generally:

Base paste (white):

   (a) low molecular-weight thiokol polymer;
   (b) inert filler (11 to 54%), e.g. titanium oxide;
   (c) plasticizer.

Activator paste (brown):

(a) oxidizing agent, e.g. lead dioxide;
(b) sulphur;
(c) an oil, e.g. chlorinated paraffin or an ester.

The **setting reaction** is a condensation reaction and occurs by chain lengthening and cross-linking of the thiokol polymer with the lead dioxide. For every increase in chain length or cross-link, a molecule of water is produced.

Advantage:

(a) high tear strength.

Disadvantages:

(a) considerable shrinkage on storage if not cast within a few hours;
(b) long setting time;
(c) the least pleasant of the elastomers for the patient and for the dentist to handle.

Silicones

Condensation silicones are so called because of their setting reaction. They were first introduced during the 1950s as an odourless alternative to the polysulphides. Because of their unpredictable behaviour (producing hydrogen gas as a by-product which caused air blows to occur in the models) their use fell into disrepute. Condensation silicones were subsequently reintroduced in the 1960s, by which time the manufacturers had altered the formulation to produce a more stable set material, with ethyl alcohol produced as the by-product instead of hydrogen. Initially, these materials were not considered as accurate as the polysulphides because a two-stage impression technique was advocated. However, when a one-stage (twin mix) impression technique is used they are in fact more accurate than the polysulphides.

Condensation-cured silicones usually have a base paste with a bottle of reactor liquid, although more recently some manufacturers have produced reactor pastes in contrasting colours to ensure thorough mixing, e.g. Lasticomp and Tewesil. They have a similar shelf life to polysulphides.

Examples: Xantopren and Optosil, Lasticomp and Tewesil.

The **addition-cured silicones** were developed during the 1960s as part of the American space programme (Armstrong walked on the moon in addition-cured silicone boots). They came into use as impression materials in dentistry during the 1970s and are recognized as extremely stable materials when set—in fact far more accurate than either the polysulphides or the condensation-cured silicones.

The addition-cured silicones come in the form of two pastes and they are produced in all consistencies. They also have excellent elastic properties when set.

Examples: Reprosil, Reflect, President, Extrude, Provil, Unosil.

The **composition** of *condensation-cured silicones* is generally as follows.

Base paste:

(a) a silicone polymer with terminal hydroxy groups, e.g. dimethyl siloxane;
(b) a filler.

Activator paste or *liquid:*

(a) a cross-linking agent, e.g. alkyl silicate;
(b) an activator, e.g. an organo-tin compound such as stannous octoate.

The **setting reaction** occurs by cross-linking between the hydroxy-terminated groups of the dimethyl siloxane and the alkyl silicate in the presence of stannous octoate. This produces the set silicone with a molecule of ethyl alcohol produced as the by-product for each cross-linkage formed.

Advantages:

(a) good handling characteristics;
(b) permanent deformation is low;
(c) reasonable setting time.

Disadvantages:

(a) very low tear resistance;
(b) shrinkage on storage if not cast within a few hours, due to loss of ethyl alcohol.

The **composition** of *addition-cured silicones* is generally as follows.

Base paste:

(a) a silicone polymer with terminal vinyl groups;
(b) a filler.

Activator paste:

(a) a cross-linking agent, e.g. organohydrogen siloxane;
(b) a platinum-salt activator, e.g. H_2PtCl_6.

The **setting reaction** occurs by cross-linking of the vinyl groups with the silane groups in the presence of a platinum salt to produce the set polyvinyl siloxane. *NB*. There is no by-product, hence addition-cured silicones are very accurate materials.

Advantages:

(a) good handling characteristics;
(b) excellent dimensional stability when set;
(c) permanent deformation is low.

Disadvantages:

(a) tear resistance is low;
(b) set is inhibited by contact with:
   (i) rubber during mixing,
   (ii) aluminium chloride-impregnated retraction cord.

Polyethers

The polyethers were produced during the late 1960s specifically for dental use. They are extremely accurate materials when used correctly. However, they suffer from distortion if they come into contact with water during setting or storage, therefore it is imperative that the set material is stored **dry**. They come as two pastes and are only produced in regular (medium) consistency.

ELASTIC AND NON-ELASTIC IMPRESSION MATERIALS

Example: Impregum.
The **composition** is generally as follows:

Base paste:

(a) an unsaturated polyether with imine end groups;
(b) a plasticizer;
(c) a filler.

Activator paste:

(a) an aromatic sulphonate ester;
(b) an inert inorganic filler;
(c) a plasticizer.

Setting occurs by a cross-linking reaction of the imine groups, i.e. cationic polymerization to form the set polyether.

Advantages:

(a) short working time;
(b) good dimensional stability if kept dry.

Disadvantages:

(a) greatest degree of thermal contraction of all the elastomers;
(b) water is adsorbed on storage and therefore the impression must be kept dry;
(c) high degree of permanent deformation;
(d) low tear resistance.

Hydrocolloids

Colloids are heterogeneous; similar to a suspension but with a smaller particle size in the range 1–200 nm. If the dispersion medium is water then they are termed hydrocolloids.

Colloids may exist in the sol or gel state. A sol can be converted to a gel by either a reduction in temperature (reversible) or a chemical reaction (irreversible).

Table 17.1
Typical composition of a reversible hydrocolloid

Constituent	Percentage	Function
Agar	13–17	Colloid
Potassium sulphate	1–2	Accelerates set of stone
Borax	0.2–0.5	Strengthens gel but retards set of stone
Alkyl benzoate	0.1	Prevents mould growth
Water	80–85	Dispersion medium
Colours and flavours	trace	Patient acceptability

Reversible hydrocolloid

Composition (see Table 17.1).

Manipulation. Reversible hydrocolloid is manipulated by heating to 100°C for 10–15 min. It is then maintained between 60–66°C, followed by tempering in the tray for 2 min at 43–46°C. Untempered material is injected around the preparation. Once the tray is seated, water coolant is passed through the tray at 13°C for 5 min.

Advantages:

(a) the material is hydrophilic.

Disadvantages:

(a) exposure to air → loss of moisture → shrinkage;
(b) should not be stored for more than 1 h in 100% humidity;
(c) must be cast as soon as possible.

Irreversible hydrocolloids (Alginate)

The typical **composition** is:

Sodium/potassium/ammonium alginate	12%
Calcium sulphate	12%
Trisodium phosphate	2%
Filler (diatomaceous earth)	70%
Potassium sulphate	small
Fluoride salts	small
Flavouring	small

On mixing water with alginate powder, the following **setting reaction** occurs:

1. Trisodium phosphate + calcium sulphate ⟶ Calcium phosphate + trisodium sulphate

This reaction does not contribute to the properties of the set material. Once the trisodium phosphate has been used up (working time), the following reaction begins:

2. Sodium alginate + calcium sulphate ⟶ Sodium sulphate + calcium alginate

The manufacturer therefore can adjust the working time of the material by varying the amount of trisodium phosphate. The dentist can decrease the working time by adding less water or warmer water.

The other constituents have the following functions: the filler strengthens the gel; the silico-fluorides improve the surface of the stone model; patient acceptability is enhanced by flavouring agents.

Advantages:

(a) fast set;
(b) hydrophilic.

Disadvantages:

(a) not dimensionally stable on storage;
(b) not accurate enough for crown and bridgework.

ELASTIC AND NON-ELASTIC IMPRESSION MATERIALS

(b) Impression technique

(i) The most accurate impression technique for all elastomers is produced using a single (twin) mix. A two-stage mix without spacer will produce an accurate impression for condensation-cured silicones, but should never be used for addition-cured silicones as the dies produced from the impression are smaller than the original. A two-stage technique with spacer is only suitable for addition-cured silicones; with condensation-cured silicones, a much larger die is produced.

(ii) All the elastomeric materials are hydrophobic, except for some of the more recent addition-cured silicones, e.g. Unosil and the new (blue) Reprosil, which are said to be hydrophilic by the manufacturers. With all hydrophobic materials it is essential that the field of operation is clean and dry.

(iii) Hydrocolloids are by nature hydrophilic and therefore require a damp field of operation.

(c) Selection of an appropriate tray and correct adhesive

(i) Elastomeric impression materials must be supported in a rigid special or stock tray.

(ii) The correct adhesive for the material must be used and allowed to dry in a thin even layer.

(iii) Elastomeric materials are best used in even thicknesses of 2–4 mm.

(iv) Ideally, an elastomeric impression tray should have occlusal stops and a good peripheral seal.

(v) A water-cooled tray is required for reversible hydrocolloid.

(d) Proportioning, mixing and loading the impression material

(i) The impression material should be proportioned according to the manufacturer's instructions.

(ii) The elastomeric impression materials and alginate should be mixed thoroughly and all air should be excluded from the mix if at all possible.

(e) Seating and stabilizing the impression in the mouth

(i) For elastomeric impression materials, when a putty-based impression technique is used, then the tray must be seated parallel to the occlusal plane, in one direction only.

(ii) All impressions must be held still in the mouth once setting has commenced.

(f) Setting time in the mouth

(i) The raised temperature of the mouth will accelerate the set of the material nearest to the tissues.

(ii) For elastomeric impression materials wait until some of the material has set at room temperature before removing the tray from the mouth as the elastic properties of elastomers improve the longer they are left in the mouth after the initial set.

(iii) All hydrocolloids should be removed from the mouth immediately the material has set.

2. Factors under the partial control of the dentist

(a) Distortion on removal from mouth

A snap withdrawal of the set material is desirable.

(b) Storage conditions of the set material

(i) After removal from the mouth, all elastomers should be washed, dried, and then stored dry. (Polyethers in particular must be stored dry as they absorb water once set.)

(ii) Hydrocolloids should be washed and cast as soon as possible. Reversible hydrocolloids must be stored in 100% humidity for a maximum of 1 h. Alginate must only be stored in damp conditions.

(iii) When sterilization of an impression is required, only the addition-cured silicones remain stable when soaked in 2% glutaraldehyde for 6 h. (Condensation-cured silicones shrink, polyethers expand, some polysulphides shrink whilst others expand, and all hydrocolloids distort.)

(c) Duration of storage

(i) The shelf-life of unused materials is limited and reduced by exposure to air; therefore punctured tubes or loosely applied tops should be avoided.

(ii) All elastomer impressions should be left for 15 min after removal from the mouth to allow elastic recovery to take place. Addition-cured silicones should be left for at least 30 min as some addition-cured silicones evolve gas during the first 20–30 min.

(iii) All elastomers should be cast within 3 h of removal of the impression. However, if the impression is to be left for more than 24 h before casting, it is advisable to use an addition-cured silicone or a polyether as these materials show minimal dimensional change on storage.

(iv) Hydrocolloids should be cast as soon as possible. Reversible hydrocolloids should ideally be cast within 15 min, but may be left up to a maximum of 1 h if stored in 100% humidity.

FURTHER READING

Brown D. (1981). An update on elastomeric impression materials. *Br. Dent. J.*, **150**, 35–41.
Combe E. C. (1988). *Notes on Dental Materials,* 5th edn, Section IV. Impression Materials. Edinburgh: Churchill Livingstone.
Phillips R. W. (1988) *Skinner's Science of Dental Materials*, 8th edn, chapters 8, 9, 10. New York: Saunders, pp. 108–56.
Wilson H. J. (1988). Impression materials. *Br. Dent. J.*, **164**, 221–5.

SECTION TWO RIGID (NON-ELASTIC) IMPRESSION MATERIALS

Impression compounds

These are thermoplastic materials containing a mixture of:

(a) resins (colophony, shellac, waxes);
(b) fillers (talc or soap stone);
(c) lubricants (stearin, steric acid).

Lower-fusing types are used for impression taking:

1. *Sheet form* (brown) — used for primary impressions in complete denture work.
2. *Brown stick composition* — used for copper band impressions.
3. *Green stick composition* — used as above and for marginal modification to special trays.

Composition is a cheap, easy-to-handle material. It has the advantage in primary edentulous impressions of being self-supporting but, being non-elastic, will not record undercuts. These tend to be labial to the maxillary ridge, buccal to the maxillary tuberosities and below prominent mylohyoid ridges in the mandible.

Manipulation

Composition must be heated for sufficient time in a water bath (55–60°C) to ensure complete softening and even flow properties in the mouth. Too long in the water and the properties of the composition may change through constituents leaching out. The material is first shaped into a suitable impression tray, then inserted in the mouth. Being viscous (mucodisplacive) in nature, over-extension of the sulcus will result unless the border of the impression is vigorously moulded. On hardening at 37°C the impression can be removed. If necessary the impression borders can be trimmed, re-softened with a pin flame and the tray inserted again, carrying out further border moulding to obtain a more accurate peripheral extension.

Brown stick composition is heated uniformly in a flame before insertion in the copper band, which is then placed over the crown or inlay preparation. Care must be taken not to volatize any of the constituents by over-heating.

Advantages:

(a) the absence of toxic/non-irritant constituents;
(b) the ability to be copper-plated — this results in a harder die surface;
(c) a long shelf-life.

Disadvantages:

(a) fine detail and undercut areas cannot be recorded;
(b) shrinkage of about 1.5% occurs on cooling from mouth to room temperature;
(c) composition is prone to dimensional changes if left, particularly in a warm room, before casting — this is due to the relief of stresses that can be set up if the composition is deformed while partially set.

Plaster

As an impression material, plaster has a limited use in dentistry. It is, however, an indispensable material in the dental laboratory for model and die construction.

Chemistry

Dental plaster and stone are chemically identical, consisting of the hemihydrate of calcium sulphate; this combines with water to form the dihydrate. Dental plaster is a β hemihydrate prepared by heating gypsum (calcium sulphate dihydrate) in air at 120°C; dental stone is produced when gypsum is heated in an autoclave at 120–130°C. They differ in that plaster (β hemihydrate) has irregular crystals while dental stones have larger crystals, leading to a stronger set material.

The chemical reaction is:

$$CaSO_4 \cdot \tfrac{1}{2}H_2O + 1\tfrac{1}{2}H_2O \longrightarrow CaSO_4 \cdot 2H_2O + \text{heat}$$

calcium sulphate hemihydrate + water → gypsum (dihydrate)

Constituents

Pure plaster expands on setting but, with the addition of 4% potassium sulphate, this is substantially reduced to 0.15–0.4%. Potassium sulphate also accelerates the setting reaction, so a retarder, borax (0.4%), is added to give a suitable working time of 2½–3 min.

Other additives include:

(a) alizarin red, a dye to contrast normal plaster during casting;
(b) flavourings;
(c) gum tragacanth, polyvinyl acetate or zinc oxide, which may be added in small quantities to improve the handling of plaster;
(d) starch, added to facilitate the removal of the impression from the model—boiling water is poured over the impression, which disintegrates through swelling of the starch particles.

Manipulation

Plaster is mixed with water to produce a smooth, bubble-free paste that sets into a brittle but stable material. Excellent recording of fine detail is obtained but, because of its rigidity when set, it has limited use where there are undercuts. It can be used for secondary impressions of edentulous arches, especially where a fibrous or flabby ridge is present. Being a mucostatic impression material, plaster will give a true representation of the mucosal tissues in the resting state. Where bony undercuts are present the plaster impression will fracture on removal. The pieces, however, can easily be reassembled. When casting the impression a separating medium must be used to prevent the model plaster bonding to the impression.

Thus the *advantages* of plaster are:

(a) accuracy;
(b) very little dimensional change during setting or storage;
(c) non-toxic;
(d) very long shelf-life.

The inability of dental plaster to record undercut areas gives it a limited use as an impression material.

Waxes

These are thermoplastic materials that have two basic forms:

(a) inlay wax;
(b) impression wax.

Inlay wax

Made in hexagonal blue sticks from a mixture of ceresin, paraffin and carnuba waxes, and beeswaxes. It softens at 42°C and hardens at mouth temperature. Inlay wax is used for direct inlay patterns in the mouth. It is first flame-softened before inserting into the inlay preparation where, upon hardening, it is easily carved to the desired contour without flaking.

The direct wax-pattern technique has the advantage of being very cheap, but more chairside time is required.

Impression wax

This contains a mixture of paraffin wax and beeswax. It can flow under pressure at mouth temperature and so is well-suited for functional impressions of mucosal-support areas for dentures.

A technique for lining partially mucosal-borne dentures, known as the Applegate or altered cast technique, uses impression wax. The partial denture framework is first constructed using a convential impression, to which is added self-curing acrylic resin in the free-end saddle region. The wax is then melted in a dish over a water bath at 60°C. This is then applied to the fit surface of the free-end saddles of the partial denture and seated in the mouth. Manual pressure is applied to the denture framework to ensure correct seating on the teeth. This is kept in place for 4 min while the wax is allowed to flow. The wax being viscous at mouth temperature will displace the supporting tissues of the free-end saddle so giving a mucodisplacive impression. Several applications of wax may be required to record the whole fit surface. The impression must be cast immediately.

The advantage of the mucodisplacive technique is that it will minimize rocking of the partial denture during function, but this results in a greater proportion of the load being transmitted to the supporting soft tissues.

Zinc oxide–eugenol impression paste

This impression material is supplied in the form of two pastes.

1. Zinc oxide in an inert oily base (e.g. olive, linseed or mineral oil) with hydrogenated rosin to improve the physical properties.
2. Eugenol with inert filler (e.g. talc/kaolin) and zinc acetate to accelerate the setting reaction. Eugenol may be substituted for a carboxylic acid.

Manipulation

Equal lengths of each paste are mixed to produce a streak-free mix.

Properties

The mix sets by chemical reaction to produce a non-elastic material. Fine detail is recorded, with little dimensional change during setting or storage. The material has a satisfactory setting time, which is accelerated by the presence of moisture and increased temperature. Impression paste is compatible with dental stone and being thermoplastic is easily removed from the model by immersion in water at 60°C.

Applications

Impression paste is usually used as a wash impression for complete dentures where no undercuts are present. This can be taken either in an existing denture or in a close-fitting special tray.

Chapter 18

Pins in restorative dentistry

INDICATION FOR PINS

Pins are indicated where there has been excessive loss of tooth substance and there is insufficient mechanical retention remaining to retain the restorative material in a cavity. They are also useful when a single cusp is missing, e.g. mesiobuccal cusp, upper first molar; for placing a core before restoring with a cast restoration; or for placement of a temporary amalgam restoration in a tooth requiring endodontic treatment under rubber dam. However, if a tooth is to be restored with a composite resin utilizing acid-etch and dentine-bonding techniques, then there is less need for pin retention.

BACKGROUND

During the 1950s a standardized technique for pin-retained amalgams was developed using 0.025 inch diameter, stainless-steel wire cemented into a pin channel which had been prepared with a 0.027 inch twist drill (cemented pins).

The mid-1960s saw the introduction of two techniques which relied on the elasticity of dentine.

1. The friction lock technique used horizontally grooved stainless steel pins which were forced into slightly smaller precut pin holes with an applicator. The pins were supplied in kit form, e.g. Unitek pins.
2. The second technique overcame the insertion problem and utilized a method of screwing threaded pins into undersized channels in dentine. The pins were marketed as the Threadmate system by TMS. Initially, pins were inserted using a hand wrench but this produced difficulties where access was limited. TMS then marketed a 10:1 reduction-gear handpiece which allowed accurate pin-hole preparation and insertion of the pins. A constriction at the shank end of the pin, combined with the force of insertion, caused the pin to shear. Hence the self-threading pin was developed. The late 1970s brought the development of the two-in-one or double shear pin, i.e. the first pin sheared on placement and the second was then inserted without the need for replacing the pin in the handpiece. However, the pins rarely penetrated to the full depth of the pin channels. To overcome this problem TMS introduced a buttress-threaded pin in the mid 1980s (Link Plus), which has greatly improved pin penetration.

METHODS AVAILABLE FOR INCREASING RETENTION

1. Retention grooves and undercuts
2. Pins
3. Bonding agents and acid-etch techniques for composite restorations
4. Posts or screws in endodontically treated teeth.

FACTORS AFFECTING PIN RETENTION

1. *Type of pin* in decreasing order of retentiveness:
    (a) self-threading,
    (b) friction lock,
    (c) cemented.

2. *Diameter of pin*: pin retention is proportional to pin diameter. However, as the width of dentine is usually in the order of 2.5 mm, a pin diameter of 0.5 mm is recommended.

3. *Pin depth:* equivalent retention can be achieved by placing the different pin types into the following depths:

Self-threading	2 mm
Friction lock	5–6 mm
Cemented	11–12 mm

2 mm is the optimum depth for self-threading pins and, as it is impossible to place pins to more than 3–4 mm without endangering the pulp or periodontal membrane, 3 mm is recommended as the practical length for both friction lock and cemented pins.

4. *Pin penetration:* most self-threading pins do *not* penetrate to the full depth of the pin channel. Pin penetration is improved by:
    (a) the use of pins with a buttress thread, e.g. Link Plus pins;
    (b) placing pins with a speed-reduction handpiece;
    (c) faceting the tip of a standard threaded pin.

5. *Number of pins:* retention is proportional to the number of pins placed. However, as pins reduce the tensile strength of amalgam, use less pins with maximum retention. In general, place one pin per lost cusp.

6. *Retention in the restoration:* important factors are:
    (a) The optimum length of pin to be retained in the restoration is 2 mm.
    (b) Serrated or self-threading pins are twice as retentive in amalgam as smoother-surfaced, friction lock pins.
    (c) Amalgam is more retentive than composite as a core material surrounding pins.
    (d) Spherical and dispersed-phase amalgam alloys provide superior adaptation to all types of pin.
    (e) 2 mm thickness of amalgam is required above the top of the pin.

7. *Material of pin construction:* pins are made of either stainless steel, stainless steel plated with gold or titanium. Gold-plated pins help to prevent the reduction in tensile strength of the amalgam which occurs when pin retention is used.

TOOTH FACTORS AFFECTING PIN PLACEMENT

1. *Dentine width:* 1 mm of dentine is required to surround the pin. Therefore at least 2.5 mm of dentine is required between the enamel–dentine junction and the pulp. As a general rule, dentine widths are:
    (a) greatest on the buccal and lingual surfaces of teeth;
    (b) narrower approximally;
    (c) widest at the cementum–enamel junction.

2. *Tooth angulation:* particular care should be exercised during pin placement when a tooth is rotated or tilted, as the possibility of placing a pin into the pulp or periodontal membrane is increased.

3. *Furcations:* although there may appear to be 2.5 mm width of dentine in these areas, dentine widths decrease apically into furcations and therefore the risk of perforation into the periodontal membrane is increased.

4. *Inter-pin distance:* dentine crazing occurs adjacent to threaded pins and increases with decreased inter-pin distance, therefore a minimum of 5 mm inter-pin distance is recommended.

PIN TYPES

1. *Self-threading pins:* the **advantages** of these are:
    (a) ease of placement especially in inaccessible areas of the mouth;
    (b) excellent retention;
    (c) pins can be bent and contoured after insertion;
    (d) pin holes can be cut accurately with a low-speed handpiece;
    (e) pins can be inserted safely and easily using a speed-reduction handpiece;
    (f) no irritant cements required.

The **disadvantages** are:

(a) expense;
(b) craze lines and stress concentration can develop about the pin.

Some **examples** of self-threading pins:

(a) TMS Minim Double Shear, Stabilock, Filpin;
(b) Link Plus pins — buttress thread;
(c) Bondent Pins — especially designed for use with composite restorations and particularly useful where there is reduced clearance with the apposing teeth.

2. *Friction lock pins:* the **advantages** of these are:
   (a) relatively easy to place but not in inaccessible parts of the mouth;
   (b) less expensive than self-threading pins;
   (c) no irritant cements required.

The **disadvantages** are:
   (a) less retentive than self-threading pins;
   (b) difficult to place in inaccessible parts of the mouth;
   (c) difficult to contour pins after placement;
   (d) pin hole must be kept dry;
   (e) the spiral drills are fragile and prone to breakage.

Example: Unitek pins

3. *Cemented pins:* the **advantages** of these are:

   (a) cheap;
   (b) no risk of tooth fracture;
   (c) pins can be exactly contoured before insertion.

The **disadvantages** are:
   (a) minimal retention gained;
   (b) pins must be pre-contoured, i.e. cannot be altered after insertion;
   (c) requires cements;
   (d) difficulty experienced in placement in some parts of the mouth;
   (e) increased risk of perforation into pulp or periodontal membrane;
   (f) leakage at tooth–pin interface.

Example: Markley pins

RISKS OF PIN PLACEMENT

Injury to (a) pulp; (b) periodontal membrane.

FURTHER READING

Bapna M. S., Lugassy A. A. (1971). Influence of gold plating of stainless steel pins on the tensile strength of dental amalgam. *J. Dent. Res.*, **50,** 846–9.

Butchart D. G. M., Grieve A. R., Kamel J. H. (1988). The retention in dentine and composite resin materials of Bondent dentine pins. *Br. Dent. J.*, **165,** 165–9.

Dilts W. E., Duncanson M. G., Collard E. W., Parmley L. E. (1981). Retention of self-threading pins. *J. Can. Dent. Assoc.*, **47,** 119–20.

Schaefer M. E., Reisheck M. H. (1981). Seating depth of three new threaded pins inserted with a contra-angle dental handpiece. *J. Prosth. Dent.*, **45,** 614–20.

Standlee J. P., Collard E. W., Caputo A. A. (1970). Dentinal defects caused by some twist drills and retention pins. *J. Prosth. Dent.*, **24,** 185–92.

Welk D. A., Dilts W. E. (1969). Influence of pins on the compressive and transverse strength of dental amalgam and retention of pins in amalgam. *J. Am. Dent. Assoc.*, **78,** 101–4.

Chapter 19

Dental amalgam

An alloy is a combination or union of two or more metals which are miscible (mutually soluble) in the liquid state. The reaction between mercury and a metal to form an alloy is amalgamation, and is unique, because mercury is a liquid, and so the alloy can be formed at room temperature.

Dental amalgam is a union of mercury with an alloy containing silver, tin, copper and sometimes zinc. This is amalgam alloy—a powder. Mixed with mercury it gives a plastic mass which hardens in the cavity preparation.

AMALGAM ALLOYS

Composition

Conventional alloys and the American Dental Association specification were designed to ensure there is sufficient silver in the alloy to prevent a significant amount of corrosion of the amalgam. Typical proportions are:

$$Ag-69\%; Sn-27\%; Cu-3\%; Zn-1\%$$

The primary constituents, silver and tin, are present in the intermetallic compound Ag_3Sn, and this is the gamma phase (see also 'The new amalgams' below).

The amalgamation of silver and mercury is too slow, so tin is alloyed with the silver to increase the reaction rate with mercury. Tin also decreases the expansion rate of the silver/mercury alloy. The tin is restricted to 25–27% because the gamma-phase Ag_3Sn exists at this composition, and amalgam made from the gamma-phase alloy has superior strength and adequate setting speed compared with alloys made from other phases in the silver–tin system.

Zinc was originally added in the manufacture to scavenge oxygen, and to prevent formation of metal oxides. It also contributed to workability and cleanliness of amalgam during trituration and condensation. It is no longer necessary and is not used, for when zinc-containing alloy is wet, delayed, excessive expansion occurs due to the release of hydrogen gas from the interaction of zinc and water.

Effects of alloy components

Silver	*increases*	strength (up to 73%) expansion setting rate (up to 76%)
	decreases	corrosion creep
Tin	*decreases*	strength (27% or more) expansion setting rate (24% or over)
	increases	corrosion creep
Copper	*increases*	strength and hardness (up to 5%) corrosion decreases creep (up to 5%) substitutes for silver
Zinc		deoxidizes reduces the brittleness of the alloy has little effect on the strength causes delayed expansion with water

High-copper alloys

These are formed in two ways:

1. Particles of Ag/Cu alloy are mixed with particles of conventional alloy — this is an admixture, e.g. Dispersalloy.
2. The three constituents, silver, tin, copper, are melted together to form a single, high-copper alloy, called a ternary alloy. Alloys of this type with four ingredients are called quaternary alloys — the added ingredient often being 1% palladium or 5% indium, e.g. Tytan, Sybralloy.

Dispersalloy is a mixture of conventional filings and particles of a silver–copper eutectic alloy. A eutectic is a two-phase alloy in which the constituent metals are separated into alternating layers. Dispersalloy was the first commercial high-copper alloy (1968).

Composition

65% conventional filings   +   35% Ag/Cu spheres   =   Dispersalloy
(69% Ag; 25% Sn; 5% Cu; 1% Zn) (72% Ag/28% Cu)   (70% Ag; 16% Sn; 13% Cu; 1% Zn)

It contains about the same amount of silver as conventional alloys, but tin is very reduced and copper increased. Clinical research shows the results are superior especially for tarnish, corrosion and creep resistance, plus marginal breakdown.

Ternary alloys (1975) — compositions:

Alloy	Ag	Sn	Cu
Sybralloy	40%	31%	29%
Tytan	60%	26%	14%

The silver content is reduced, and the tin content stays the same. They again fare better than the conventional alloys, which is due to a better understanding of the mechanism of corrosion.

High-copper alloys are considered further under 'The new amalgams' below.

Particle size and shape

As well as differing in chemical composition, alloy powders differ in the size and shape of their particles. These factors greatly influence the handling and physical properties and often form the basis of selection for clinical use.

The two shapes are **filings** and **spheres**.

Filings are irregular shapes produced by the cutting action of a lathe on the alloy ingot (lathe-cut or conventional alloys). Spherical alloys were developed in 1962. Spherical alloy particles are made by atomizing the molten metal into a closed chamber filled with inert gas or water. The alloy droplets solidify and drop to the floor. They are graded and blended to give size distribution.

Filings give a firm packing resistance and are marketed in three size grades:

(a) regular: greater than 50 μm;
(b) fine cut: 35 μm;
(c) micro cut: 26 μm.

These are averages distributed in the particles. Fine cut is the most popular and the particles range from 5–40 μm.

Smaller particle size has been a major advance, as large particles require a long setting and hardening time with mercury. Early amalgams took up to 7 days to set! New amalgams reach 90% of final compressive strength in 8 h and some high-copper ones are faster still. As the rate of reaction increases with the surface area available to the mercury, small particles with high specific surface areas set faster.

The advantages of small-particle alloys are:

(a) faster amalgamation;
(b) greater early strength;
(c) more plastic mix — easier condensation;
(d) smoother surface;
(e) increased setting contraction, less mixing time required to reduce expansion;
(f) lower mercury/alloy ratio required to give a plastic mix.

Advantages of spheres over filings

The major advantages of spherical alloy particles are:

(a) more rapid and complete amalgamation;
(b) greater early compressive strength;
(c) lower mercury/alloy ratio;
(d) less sensitive to poor manipulation;
(e) smoother surface.

The ultimate strength of spherical alloys of standard composition is no greater than lathe-cut ones, but they handle differently.

THE AMALGAMATION REACTION

Mercury reacts with the gamma-phase Ag_3Sn to produce dental amalgam, which has a cored structure consisting of unreacted gamma-phase particles surrounded and bound together by a matrix of two new phases — gamma-1 = Ag_2Hg_3, and gamma-2 = Sn_8Hg. Thus:

$$Hg + Ag_3Sn \rightarrow Ag_3Sn + Ag_2Hg_3 + Sn_8Hg$$
$$\text{gamma} \quad \text{gamma} \quad \text{gamma-1} \quad \text{gamma-2}$$

The amount of each phase varies from product to product, and with manipulation, but the average for the final amalgam is:

gamma = 30–35%; gamma-1 = 60–70%; gamma-2 = 1–10%

The composition of amalgams made from high-copper admixtures is different. In addition to gamma and gamma-1, the silver–copper eutectic spheres are present, along with a 'reaction-ring' of Cu_6Sn_5 on the surface of the spheres. Very little, if any, of the gamma-2 is present in either admix or ternary forms. Tin reacts preferentially with copper to form Cu_6Sn_5 — rather than with mercury to form the gamma-2 phase. The steps are:

(a) 'wetting' of the alloy particles by the mercury;
(b) dissolution of silver and tin in mercury;
(c) diffusion of mercury into the alloy;
(d) precipitation of gamma-1 and gamma-2 from the liquid phase;
(e) crystal growth of gamma-1 and gamma-2.

The alloy must be well mixed to obtain the initial 'wetting'. A plastic mass with slippery particles is produced.

The setting curve of amalgam exhibits a slight initial contraction, followed by expansion, then small, slow contraction. The initial contraction is due to diffusion of mercury into the alloy particles. During this diffusion, the mercury–silver–tin solution becomes supersaturated with respect to silver and tin, so that the two new phases, gamma-1 and gamma 2, precipitate.

The precipitation and growth of these crystalline phases results in expansion and hardening of the amalgam. The final contraction is caused by slow diffusion of remaining free mercury into the unreacted portion of the alloy particles.

Properties of the phases

Gamma (untreated particles):

(a) strongest phase;
(b) intermediate corrosion resistance.

Gamma-1 (Ag_2Hg_3):

(a) intermediate strength;
(b) highest corrosion resistance.

Gamma-2 (Sn_8Hg):

(a) lowest strength;
(b) greatest creep;
(c) lowest corrosion resistance.

The best properties are from an alloy with maximum amounts of unreacted particles, minimum matrix and the least gamma-2 phase.

THE NEW AMALGAMS

This section does not set out to deal with the basic constituents and properties of amalgam, which have been considered above, but will look at the significance of an advance in the material which is more recently available commercially.

Whether or not we should still be using amalgam as a dental restorative material is open to question but, until composite resin, glass ionomer or some other new material has been shown to have an equivalent clinical performance in everyday use, and until it has been shown conclusively that mercury from dental amalgams is the causative agent in either some local or systemic disease, its use is likely to continue.

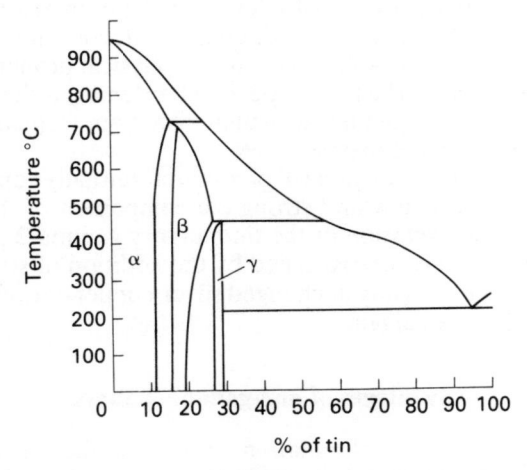

Fig. 19.1 *Constitution (α, β, γ) diagram of the silver–tin system.*

Spherical particle alloys (see above) have been commercially available for 20 years and, despite the known advantages of using these, they have not been widely adopted by the profession in routine general practice. Non-gamma-2 alloys appear to be receiving the same response which, given the benefits to be derived from their use, must relate to short-term considerations of cost.

What is a non-gamma-2 alloy? (Fig. 19.1)

Disregarding other minor constituents, we have seen that the basic dental amalgam alloy is composed of silver and tin in the approximate proportions of 75% silver to 25% tin. When silver and tin are melted together the resultant metal will assume different alloy forms depending upon their relative proportions, and categorization of these alloys has conventionally used pure silver as a baseline. As proportionately more tin is contained in the alloy, a series of different alloys is formed: 1–11% tin gives the alpha alloy, 14–18% tin gives the beta alloy, 25–27% tin gives the gamma alloy, and proportions between those quoted contain a mixture of the two adjacent alloys.

The gamma form is the main constituent of dental restorative alloys, but there is also likely to be some beta alloy included.

As outlined under 'The amalgamation reaction' above, when the gamma alloy is mixed with mercury to form amalgam, two new alloys are formed by the combination of the mercury with silver and tin respectively: the silver/mercury alloy is named gamma-1 and the tin/mercury alloy is named gamma-2. These form a matrix around remnant unchanged gamma particles so that all three components are present in set amalgam.

The unchanged gamma particles form the strongest component of the set amalgam, the gamma-1 component of the matrix is only slightly less strong, and the gamma-2 is the weakest by a factor of 10.

In the early 1960s, attempts were made to strengthen amalgams by applying the theory of dispersion hardening, which is a well-established principle in metallurgy. Dispersion hardening is produced by the inclusion of a large volume of fine filler particles (usually less than 1 pm in size), which is then dispersed throughout the metal. A silver/copper eutectic alloy was used as this 'dispersed' phase with favourable results in the physical properties. However, this was soon realized not to be true dispersion hardening as the copper was not entirely retained as a separate fine particulate phase but formed a new reaction product within the amalgam matrix.

The spin-off was that the 'dispersed' phase preferentially combined with the tin in the alloy to form a new and strong eta component of the set amalgam matrix (Cu_6Sn_5) to the exclusion of the tin/mercury gamma-2 phase.

Composite materials are strengthened by the addition of strong fillers, and the new eta component and any unchanged silver/copper particles act as strong fillers in a high-copper amalgam.

Advantages of non-gamma-2 alloys

The prime advantage is the elimination of what is the weak phase in the amalgam matrix. The eta component further strengthens the amalgam by forming crystals across grain boundaries and thus helping to prevent slip between these grains. The net effect of including the additional copper is to produce a stronger amalgam which has less tendency to creep.

This hardening effect was concurrently and serendipitously discovered by general practitioners who, seeking to gain an antibacterial effect from the inclusion of extra copper, added copper to their standard amalgam alloys. In certain proportions it was coincidentally found that these higher copper alloys were self-polishing with use in the mouth and retained a high lustre. By elimination of the gamma-2 phase, amalgam alloys are rendered less liable to the corrosion that this component suffers.

Clinical trials have shown that certain non-gamma-2 alloys produce amalgams which have very little marginal breakdown by comparison with conventional alloy amalgam.

Presentation of the alloy

To recapitulate, dental amalgam alloys can be either lathe-cut particles, spherical particles, or a mixture of the two.

Both the lathe-cut and the totally spherical particle alloys (single composition) have an even distribution of the high copper content. Mixed particle alloy (admixed) usually has the high copper content only in the spherical component, which is the silver/copper eutectic, although alloys are available of this type that have an even distribution of the copper through both components.

Single-composition alloys generally have a copper content which ranges from 13% to 30% by weight, while the copper content of the spherical component of the admixed alloys is 28% and gives an overall content of between 9% to 20% by weight depending upon the proportion of this component in the alloy. Admixed alloys usually contain between 30% and 55% of spherical particles by weight.

The reaction

The essential features of this have been outlined above. As with alloy/mercury reactions in general the resultant amalgam has unchanged particles of the original alloy in a matrix formed from the reaction products, and the set amalgam has the form of a composite material with these unchanged particles acting as the strong filler.

Amalgams from single-composition alloys will contain unreacted beta and gamma particles and some unreacted copper/tin alloy of the form Cu_3Sn, in addition to the matrix phases of gamma-1 and eta. The eta tends to form a mesh on the surface of the unchanged alloy particles and thus helps to bind them into the matrix, which itself is strengthened by smaller numbers of eta crystals traversing its grain boundaries. The eta particles formed from single-composition alloys are much larger than those formed from admixed alloys.

Amalgams from admixed alloys contain unreacted particles of beta and gamma alloys and the silver/copper eutectic in a matrix of gamma-1 and eta. The eta component tends to form crystals around the particles of silver/copper, although they are also found amongst the gamma-1 matrix.

It has been estimated that at least 12% by weight of copper is required in an amalgam alloy to ensure that no gamma-2 phase is formed in the subsequent amalgam.

Which type of non-gamma-2 alloy should I use?

The evidence of laboratory and clinical research does not clearly answer this question, with its dependence on differing copper content, quality control in manufacture, presence of other trace elements, comparability of examination criteria, and clinical variables in addition to considerations of alloy type. There is reasonable evidence to indicate that single-composition alloys are capable of producing very high strengths in bench testing and that some admixed alloys have very good records in clinical use.

There is also some statistical evidence that high-copper alloys that are also zinc-containing have a better clinical performance than those that are not.

The criteria for assessment which are available to the general practitioner remain very subjective, but a brief survey of the literature on amalgam does tend to highlight certain brand names which seem to maintain an above average performance whatever the tests applied.

SOME WORDS ON THE HANDLING OF MERCURY

It is undoubtedly safer to use dental amalgam alloy and mercury in pre-dispensed capsule form as this avoids the danger of mercury spillage. Mercury is volatile at room temperature and small amounts can give a high atmospheric content. Inhalation of mercury vapour is the primary route by which it is likely to enter the bodies of dental staff.

Do not assume that just because alloy and mercury are encapsulated that there will be no leakage. Mercury can be vaporized by the high energy of mechanical mixing, and capsules can allow the escape of liquid mercury if the caps are not properly fitting. Self-activating capsules are probably more reliable, but all capsules should be checked periodically by mixing with some adhesive tape around the junction of the cap with the capsule to see if any mercury reaches the sticky surface of the tape.

Use of amalgam in capsule form is not necessarily wasteful and many manufacturers would argue that the variety of measure available for any one amalgam should make the format more economical once the dentist has become accustomed to the spill size. All unused amalgam should be kept under water in a closed jar.

It has been shown that a high concentration of mercury vapour is produced in the area immediately around the patient's mouth when old amalgam is being removed with a high-speed drill, and that the effective method of minimizing the presence of this vapour is to cut under copious water spray with the help of high-volume aspiration. Use of a face mask to protect the dental staff may not necessarily be beneficial, as the mercury vapour can recondense in the fabric of the mask and prolong the effective risk. Special face masks have been produced which will de-activate the mercury on contact.

Mercury vapour can also be produced by the use of high-frequency packing devices and these should thus be avoided.

Chapter 20

Post crowns

ANTERIOR TEETH

When a root-filled tooth requires subsequent crowning it is generally recommended that this takes the form of a post crown. This is usually for the following reasons:

1. If the remaining natural tooth core is used for the porcelain jacket crown preparation, the amount of tooth substance removed by this preparation and that lost internally by the root canal procedures usually means that the remaining tooth will be very weak and the core may well fracture off under normal incisal loading.
2. Dentine is considered to become more brittle in the non-vital tooth, further increasing the risk of failure in a natural tooth core.
3. The configuration of the fracture line occurring in a tooth usually shows an oblique downturn running subgingivally on the side opposite to the applied force. An oblique fracture of this kind is typical of brittle materials. Enamel is a brittle substance but will tend to fracture along the natural cleavage lines between prisms. Dentine is not brittle but can act as such under a rapid rate of force application, thus producing the awkward 'tail' seen in many dental fractures.

If a root-filled tooth is likely to fracture more readily it is argued that it is better for the dentist to decide on the line of fracture by removing the clinical crown.

Arguments against decoronation

1. Post preparation is considered to weaken the root, and the further apically the full diameter is placed the greater is the potential weakening effect and the greater the risk of lateral perforation. If, on the other hand, the bulk of the coronal dentine is retained, then either the use of a post will not be necessary or, if one is used, the same length of post will be less apically placed. The post and part core in this latter situation can then be designed to strengthen and protect the remaining dentine core and there is generally more root dentine retained around the intraradicular preparation.
2. There is less chance of perforation with a more coronally placed post.
3. Clinical procedures are simplified if no post is used.

Because of the complex nature of the clinical situation to be investigated very few hard and fast, scientifically substantiated criteria have emerged to govern the use and design of post/core systems. However, the literature is frequently dogged by subjective assessments and rules of thumb.

Questions which may still require an answer

1. How frequently do roots fracture simply because of post design?
2. Does root dentine become brittle after devitalization and with age?
3. What is the ideal post length and diameter for any tooth root length and diameter? Should the post be as long as possible? Should the post length relate to crown length?
4. Is it best for the post to mimic the external root shape? How realistic is the danger of a parallel-sided post perforating if it is centrally placed in the root? How often does a parallel-sided post weaken the root apex?
5. Does a post act as a root strengthener? Can partial cores actually protect remnant tooth crown dentine?
6. Is a root actually strengthened by a diaphragm and collar?
7. Does the post have to fit the root preparation in its entire length?
8. Is anti-rotation best achieved within the root preparation or should it be on the surface of the root face?
9. What are the long-term effects of normal loading?
10. What are the clinical effects of back pressure of cement during placement of the post? Do roots fracture during cementation? Can the cement actually be compressed so as to produce rebound of the post if pressure on it is not maintained?
11. Is gold really the best material for a post/core?

What are the facts, and what has research shown?

1. For a given post diameter, gold is weaker than steel which, in turn, is weaker than nickel chrome or titanium.
2. The general resistance to dislodgement by an axially applied tensile force has been studied for the main post configurations. Threaded posts are more retentive to axially applied extraction forces than parallel-sided smooth posts which, in their turn, are more retentive than tapered posts.

Long posts are more retentive than short posts, but there is no need for the retentive value of the post to exceed that required to extract the tooth. The minimum length of a smooth parallel-sided post should be 5 mm.

The larger the post diameter, the more the retentive value. Cement type and thickness affect post retention.

3. Recent research into the physical properties of dentine has answered some of the issues concerning brittleness. There would appear to be no change in the elasticity of dentine with age, nor with loss of tooth vitality.

Dentine from the female tooth has been shown to be less elastic than that from the male!

4. Crack propagation in brittle substances is well described in the engineering literature. The stress generated at the tip of a surface notch when a force is applied to the body containing the notch is inversely proportional to the

diameter of that tip, and so scratches and indentations should be avoided in any brittle object to which large forces are to be applied. Even if dentine only assumes brittle characteristics under the fast application of a load, this would still indicate that the small notches produced by threaded posts should be avoided where adequate retention can be obtained with other systems.

5. Studies into the resistance of posts/cores to laterally applied forces indicate that the longer a cylindrical post is the better is its resistance to dislodgement, up to a maximum of 8 mm. The resistance of the root to fracture under such loading is proportional to the dentine thickness of the root in the area opposite to the applied force. Collars placed around the coronal end of the root actually diminish the resistance to applied forces if the accommodation of the collar means that a diminution in root-face dentine diameter is incurred.

6. A closely fitting post can exert considerable internal pressure during cementation owing to cement entrapment and incompressibility. This would indicate the need for cement release channels along the length of the post.

7. The post should be placed after filling the canal with cement as this is the best way of ensuring a complete cement layer.

8. The stress distribution exhibited by certain post shapes when they are under load and in situ has been studied by photoelastic stress analysis. These studies depend upon model systems being designed on the basis of the known structure and properties of the components to be examined; since, in the main, these are either unknown or difficult to replicate for dental situations the results can only be considered to be approximate.

9. Posts with cores of different material may be subject to corrosion by electrolytic activity between the two components.

10. Study of the tooth anatomy has indicated that, given an axial placement of the post, the end would have to be within 2 mm of the root apex of an upper lateral incisor before perforation would occur with the largest prefabricated post diameter available (2 mm).

11. Specific consequences of a threaded post system:

(a) Because the post is threaded and has to be inserted with a screw action it is impossible to predict where the core will come to rest against the root face. The core, therefore, has to be circular in cross-section and has to be trimmed in the mouth after insertion.

(b) Because of the circular nature of the system it is difficult to include an anti-rotational device.

(c) Forces generated during thread preparation within the root canal are potentially damaging.

In the light of what is already indicated from research findings **the probable criteria for post/core systems** should be:

(a) parallel-sided post;
(b) length between 5 and 8 mm;
(c) non-threaded, but not completely smooth;
(d) having a release vent for the cement;
(e) as narrow as possible commensurate with rigidity and strength;
(f) conforming to standard instrument sizes;
(g) general core shape catering for the majority of teeth;

(h) simple and effective anti-rotational device at the root face;
(i) non-corrodable;
(j) simple and cheap to manufacture;
(k) simple and quick to fit in the mouth;
(l) removable in the event of failure.

Specific post systems

The following specific post systems have been chosen because they are typical of the different post design trends or because they are felt to have a majority regional use — the list is not intended to be in any way comprehensive of all the post or post/core systems in use in dentistry.

The cast gold post

Advantages —

1. It can be used in any situation regardless of root size, shape or angulation.
2. Both direct and indirect techniques can be used.
3. Core can be complete or partial, and can include shoulder extensions to make up for tooth loss (diaphragm).
4. Accessory pin retention can be used and this will serve also as an anti-rotational device.
5. Since it can conform to irregular shapes, compromised canals require the minimum of preparation and usually provide their own anti-rotation.

Disadvantages —

1. Dependent upon accurate impression techniques.
2. Dependent upon good technical back-up to achieve accurate post reproduction and appropriate core size and shape.
3. Temporary crown retention can be difficult, and danger of leaving cement in prepared post hole.
4. Two-stage technique, so danger of slight lack of fit of one component influencing the fit of the other if both post/core and crown are made at the same time.
5. Gold is not adequately strong in some circumstances.

The Charlton post (Fig. 20.1)

Description —

1. High quality cylindrical, unthreaded steel posts 1.3, 1.4, 1.5, and 2.00 mm in diameter.
2. Cores either untrimmed or pretrimmed in normal, proclined and retroclined versions.
3. Cores have parallel mesial and distal aspects to locate in simple anti-rotational groove.

Advantages —

1. Cheap and uncomplicated.
2. Basically strong.

POST CROWNS 221

3. Conform to standard bur sizes for post hole preparation, but better to use hand drills of corresponding size (Panadrills).
4. Core shapes cater for most crown/root angulations.
5. Minimal core dimensions allow for stronger covering crown.
6. Cores trimmed out of mouth.
7. Special shape for lower incisors.
8. Non-corrodable.

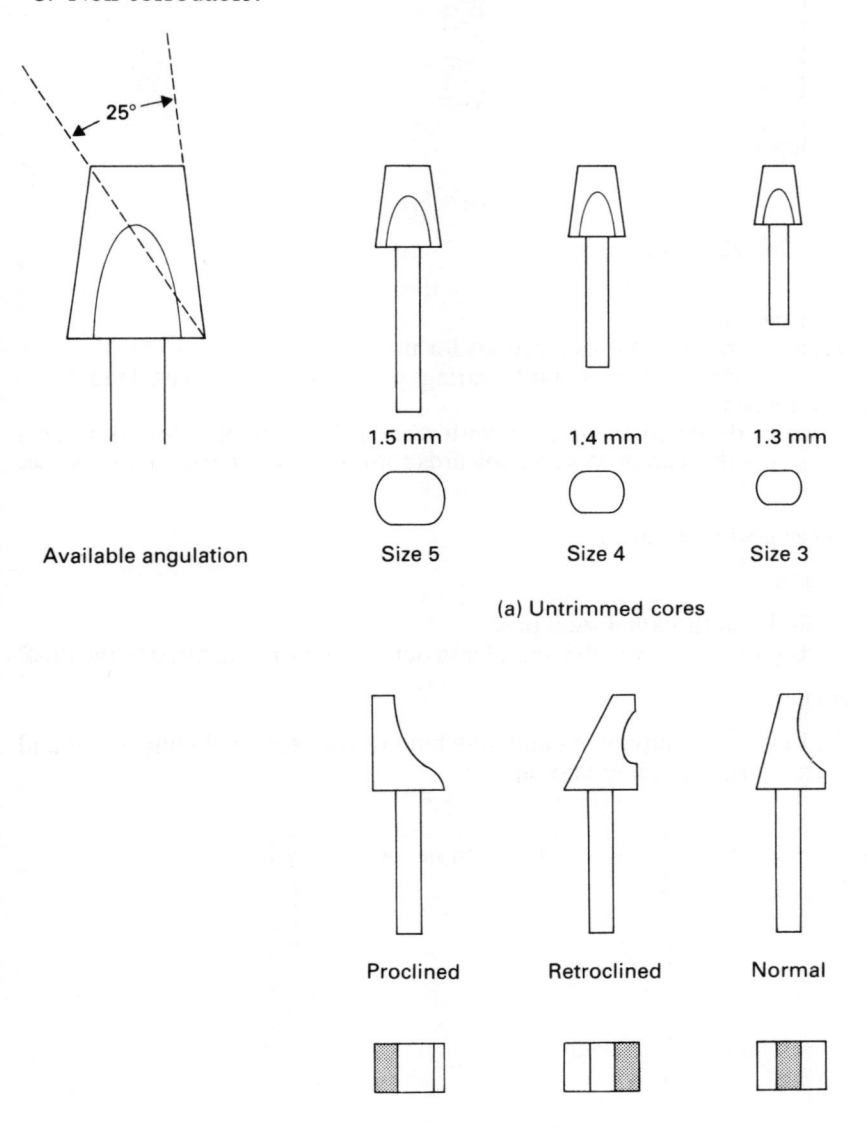

Fig. 20.1 *The Charlton post: untrimmed and pretrimmed cores.*

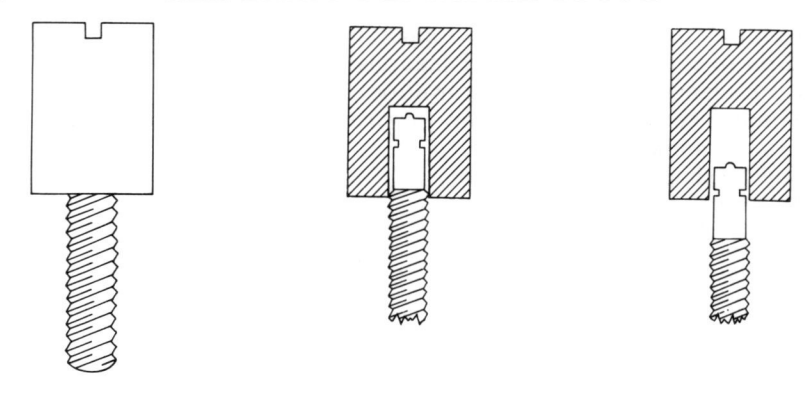

Variable post fit in core

Fig. 20.2 *The Kurer post system.*

Disadvantages —
1. Lacking in adequate instructions for use.
2. Have suffered from manufacturing problems in the past leading to weakened posts.
3. Initially designed to be used with standard dental burs for root canal preparation — this can predispose towards root perforation with careless use.

The Kurer post (Fig. 20.2)

Description —

1. Cylindrical threaded steel post.
2. Softer metal core which is circular in outline and friction fitted to the post.

Advantages —

1. Full kit of accompanying and matching instruments including initial and final twist drills, root facer and tap.

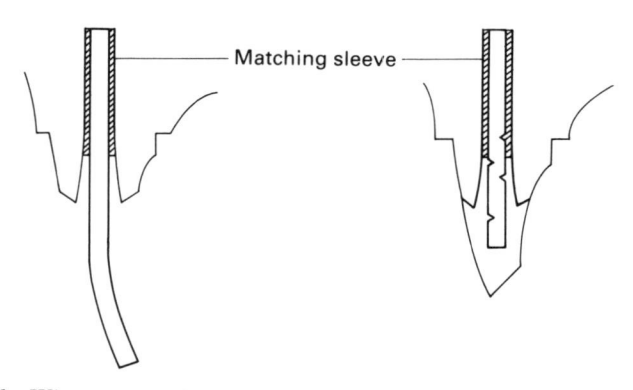

Matching sleeve

Fig. 20.3 *The Wiptam post system.*

POST CROWNS

2. Excellent retention.
3. Can be used to stabilize teeth with root fractures in coronal one-third.

Disadvantages —

1. Injudicious use of tap can split root.
2. Core has to be trimmed in mouth.
3. Thread profile can generate high stress in the root.
4. Differential metals can corrode.
5. Friction fit of core gives variable attachment to the post.
6. No anti-rotation.
7. Root facer has uncomfortable action due to small number of cutting edges.

The Wiptam post (Fig. 20.3)

Description —

1. Based on the use of nickel–chromium–cobalt wire and matching tubing.
2. The post is strong and rigid, but cores have to be cast on by direct or indirect impression methods.

Advantages —

1. Strength and rigidity of posts.
2. The matching metal sleeve allows accurate placement of post and ease of its withdrawal from working models when the indirect technique of core preparation is used.
3. Panadrills for post hole preparation match post diameters.
4. Minimal use of specialized instrumentation and thus inexpensive.

Disadvantages —

1. Different metals can lead to corrosion of system.
2. Preferred tooth preparation may be weakened by provision of internal anti-rotational geometry.
3. Core attachment to the post may not be secure.
4. Advised that the post should be '... the largest ... suitable for the diameter of the root' with no guide as to the criteria to be applied.

The Parapost (Fig. 20.4)

Description —

1. Cylindrical posts in five sizes which are serrated and vented.
2. Prefabricated posts in steel, and plastic formers for cast posts.
3. Anti-rotation achieved by accessory pin placement.

Advantages —

1. Well presented and comprehensive.
2. Well matched drills and posts.

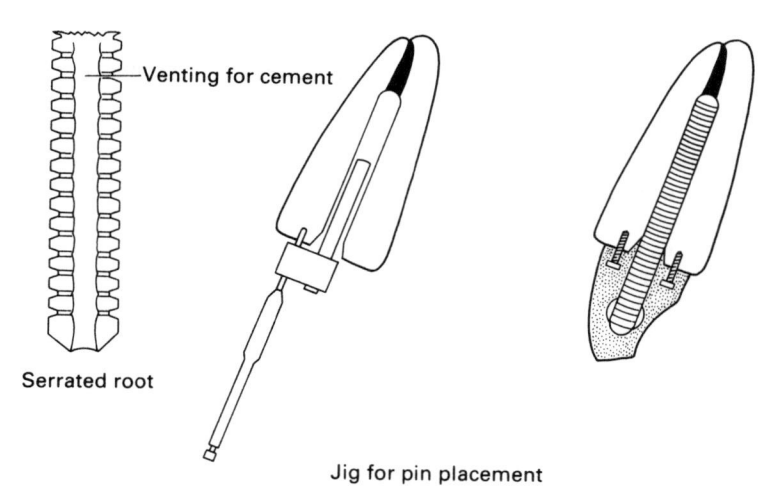

Fig. 20.4 *The Parapost system.*

3. Serrated post gives good cement locking.
4. Venting allows release of cement with no pressure.

Disadvantages —

1. Expensive.
2. Dissimilar metals in system, if core is cast onto prefabricated post.
3. Cast core may have limited retention on prefabricated post.
4. Cast post may be difficult to cast and, since the maximum thickness excluding the serrations is 1.5 mm, the gold may not be strong enough in some situations.
5. Anti-rotational pin preparation may craze and weaken the root face.

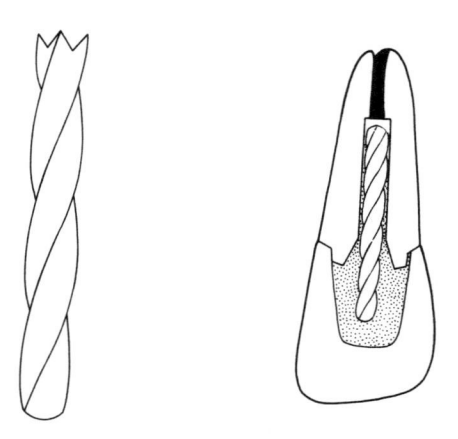

Fig. 20.5 *The Master post system.*

The Master post (Fig. 20.5)

Description — formers provided for cylindrical, fluted posts.

Advantages —

1. Inexpensive and uncomplicated.
2. More than adequate cement sluiceways.

Disadvantages —

1. Post cross-sectional content markedly diminished by fluting.
2. Commitment to gold will give relatively weak post compared to similar sized posts of steel, nickel–chromium–cobalt or titanium.
3. Poor presentation — simply a variation on the Tical rod cast-post concept with a different solution to preventing cement pressure build-up.

The Radix–Anker (Fig. 20.6)

Description —

1. Cylindrical posts in steel or titanium 1.15, 1.35, and 1.6 mm in diameter.
2. Each post has a fine, high-profile thread in its middle section and vertical cement release channels.
3. The cores are also cylindrical in overall section and are finned and shaped to accommodate a screwing spanner.

Advantages —

1. Excellent engineering and presentation.
2. All components work simply and well.
3. Can be used in most situations.
4. Very 'user friendly'.

Disadvantages —

1. Thread profile predisposes to high internal stress concentration in root.
2. Core has to be built and shaped in the mouth.

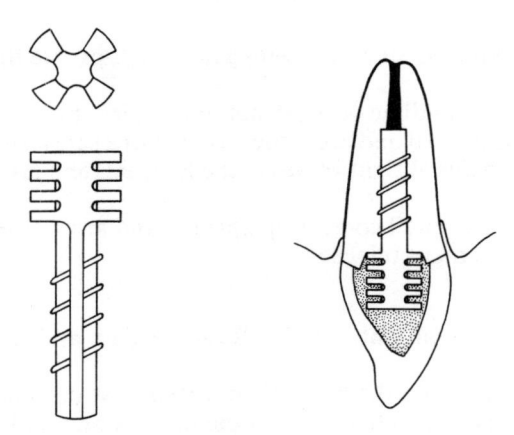

Fig. 20.6 *The Radix–Anker post system.*

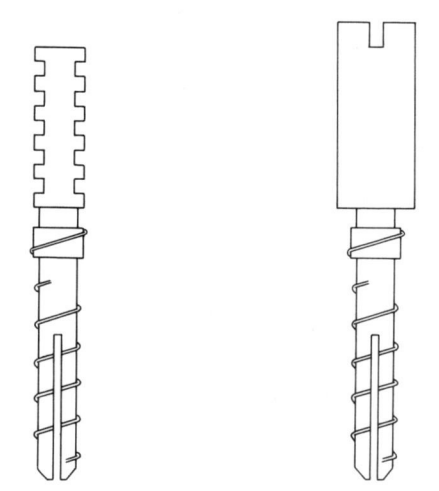

Fig. 20.7 *The Flexipost system.*

3. Attempts at removal can result in core collapse because of loss of its substance during trimming and because remnant composite or amalgam will prevent derotation.

4. When failure of the post occurs, the fracture tends to be just coronal to the threaded section, which renders the post fragment inaccessible and difficult to remove.

5. Because of the screw insertion the core has to be circular and thus requires a circular seating.

6. The post *must* be cemented in place otherwise normal biting pressure will cause the very sharp thread profile to cut further into the root preparation, loosening the post and leading to internal root dentine decay and breakdown.

The Flexipost (Fig. 20.7)

Description —

1. Cylindrical stainless-steel post with a fine, high-profile thread in its entire length.
2. Each post has a midline vertical slot in its apical two-thirds.
3. Cores are cylindrical and are either solid with a screw slot on the head or have small but solid fins at right angles to the long axis and are shaped to take a spanner.
4. All posts have a small conical tip apically and are vented in the coronal one-third to allow cement release.

Advantages —

1. These posts are variants of the Radix–Anker and are similarly well engineered.
2. They are designed on the basis of photoelastic stress analysis studies and claim to be sufficiently retentive without the threads causing high internal root stresses.

3. The apical configuration limits stress concentration in this potentially weakened area of the root.

Disadvantages —

1. The solid coronal one-third of the post is the part most likely to bend under bite pressure and thus exert internal root forces and, since this is an area where the threads will self-tap, the 'notch effect' will still be an important consideration in the resistance to applied loads.

2. The apical two-thirds of any screw post are the least important in the retention of the post. Either the threads will tap into the tooth surface and produce fine notches or they will not and thus have no specific function other than to provide cement locking by their configuration.

3. The core is potentially less retentive of restorative material than that of the Radix–Anker.

There are many more individual post/core systems available, but the above examples illustrate the main design trends that have been used. The only remaining system that warrants consideration is the cast gold post/core as it can be custom-made to any situation.

POSTERIOR TEETH

The majority of systems can be used for both anterior and posterior teeth, and there are some variations of the main post/core designs that are specifically for the posterior situation.

The Charlton post

This system (see above) is primarily for anterior teeth, although posts with the untrimmed version of the core can be used successfully in lower premolars.

Where the root face contour is flat buccolingually anti-rotation is achieved by recessing the base of the core circumferentially.

The Kurer post

This has a variant, the Crown Saver, which has a smaller or finned core which may be more appropriate to posterior teeth in that it allows a composite or amalgam core build-up to suit the clinical circumstances.

The standard Kurer Anchor can be used in lower premolars.

The Parapost, Wiptam and Master posts

These systems can all be used with custom-made cores cast on to the basic post and can thus be used in any posterior situation where there is a good straight canal available.

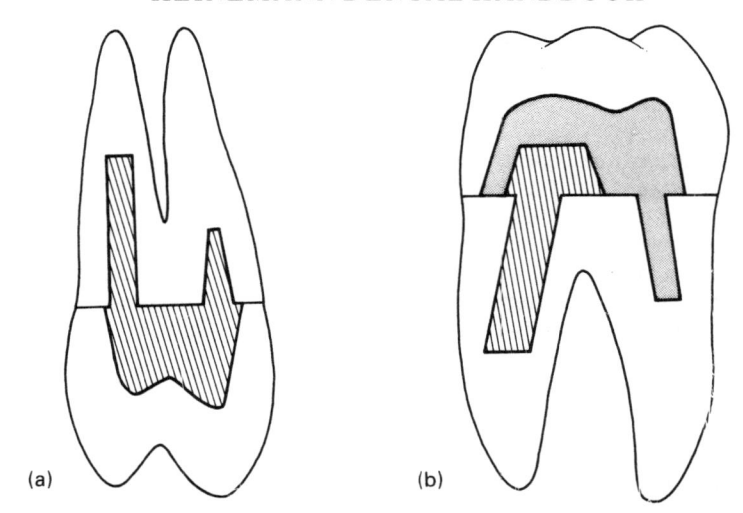

Fig. 20.8 *Cast gold posts in posterior teeth.*

The Radix–Anker and Flexipost

These can be used in any posterior teeth, including those with divergent root canals, as the core is built up in plastic filling material after placement and this may be their particular function.

Dr Spang, who designed the Radix–Anker, has also designed a root post system which has a smaller core size and this will be more easily placed where the root canal apertures converge occlusally (RS root posts).

The cast gold post (Fig. 20.8)

This lends itself particularly to posterior teeth. Upper premolars can be prepared by choosing one canal as the main one for retention and using the other

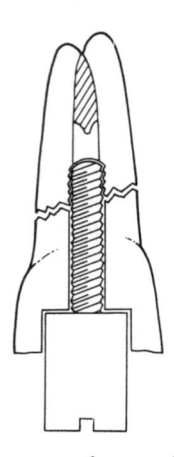

Fig. 20.9 *Post crown placement in a root-fractured tooth.*

as far as parallelism can be obtained for anti-rotation and accessory retention (Fig 20.8a).

Molar teeth can be saved by using a two-stage post/core technique. The first stage is to place a post in the major canal which has a small half core. This is then overlaid to establish a full core by a second casting which makes use of the remaining minor canal/s for retention (Fig. 20.8b).

Despite the statements that have been made for and against the quoted systems, ultimately the most important variable is the operator. Any of the major systems will work well in the majority of cases as long as care is taken with case selection and the meticulous use of the technique.

SPECIAL CASES

1. Where there is a short root and an open apex it is reasonable to use the post as the root filling so that adequate length and retention is achieved. In this case it should be explained to the patient that this is probably a last ditch procedure and that further failure will probably mean extraction.

2. Where the root has been fractured (Fig. 20.9) it is possible to stabilize the situation as long as the fracture is in the coronal third of the root. The main problem is that a repair of this sort is only considered late in the day and there has usually been movement of the two fragments and ingrowth of vascular tissue between them.

The tooth is root-filled and a sectional point cemented, if possible. The remaining canal is prepared after partial decoronation to take a Kurer anchor, so that the post is equally placed in both tooth fragments. The coronal fragment is then prepared further to remove the threads and slightly expand the hole diameter. This coronal section then becomes effectively a washer between the base of the core when it is screwed in and the apical root fragment. Bleeding is controlled as much as possible, cement is spun up the prepared hole and the post is screwed finally into position to compress the entrapped vascular tissue as much as possible.

The core and remaining clinical crown are then prepared to take a porcelain jacket crown.

Chapter 21

Dental cements

Cements are used for:
(a) cavity linings: thermal/chemical/electrical protection of the pulp;
(b) luting, i.e. sealing the gap between castings and prepared teeth;
(c) temporary fillings;
(d) pulp capping;
(e) root canal sealing;
(f) retention of orthodontic brackets.

TYPES OF CEMENT

Zinc oxide – eugenol (unmodified)

A white powder (zinc oxide) with yellow liquid (eugenol — oil of cloves). Mix to a thick paste. Powder/liquid, 3:1. Takes 24 h to harden, accelerated in moist atmosphere. For temporary fillings where an obtundent effect is required.

Accelerated zinc oxide – eugenol

White powder (zinc and magnesium oxides and zinc acetate (accelerator) plus eugenol. Powder/liquid ratio, 3:1. Sets to form zinc eugenolate. For cavity lining (except under polymer restorations — discoloration) and for temporary fillings.

Resin-bonded zinc oxide – eugenol

White powder (90% zinc and magnesium oxides, 10% hydrogenated resin) plus yellow liquid (90% eugenol, 10% polystyrene). Powder/liquid ratio, 4:1. For cavity lining (except for polymer fillings). Endodontic applications.

EBA (ethoxybenzoic acid) cement

A white powder (65% zinc oxide, 30% quartz, 5% hydrogenated resin) plus pink liquid (37.5% eugenol, 62.5% O-ethoxybenzoic acid). Mix with Co–Cr spatula to form a thixotropic paste. Powder/liquid ratio, 7:1. For luting of inlays, crown and bridge work. Cavity lining (not under polymer fillings).

Zinc phosphate

White powder (zinc and magnesium oxides, plus traces of calcium and aluminium hydroxides), with clear liquid (50% aqueous solution of phosphoric acid, buffered with some zinc and aluminium ions). Mix by slowly incorporating the powder and liquid: slower mix — slower set. Thick paste for lining or creamy paste for luting. Liquid must be stoppered to prevent loss or gain of water. Sets to form zinc phosphate. Potential hazard to pulp with low pH at early stages of set. Can be used over calcium hydroxide lining for reinforcement. For lining under all filling materials and luting for crown and bridge work, especially for post/core cementation. Very strong.

Copper phosphate

Cupric, cuprous and silver oxides reacting with phosphoric acid to produce setting cements. Mix rapidly on chilled glass slab and use instantly. Very low pH. For silver cap splints in oral surgery.

Zinc silico-phosphate

Pigmented opalescent powder. Zinc and magnesium oxides and fluoroaluminosilicate glass, sometimes fused together, sometimes containing small amounts of mercuric ammonium chloride as a potent bacteriocidal agent. With a clear liquid: 50% aqueous solution of phosphoric acid with zinc and aluminium ions. Mix powder and liquid in increments. Pulpal irritation. Fluoride leaches out. For cementing porcelain jacket crowns, children's fillings, cementation of orthodontic brackets, production of dies.

Zinc polycarboxylate

Type A. White powder (zinc and magnesium oxides) with clear, syrupy liquid (40% aqueous solution of polyacrylic acid, or an acrylic acid copolymer with other unsaturated carboxylic acids).

Type B. White powder (zinc and magnesium oxides plus dehydrated polyacrylic acid or acrylic acid copolymer) mixed with water only. (Anhydrous form — more popular.)

Sets in 5 min to form zinc polycarboxylate. Adheres to clean, dry enamel and stainless steel.

Uses

1. Cavity lining under all fillings (very thick for a base).
2. Luting cement for crown and bridge work.
3. Temporary fillings.
4. Cementation of orthodontic stainless-steel brackets.

Glass-ionomer

Type A. Pigmented, opalescent powder (fluorocalcium aluminosilicate glass) with clear, viscous liquid (50% aqueous solution of polyacrylic acid and polyalkenyl carboxylic acids).

Type B. Pigmented opalescent powder (fluorocalcium aluminosilicate glass plus dehydrated (freeze-dried) polyacrylic acid and polyalkenyl carboxylic acids). Mix with distilled water.

Sets in 7 min. Adheres to clean, dry enamel and dentine if cleaned with pumice and water and conditioned with a dilute solution of polyacrylic acid.

Uses

1. Cavity lining — on top of calcium hydroxide base.
2. Luting for crown and bridge work.
3. As a filling material, with e.g. amalgam alloy particles incorporated.

Calcium hydroxide

Comes as two pastes:

1. Calcium hydroxide plus inert fillers, e.g. zinc oxide plus barium sulphate as a radiopacifier, in a fluid, non-active carrier containing ethylene toluene sulphonamide.
2. Reactive polysalicylate acid fluid plus inert fillers and radiopacifiers.

Also as visible light-cured (VLC) form: one paste of calcium hydroxide plus barium sulphate dispersed in a biocompatible urethane dimethacrylate resin. It is light-cured.

The two-paste system sets by an acid–base reaction to form an amorphous calcium disalicylate complex with an excess of calcium hydroxide. Setting occurs from outwards to inwards, and is accelerated by moisture. pH = 11, even when set.

Uses

1. Cavity liner — thin films only, near pulp, as first layer.
2. Pulp capping.
3. Protection of freshly cut dentine during acid-etching. Especially VLC variety, which shows superior resistance to acid solubility.

Non-setting variety

For pulp capping, a glass syringe of paste containing calcium and magnesium hydroxides plus barium sulphate (for radiopacity), in a casein base. Syringed out of tube to form a thin layer in root canal or base of cavity. As these cements have no structural strength, their effects are purely biological.

Uses

1. Pulp capping deciduous teeth.
2. Settling down infected root canals.
3. ? Causing calcification to continue in traumatized anteriors as an alternative to root canal therapy in the young patient.

Bowen's resin (dimethacrylate)

Comes as two pastes; they are lightly filled and of low viscosity. One has a dimethacrylate resin and an initiator (usually benzoyl peroxide), and the other, an activator (usually a tertiary amine). Some have components which promote the formation of a bond to clean metal surfaces. Low exothermia, less shrinkage, neutral pH.

Uses

1. Luting—crown and bridge work.
2. Retention of polymeric and metallic orthodontic brackets.
3. Retention by flow into the pits etched onto the fit surface of the base metal framework of Maryland bridges.

Temporary luting cements

Two tube paste system: one tube containing zinc oxide in an oily base; the other, eugenol and an inert filler.

Used for cementing temporary crowns and bridges, the main advantage here being the clean separation from the tooth preparation on removal of the temporary crown.

Chapter 22

Enamel and dentine bonding agents

Many restorations are adhesive in nature—for example, the restoration of an incisal tip, or the placing of a composite resin restoration in an anterior or posterior tooth. All such restorations rely on the bond between the enamel and/or dentine and the restorative material. It is important to know which materials are available for use in these situations, so that the correct one can be chosen for the job.

For the purposes of this chapter, the glass-ionomer cements will not be considered and the focus will be on the resin-based systems, looking in particular at the substance which acts as the intermediary between the enamel/dentine and the composite resin. Bonding agents and composite resins themselves can be chemical cured, or 'command set' by a light source. The latter system is more in favour at present because of:

(a) the easier way the materials handle;
(b) a longer manipulation time before setting;
(c) (for anterior restorations) a better aesthetic result due to a different setting reaction, which leads to better colour stability of the finished restoration.

ENAMEL BONDING AGENTS

These consist basically of:

1. A methyl methacrylate fluid monomer, although some newer systems are using a diacrylate. The basis of the former systems is the traditional Bowen's resin.

This is the bis-GMA compound, formed by the reaction between bis-phenol A and glycidyl methacrylate. The latter systems use either an aliphatic or aromatic diacrylate as their monomer.

2. There has to be an initiator to start the polymerization reaction. In the chemically activated systems this is usually benzoyl peroxide. For the light-activated systems the initiator depends on the wavelength of light used.

3. An activator to stimulate the initiator, e.g. dimethyl-p-toluidine for the chemical cure, or visible or ultraviolet light. The light-cured systems contain an alpha-diketone and an amine, which under the influence of blue light (wavelength 440–480 nm) produces the necessary free radicals.

4. Minor additions such as stabilizers, etc. to give adequate shelf-life, etc.

(If you add an inert filler to these basic types, you will obtain the 'composite' itself, which forms the major part of the restoration.)

The above substances will bond to freshly acid-etched enamel, and not to dentine.

The most important fact to note here is to line any exposed dentine, or freshly cut tubules, because with the subsequent use of phosphoric acid, the tooth can easily become devitalized.

A calcium hydroxide-based material is the lining agent of choice which, when set, does not dissolve to any significant degree under the acid attack. It comes as two pastes:

1. Calcium hydroxide plus inert fillers, e.g. zinc oxide, and barium sulphate as a radiopacifier. These are in a fluid, non-reacting carrier containing ethylene toluene sulphonamide.
2. Reactive polysalicylate fluid with inert fillers and radiopacifiers.

VLC (visible light-cured) one-paste lining materials are now available, and their supposed advantages include:

(a) less acid solubility;
(b) greater compressive strength;
(c) better colour under composites, being a less 'yellow' hue than the two-paste systems;
(d) a greater resin content — a more integral part of the restoration, in that it will 'bond' to the subsequent composite restoration.

Its one paste consists of calcium hydroxide and barium sulphate dispersed in a biocompatible urethane dimethacrylate resin. It is placed in the cavity in the normal way, and light-cured for 40 s.

Next, we can look at the **phosphoric acid** used. A 37% solution has been found to be the most reliable in providing the best acid-etch pattern on enamel, and most of the liquids now contain somewhere around this amount. The gels are made 'gel-like' by the addition of small polymer particles, and these allow the diffusion of acid through the material so they do not have to be stirred on the tooth surface like the original gels.

AGENTS THAT WILL BOND TO DENTINE

These agents will bond to etched enamel and to dentine, and so are more versatile than the above categories of materials. There are now various types, as follows.

Phosphonate derivatives (e.g. Scotchbond)

This is a two-part liquid system. Resin A contains a mixture of phosphorous esters of bis-GMA, diluent resin and benzoyl peroxide (the initiator). Liquid B is an alcoholic solution of a tertiary amine and a sulphinic acid salt. The mixed Scotchbond has a pH of 1, and so very rapidly dissolves some of the apatite when applied to the tooth surface. The resin in the liquids is activated upon mixing.

The tooth surface is dried, the mixed 'resin' is then painted on, blown dry gently, and a second layer applied. This is again blown dry. The addition of the filled composite will then eliminate oxygen from coming into contact with the resin, and the whole will polymerize, with the aid of a light source if the system is so geared. The calcium and the phosphate in this 'micro-emulsion' reprecipitate to form a part of the surface apatite again — thus the whole layer consists of an ionic copolymer bonding the composite to the tooth. The material is now available in a light-cured form as Scotchbond 2.

In order to achieve adhesion of a dentine bonding agent, one of four techniques have been employed:

1. The smear layer could be removed with acid.
2. It could be infiltrated, as was the case with Scotchbond.
3. It could be fixed with glutaraldehyde.
4. It could be removed and replaced with a precipitate.

The last technique is that for Scotchbond 2. If the smear layer is to be removed, then a 1% solution of hydrochloric acid in ethanol is less traumatic to the dentine than 37% phosphoric acid. EDTA (ethylenediaminetetra-acetic acid) could also be used.

Glutaraldehyde/hydroxyethyl methacrylate systems (e.g. Gluma)

Use is made here of the amino acids of dentinal collagen. A bond is formed by removing the smear layer of dentine with a weak solution of EDTA. The glutaraldehyde forms a bond on the one side with the collagen and also, on the other, with the HEMA (hydroxyethyl methacrylate). The selected filled resin is then applied, and a chemical reaction will take place with the diacrylate resin it contains. The composite can be light- or chemically cured.

The enamel bonding agents are used in the conventional way, with the enamel being cleaned, dried, etched with the acid, and the resin applied with a brush, left to set or light-cured as appropriate.

Scotchbond is used in a different manner. The tooth is cleaned as before, washed and dried. Enamel is etched with a gel, so as not to allow it to go over the dentine, then washed, dried, etc. The liquids are mixed, and a thin layer is brushed over the etched enamel and the dentine. This is then 'dried' for a few seconds with the air spray, and then a second layer of the mixture brushed on again. This is dried in the same way. The composite resin is then placed and the whole restoration is cured, either chemically or with the light source. There is a resin/alcohol/acid emulsion, and as the alcohol is evaporated by the air spray, the initiator is activated. The resin polymerization is inhibited by the oxygen at its surface. The calcium and phosphate ions are displaced into the emulsion by the acid, and as the alcohol evaporates, the composite layer is added, thus eliminating the oxygen and helping the polymerization of the resin. Calcium and phosphate ions are incorporated into the dentine structure, and a bond is formed.

From the above information, one should be able to assess the clinical situation more clearly, and decide whether to use a lining, a conventional enamel bonding agent, or an enamel/dentine bond, and have some idea of the chemistry going on around the restoration as one completes it.

Chapter 23

Light-activated composite materials

The setting chemistry of two-paste systems centres around a polymerization reaction which begins the minute the pastes are mixed together. It ends about 5–10 min later, and during the process the molecules within the resin start to join together and the viscosity (fluid stiffness) increases. To get a well-fitting restoration, the material has to be placed quickly, and under pressure, otherwise leakage and marginal discoloration occur. Two things can help eliminate these problems:

1. Acid etching — which with a bonding agent forms a seal.
2. Light-activated systems. These give longer working time, and with the liquid phase give it more time to enter the pits created by the acid. With two-paste/liquids they are polymerizing and stiffening on mixing. There is also no air incorporated in the composite — no mixing — so less porosity that otherwise reduces the strength and abrasion resistance of the set material.

DEVELOPMENT OF LIGHT-ACTIVATED RESINS

Visible light is only a fraction of the electromagnetic spectrum, and only two wavelengths are used for activating dental materials:

(a) ultraviolet (UV) — 365 nm;
(b) visible blue light — 470 nm.

Ultraviolet

Used in the 1970s, it fell out of favour for three reasons;

1. UV lamps age quickly, so results were variable.
2. Potential tissue damage from UV light.
3. Research developed light-activated materials.

Visible light-activated resins

These were introduced in the early 1970s, and have become ever more popular since. They are easier to use and manipulate, and the advances in manufacture, plus the variety of shades and viscosities now available, will ensure that popularity continues.

LIGHT-ACTIVATED RESIN SYSTEMS

Unfilled or lightly filled systems

These are 0–10% by volume of filler particles. Mainly used for fissure sealing.

Moderate to highly filled systems

These are 20–70% by volume of filler. These cover all the available makes, and are divided into:

1. *Traditional composites* — particles of ceramic or glass; 10–20 μm originally, now down to 2–5 μm.
2. *Microfines* — particles of pyrolytic silica (SiO_2) produced by ignition of silica compounds. Size: 0.01–0.05 μm. They cannot be made radiopaque, which is a distinct disadvantage. The pyrolytic silica is incorporated into the unpolymerized resin by, firstly, diluting the resin with a solvent; this will make it more fluid. It is then made viscous again by the addition of the silica dust. The whole is then heat-polymerized, and the resultant block splintered to make the composite filling material when incorporated into the resin.
3. *Hybrid composites* — a mixture of particles of ceramic or glass, some radiopaque, average particle size 2–10 μm, together with some pyrolytic silica incorporated into the unpolymerized resin. These have a greater amount of inorganic filler.

The setting of composite materials

Resins set by addition reactions, i.e. small molecules of low molecular weight (monomers) join together to produce large molecules (polymers). This increase in the molecular weight causes changes in the mechanical and physical properties. In this way, fluids become rigid solids.

Monomer molecules require an initiator; they do not join together on their own so a special molecule is needed to start the reaction. In two-component composites, this is dibenzoyl peroxide, and it is activated by coming into contact with an activating compound — an amine (peroxide–amine reaction)

In light-activated resins, the reaction is more complex, but still requires the stimulation of the initiator. There are two components which are produced from a reaction between a light-activated compound, called an alpha-ketone, and an amine, once the alpha-ketone has absorbed some energy from the light.

In two-paste systems, mixing means a set throughout the material, even in the base of the cavity. In light-activated materials, the blue light wavelength must activate the alpha-ketone or no reaction occurs, and the final composite must be hard, rigid and cured throughout the bulk. If not, a 'soggy bottom' remains. This is bad for the following reasons:

1. Hazard of free monomer; this is a danger to the pulp.
2. Free monomer can react with cements present, e.g. zinc oxide/eugenol, polycarbonates, etc., and affect aesthetics.

3. Soggy base: this provides no support for the restoration, and fracture can occur, along with subsidence and leaking.

Factors influencing curing

1. *Optical variables*. These are often set by the manufacturers and cannot be varied. The shade can influence the depth of polymerization. Dark pigments inhibit the passage of light—the darker the shade, the longer the polymerization.
2. *Light-source variables*. The lights are low-voltage tungsten–halogen lamps. There are three varieties of light-guide:
  (a) liquid gel, in flexible tube;
  (b) fibre-optic in multiple sheath;
  (c) single-light connecting rod.

The diameter of the rod is important. For the larger posterior composite restoration, the light source may only 'shine' directly on half of the area to be cured. Two or even three applications of the light source may have to be applied, as well as limiting the depth of material to be cured, to ensure a full cure of the composite resin. The lamps lose efficiency, so the output is reduced as the bulb gets older. Dust etc. collects around the reflector, thus cutting down the efficiency of the light. Internal damage to the carrying medium, breakage of some fibres in the fibre-optic system, scratching of the tip, left-over composite stuck to the tip, etc., all help to make the light source less efficient.

3. *Manipulative variables*. These involve:

   (a) Proximity—the further away, the less the power, the longer the cure required. Check for shadows, etc. cast by cusp angles. Cure in small layers.
   (b) Manufacturer's data—read and double.
   (c) Temperature of the composite—should be room temperature.
   (d) Layer technique—although there is a weakness between the layers of composite, this is better than a 'soggy bottom', so use this technique if in doubt.
   (e) Use of bonding agents—seal the cavity with resin by the acid-etch technique. Use unfilled or bonding resin between tooth and composite. Flow it over the base etc., but don't 'puddle' in the line angles. If there is a 'puddle' of non-filled resin in a part of the cavity, this will not be radiopaque, and may show up on a subsequent radiograph mimicking secondary caries. Set with the light, or if using a bonding agent that is not light-cured, place the composite over it and the exclusion of air lets it harden as the composite sets.

POSTERIOR COMPOSITES

These are mostly hybrid systems with small particle size. They are light-activated, radiopaque and of high strength. Many are now available in a variety of shades. These radiopaque and pigmented types require longer exposure to the light. Poor access of the light-tip to certain parts of the restoration may result in poor cure and 'soggy bottom', so careful technique is required. Some areas may be as far as 5 mm away from the light source, e.g. base of Class II boxes.

ADDITIONS AND REPAIRS

These are only possible at the time of curing. Water is absorbed by the polymer systems in the mouth, and joining up to saturated polymer systems is not good. So any repairs have to be mechanically retentive. Dry very thoroughly, apply bonding agent before the new composite.

SHADE MATCHING

Do not mix shades, as this destroys the one-paste system and lets in air. In addition to the porosity, the oxygen in the air acts as a polymerization inhibitor, and both features reduce wear and strength of the composite.

SENSITIVITY TO OPERATING LIGHT

Light-activated composites require blue wavelengths to cure, and these are in daylight and operating lights. So do not leave pots open, or the material will stiffen prior to placement. A yellow/orange filter is available to go on the operating light.

HAZARDS FROM CURING LIGHT

The light is very bright, and a cumulative effect from the light scattered by the enamel and dentine can be harmful. Filtered shields are available, as are glasses for dentist and patient.

LATEST DEVELOPMENTS IN DENTAL RESTORATIVE MATERIALS

As technology progresses, new forms of materials will supersede the older ones, just as light-cured composite resins have virtually replaced the chemically cured varieties. (Except for certain cases, e.g. cementation of metal-winged acid etch-retained bridges.) Thus, in time, other well-known materials will be improved.

The use of visible light-cured (VLC) products will increase. Calcium hydroxide base linings can now be light-cured, and as a further development, a lining material is available which contains a phosphate dentine-bonding agent, along with a urethane dimethacrylate resin. This means that the lining/base will bond to the tooth and to the restoration. For good measure, the lining will release fluoride.

The urethane resins are again to the fore in the new light-cured impression materials. A polyether urethane dimethacrylate resin with silicone dioxide fillers, VLC photoinitiators and accelerators, has been combined with the usual coupling agents, plasticizers, etc. to form an impression material suitable for crown and bridge work. The material is a wash and heavy-bodied system. A similar urethane material is used as a periodontal dressing after any form of periodontal surgery.

Composite materials are used for luting cements, VLC for veneers etc., and chemical-cured forms for the placement of crowns. These latter types have a film thickness of less than 25 μm, and are said to be better tolerated by the tissues than other cements. Each year new materials will evolve, and the dental surgeon will face the process of keeping up to date with technology.

Chapter 24

Castable ceramics

Castable ceramic material is now used for the construction of full coverage crowns, onlays, inlays and facings. The main type available in the UK is Dicor, manufactured by DeTrey/Dentsply. Research started in 1977 in the USA, after glass-ceramics had been used for cooker tops, floor tiles, etc.; all these were a spin-off from the space technology of a few years before.

The castable ceramic material itself contains the oxides of silicon, potassium and magnesium, with minor amounts of aluminium and zirconium oxides incorporated for durability. A fluorescing agent is added for aesthetic reasons, and magnesium fluoride is included to act as a nucleating agent, which aids in the transformation between the different states of the process, and to help provide the fluidity required when the ingot melts. This ensures that the investment mould fills completely. Fluoride ions are an essential component of the crystalline phase.

THE CLINICAL PREPARATION OF TEETH TO TAKE A CROWN

At least 1–2 mm of tooth substance have to be removed from all surfaces. The preparation is more extensive than for a bonded crown, where only about 1.5 mm are removed labially and there is a minimal palatal chamfer. The reason for this more extensive preparation lies in the optical properties of the material, sufficient thickness of which has to be present in order to get a good aesthetic result. A small ball-ended instrument is made, called a gauge, which has a 1.5 mm ball on one end and a 2 mm ball on the other. By placing it on the shoulder, or between the teeth, one can assess the depth of cut. The preparation must include a shoulder with a rounded gingivoaxial line angle, or a deep 120° chamfer. The preparation must not have sharp angles, feather edges, slices, etc.

Impressions are taken in the usual way with whatever material is preferred.

In the laboratory, a die is made in the usual way, and a wax-up is made of the crown form. The glass is made in small ingots, and after the wax-up has been invested and burnt out, the ingot is used to cast the crown centrifugally in a special casting machine. The investment is a special phosphate-bonded type. The glass ingot is placed into a crucible which fits specifically into the furnace. The crucible can only be used once, but you can cast multiple units. The casting process takes a few minutes, as the glass is quite viscous in the molten state and has to be allowed to cool naturally. The investment is cleaned off the crown with grit abrasion (25 μm alumina) and inspected. The crown at this stage is transparent, and is then re-invested and placed in the ceramming oven. The oven 'heat-treats' the crown through the cycle, until it is converted into a partially crystalline state. The mica crystals appear at 650°C and an interlocking microstructure forms within a matrix of the parent glass, of which about 45% remains. This microstructure gives light-scattering properties to the ceramic, similar to those of enamel prisms. The crown is cleaned again and replaced on the model. Body and enamel porcelains are then added to the shaped crown, and fired on in a normal porcelain furnace at 940°C. This is about 430°C lower than the casting temperature of the crown, so multiple firings can take place.

The finished crown is then ready for fitting. If the shade is incorrect, the porcelain surface layer can be removed and a new shade added. The shade of the tooth beneath the preparation is vital for the coloration of the finished crown, and this is cemented with a special range of cements, or with light-activated composites. There are five different colours, and they are matched to the porcelain shades. The die will have been covered with a spacer to match the estimated colour of cement. This gives the technician a chance to assess the colour during the build-up of the shading.

Chapter 25

Veneers

INTRODUCTION

During the past decade, veneers or facings have provided a conservative treatment alternative to crowns for many unsightly upper anterior teeth.

More recently, improved materials have led to an extension of the use and techniques of veneering. These include labial veneers for teeth other than upper anterior teeth, protection of worn palatal surfaces of upper anterior teeth, and restoration of occlusal surfaces of posterior dentitions.

Definition

Veneers are thin facings of dental restorative materials bonded on to a surface of a tooth.

They may be constructed either:

(a) directly on the tooth in the clinic; or
(b) indirectly on a model in the laboratory.

The tooth may remain unprepared or may have been minimally prepared or modified.

TYPES OF VENEERS

Composite veneers

Composite veneers are of two types:

1. *Direct*. Materials have improved markedly and most workers now favour:

   (a) a microfilled resin (Chapter 23) for surface translucency and good finishing properties;
   (b) a small-particle resin (Chapter 23) for strength and opacity.

2. *Indirect.* Clinic- and laboratory-constructed indirect veneers are usually filled resins cured either by additional heat and pressure or by additional light. These new composites have much improved qualities and some of them have natural fluorescence.

Advantages of composite veneers

Treatment can be restricted to the clinic without the necessity for laboratory procedures; and the method is cheap.

Disadvantages of composite veneers

The major drawbacks are:

 (a) polymerization shrinkage;
 (b) thermal dimensional change;
 (c) staining and poor wear resistance, particularly if easy-flow materials with low filler contents are used;
 (d) incisal chipping.

Despite the above disadvantages, composite veneering systems provide a very useful, simple, economical and effective treatment alternative for many situations and in patients of all ages.

Acrylic veneers

Acrylic veneers were introduced in order to attempt to overcome some of the shortfalls of the direct composite veneers. However, with the improvement in composite materials and other veneering techniques, they have been largely superseded.

Acrylic veneers are of three types:

1. Custom-made in the laboratory.
2. Hollowed-out denture teeth.
3. Prefabricated laminate veneers—these are <0.25 mm thick; they come in a variety of moulds and sizes and can be trimmed either in the clinic or in the laboratory. In the laboratory they can additionally be heat-moulded.

Acrylic veneers must be bonded on to the surface of the tooth. Most commonly, composite materials have been used for bonding.

Acrylic veneer primers

In order to achieve a bond, the acrylic veneer first requires priming with one of the following:

 (a) ethyl acetate;
 (b) methylene chloride;
 (c) methylmethacrylate.

These veneer primers provide:

(a) a chemical bond between the veneer and the luting resin;
(b) a mechanical bond between the veneer and the etched tooth.

However, chemical bonds between composites and acrylics are poor, and debonding at the interface between the laminate veneer and the composite has been the most common cause of failure.

Advantages of acrylic veneers

They are cheap and comparatively simple to use.

Disadvantages of acrylic veneers

The major disadvantages are:

(a) weak chemical bond between composite and acrylic;
(b) bulky restoration;
(c) poor wear resistance;
(d) poor surface staining resistance;
(e) subject to long-term stress relief fracture if heat-moulded;
(f) dull and monochromatic appearance.

At present, acrylic veneers may have a place in children's dentistry, providing a cheap and non-invasive alternative treatment to more costly veneers or crowns. This treatment may be carried out as an interim measure.

However, as improved acrylics are developed, together with improved bonding between acrylics and tooth substance, acrylic veneers may gain in popularity.

Porcelain veneers

Porcelain veneers have gained in popularity since the early 1980s.

Techniques involved in laboratory construction

1. Porcelain built up on a platinum foil matrix.
2. Porcelain built up on refractory dies.

The fitting surface of the porcelain veneer, once fabricated, should be etched in the laboratory with hydrofluoric acid (or an hydrofluoric acid substitute), or sand-blasted with aluminium oxides.

Silane coupling agents

The major advance that led to the success of the porcelain veneer was the development of a silane coupling agent acting as a chemical bonding agent between the porcelain and the composite lute. Additionally, there may be some mechanical retention from etching or sand-blasting the porcelain.

Silane coupling agents have the following chemical composition:

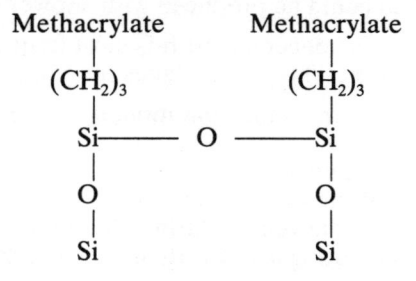

$$\begin{array}{ccc}
\text{Methacrylate} & & \text{Methacrylate} \\
| & & | \\
(CH_2)_3 & & (CH_2)_3 \\
| & & | \\
Si & \!\!\!\!-\!\!\!\!-\!\!\!\!- O -\!\!\!\!-\!\!\!\!-\!\!\!\!- & Si \\
| & & | \\
O & & O \\
| & & | \\
Si & & Si
\end{array}$$

Action of the silane coupling agent

1. Polymerization occurs between the composite resin and the methacrylate group.
2. Siloxane linkages form to the silicon in the ceramic.
3. Additionally there is cross-linking of the coupling agent itself.

Low-shrink porcelains are generally used for veneering techniques. Porcelain veneers are generally between 0.5 mm and 0.8 mm thick.

Advantages of porcelain veneers

1. Porcelain is inert and oral tissues are subsequently very tolerant of porcelain when it is used as a dental restorative material.
2. Good masking of discoloration can usually be achieved.
3. Using the silane coupling agent, bonding is excellent.
4. Once cemented, a porcelain veneer has adequate strength even though it is often very thin.
5. Good translucency can be achieved.
6. Porcelain veneers are usually complete labial veneers but they can be shaped like acid etch-retained composite restorations covering only part of the tooth surface.

Disadvantages of porcelain veneers

1. Porcelain veneers are technique-sensitive both in the clinical situation and in the laboratory situation:

   (a) veneer must be kept dry and free from contamination for good bonding;
   (b) veneer must be handled with extreme care as it is very brittle, and subject to fracture — during cementation the veneer requires particularly careful handling.

2. Care must be taken in production of thin porcelain veneers to ensure that there is sufficient translucency but that masking is adequate.
3. The final colour of the restoration is often dependent on the thickness and colour of the cement lute.

4. Porcelain is highly abrasive to opposing natural teeth so it would be desirable if a porcelain could be produced with a lower coefficient of friction.

If failure of a porcelain veneer occurs it is most frequently due to the faulty technique of the operator. This usually takes the form of:

(a) inadequate attention to the conditioning of the tooth surface for successful bonding;
(b) lack of moisture control;
(c) contamination of the surface of the veneer;
(d) rough handling of the veneer during placement;
(e) use of composite luting agent with insufficient flow characteristics and subsequent fracture of the veneer.

Castable glass ceramic veneers

Castable glass ceramic veneers require special facilities from the dental laboratory.

Advantages of castable glass ceramic veneers

An excellent appearance can be achieved, and the veneers are strong.

Disadvantages of castable glass ceramic veneers

1. Recontouring after glazing can lead to poor appearance since the colour matching and characterizing of castable ceramic veneers is largely incorporated into the surface glazes.
2. Colour matching involves matching the luting cements as well as shading the ceramic veneers and this can lead to difficulties in achieving a good match.
3. Cost.

INDICATIONS FOR VENEERS

1. Masking surface defects and strengthening weak coronal tooth substance caused by:

(a) defects in calcification;
(b) tooth wear, in particular abrasion and erosion;
(c) structural loss caused by trauma;
(d) abnormal development, i.e. peg-shaped laterals.

2. Masking discoloration caused by:

(a) trauma;
(b) loss of vitality;
(c) tetracycline staining.

3. Improving appearance when orthodontics is not feasible:

(a) rotated or lingually inclined incisors;
(b) diastemas or generalized spacing — so long as the spaces are not too great.

CONTRAINDICATIONS TO VENEERS

1. Poor quality tooth substance for bonding.
2. Insufficient sound tooth substance for bonding.
3. Insufficient tooth substance to support the veneer.
4. Rotated or overlapped teeth can present problems in the placement of the veneers.
5. Traumatic occlusion.
6. Poor oral hygiene.

GENERAL CONSIDERATIONS

1. It is difficult to get a good colour match for single teeth.
2. Veneers are thin sectioned and they have a tendency towards being monochromatic.
3. Veneers rely to a great extent on reflecting colour either from the natural tooth or from the coloured bonding resin cements.
4. Successful placement of veneers is very technique-sensitive.

PREPARATION OF THE TOOTH

Unprepared teeth

Some workers prefer to leave the tooth unprepared since the procedure is then totally reversible.

However, unprepared teeth give some periodontologists cause for concern because bulky teeth can lead to plaque retention and subsequent stagnation areas, particularly at the gingival margin regions.

Prepared teeth

The operator should aim to remove only 0.5 mm of enamel. In the cervical region, where the enamel is very thin, less enamel should be removed if possible. If conventional composites are used for cementation, attempts should be made to avoid finishing the preparation on root dentine. New materials allowing for bonding between porcelain and dentine will extend the use of veneering techniques.

Tooth preparation can be carried out using tapered high-speed burs. A round-ended tapered bur aids establishment of a suitable finishing line cervically and interproximally. The preparation should be finished with superfine high-speed burs, and conventional finishing burs and polishing points.

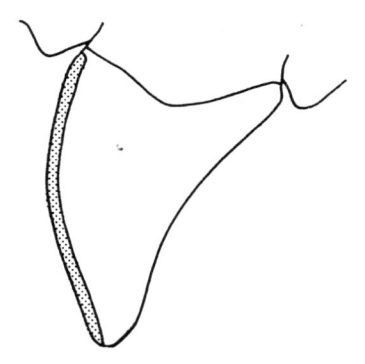

Feathered incisal edge preparation

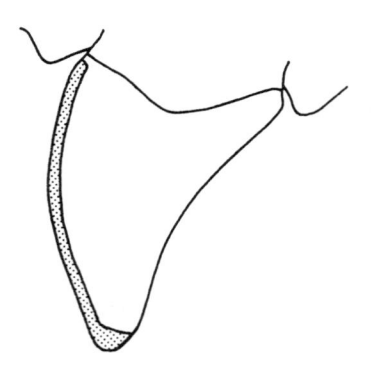

Incisal bevel preparation

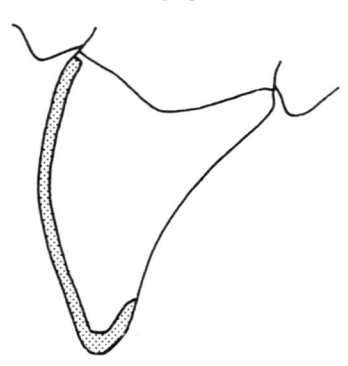

Overlapped incisal edge preparation

Fig. 25.1 *Incisal edge preparations.*

Tooth reduction

Establishment of the finishing line

Interproximal and gingival cervical finishing lines should be achieved using a round-ended tapered bur. This bur should provide a chamfered margin.

1. *Interproximal region.* The interproximal region should be extended into the embrasure area but should remain labial to the contact point.
2. *Cervical region.* If there is no discoloration, the finishing line may be supragingival. However, in most instances when a labial veneer is constructed, it will be necessary to extend the finishing line subgingivally in order to achieve a good appearance and mask discoloration.

Reduction of the surface to be veneered

A uniform 0.5 mm enamel should be removed. Care should be taken not to penetrate the enamel. Any dentine that is exposed should be protected with glass-ionomer.

Some workers carry out enamel reduction by cutting a series of tracer cuts in the surface of the tooth and then removing the intervening enamel. This technique can help ensure that not too much enamel is removed but great care has to be taken to ensure that the resultant prepared surface does not appear corrugated.

Incisal edge reduction

There are three commonly accepted designs for tooth preparation (Fig. 25.1):

1. *Feathered incisal edge preparation.* This is a conservative preparation but may:

    (a) lead to the incisal edge being weakened;
    (b) create difficulties in producing a veneer with a translucent incisal edge.

2. *Incisal bevel preparation.* This is a popular finishing margin.
3. *Overlapped incisal edge preparation.* This preparation has advantages in certain situations; it increases retention and is useful when the veneer is also repairing a fractured incisal edge.

IMPRESSION OF PREPARATION

An impression should be taken with an elastomeric impression material.

If possible, retraction cord should be avoided in order to reduce damage to the gingival tissues. Retraction should not be necessary unless the tooth has been prepared subgingivally.

TEMPORARY COVERAGE OF THE PREPARATION

This is only required if the appearance is unsatisfactory after tooth preparation, or if the tooth is sensitive.

In most instances sensitivity is not a problem as the enamel should not have been penetrated. Gingival health will be most readily maintained if the preparation is left without temporary coverage.

If temporary coverage is required, this can be achieved by placing a composite on the tooth surface without etching the tooth. This will usually last for a couple of weeks prior to cementation of the final restoration.

A composite temporary can be achieved in two ways:

1. Building the composite on to the tooth surface directly.
2. Taking an impression before preparation of the tooth. This impression can be used as a template to form a composite facing conforming to the original form of the unprepared tooth. This is then cemented with composite on to the unetched enamel.

A temporary restoration may cause some degree of gingival reaction as a result of chemical and physical irritation. The temporary restoration should be kept well clear of the gingival margins in order to minimize detrimental effects on the gingival contour of the final restoration.

VENEER CEMENTATION

Types of cements

1. *Catalyst cure*.
2. *Light cure*: There is some concern that curing through the veneer may be insufficient.
3. *Dual cure*: These cements can be light-cured but will additionally continue to cure via a catalyst reaction if there is any uncured catalyst left after light-curing.

Cementation procedure

The veneer should first be tried in place. Extreme care must be taken by the operator since the veneers are very delicate and fragile. The veneer should be checked for seating and appearance. If at all possible, minor adjustments should be made once the veneer is finally cemented.

Trial shading can be carried out in the following manner:

(a) clean the veneer with alcohol;
(b) apply try-in paste or composite without catalyst to the veneer and place on the tooth in order to assess for suitability.

Once a satisfactory cement has been selected the veneer cementation procedure can commence:

(a) clean veneer in ethyl acetate or acetone and additionally blast with aluminium oxide if laboratory equipment available;
(b) thoroughly wash in water;
(c) dry.

The fitting surface of the veneer should not be contaminated prior to the application of the silane bonding agent.

Isolation and treatment of the tooth surface

1. Isolate with rubber dam or cotton wool rolls.
2. Thoroughly clean with pumice and water.
3. Dry tooth with oil and water free air supply.
4. Follow detailed instructions of particular bonding system selected. This will generally involve the following stages:

    (a) etch enamel;
    (b) wash tooth;
    (c) dry tooth;
    (d) isolate tooth with matrix strip;
    (e) apply thin film of unfilled resin;
    (f) line fitting surface of veneer with cement taking care not to entrap air and position on the tooth surface;
    (g) remove gross excess;
    (h) cure.

Only essential finishing should be carried out at this appointment if the coupling agent takes time to achieve its maximum strength.

The occlusion should however be carefully assessed and adjusted if necessary at this visit.

Review visit

Any final finishing should be carried out at this visit.

Superfine diamond instruments can be used to contour the margins if necessary. Any adjusted areas should be thoroughly polished using silicon points and finished with fine polishing pastes.

The patient should be advised of the importance of meticulous home care of these restorations.

CONCLUSION

Veneers are now offering a viable alternative to crowns. As materials and bonding systems improve, the life expectancy of these restorations should increase and it is likely that there will be be a wider application of the technique in the future.

Chapter 26

Glass-ionomer cements

DEVELOPMENT

The glass-ionomer (polyalkenoate) cements were patented in 1969 and first described in the dental literature in 1972. They have been known by the acronym ASPA, derived from their major constituents, aluminosilicate glass and polyacrylic acid.

In their development from silicate cement powder and polycarboxylate cement liquid they combined the desirable properties of fluoride release and adhesion to enamel and dentine.

COMPOSITION

Current self-setting commercial glass-ionomer cements have three essential components: the glass powder, the polymeric acid, and tartaric acid to sharpen the setting reaction.

The basis of the powder is an acid-decomposable calcium aluminosilicate glass with a high fluoride content.

PRESENTATIONS

Powder liquid form

The glass powder is a calcium aluminosilicate glass and is mixed with a 50% aqueous solution of polymeric acid (e.g. a copolymer of acrylic/itaconic acids or acrylic/maleic acids) with 5% tartaric acid.

Some brands are encapsulated.

Water-hardening (anhydrous) forms

1. The glass powder is blended with the freeze-dried polymeric acid (e.g. a copolymer of acrylic/maleic acids).
The liquid is a dilute aqueous solution of tartaric acid.
2. The glass powder is blended with the freeze-dried polymeric acid (e.g. acrylic acid homopolymer or acrylic acid/itaconic acid copolymer) plus the freeze-dried tartaric acid.
The mixing liquid is simply distilled water.

SETTING REACTION

On mixing, the acids leach calcium and aluminium ions from the glass and these produce cross-linking of the polymer acid chains.

The initial set is produced by the faster reacting calcium ions; the slower aluminium ion exchange is responsible for further hardening. In the set cement both salts are present in equal amounts. Hardening continues for 24 h and a slow maturation (over months) increases the strength and rigidity of the cement and renders it less vulnerable to water loss or gain.

Only about a quarter of the glass at the surface is used in setting and the set cement consists of the unreacted core particles surrounded by partially dissolved glass embedded in a cross-linked matrix of polymeric acid.

ADHESION

Glass-ionomer cements bond to enamel, dentine, and the smear layer of cut dentine, amalgam and base metals, but not to porcelain.

The bonding to tooth substance is attributed to the reaction between free carboxylic acid groups in the cement and hydroxyapatite. Thus higher bond strengths (up to 9.6 MPa) are recorded to enamel than to dentine (up to 4.5 MPa), which has a lower inorganic content, and the bond to dentine falls as the pulp is approached.

The role of conditioning agents is disputed and although conditioning tooth surfaces with 25% polyacrylic acid for 10 s may enhance bonding, it opens the tubules and could cause sensitivity, which is also true for citric acid. Citric acid conditioning has been found not to increase the clinical retention of a water-hardening glass-ionomer restorative in non-undercut cervical margin lesions.

Phosphoric acid-etching removes hydroxyapatite and is detrimental to bonding, as also is EDTA (ethyldiaminetetracetic acid), which is not compatible with glass-ionomer cements. Acid conditioning should not be used on deep cavities.

BIOCOMPATIBILITY

The pulpal toxicity of glass-ionomer cements is controversial but they are generally considered mildly irritant to the pulp.

In histological studies on human teeth, glass-ionomer cement caused more inflammation than zinc oxide–eugenol cement but the response resolved in 30 days. A water-hardening cement produced less irritation than early powder/liquid materials.

Restorative cements were less irritant than luting cements, which have been associated with clinical reports of post-cementation sensitivity.

The luting cements remain acidic longer after mixing and the effect may be exacerbated by the large number of tubules opened under extensive preparations. In deep cavities, only areas of dentine estimated to be less than 1 mm thick should be lined with calcium hydroxide, leaving the maximum area of dentine available for bonding.

Glass-ionomer cements may be relatively bland to the pulp because:

1. Polymer acids are weak acids.
2. The high molecular weight of the acids restricts diffusion down the tubules.
3. The acids tend to bind to the hydroxyapatite.
4. Hydrogen ions dissociate less readily from the polymer chains than from simple acids.
5. Only a minimal temperature rise occurs on setting.

Properly finished glass-ionomer restoratives are well tolerated by the gingival tissues.

METAL REINFORCEMENT (CERMETS)

When silver amalgam alloy particles are simply admixed with the glass powder the flexural strength is increased but appearance is poor and resistance to abrasion is reduced.

When silver (or gold) is sintered with the glass powder at high temperature the so-called cermet–ionomer cement powder is formed. This enhances the wear resistance, radiopacity and surface smoothness of the set cement. White titanium oxide may be incorporated to improve the colour.

Cermets are intended for use as replacements for small posterior amalgams, core build-up or as a base beneath posterior composites.

OTHER PROPERTIES

Radiopacity

The early glass-ionomer cements were radiolucent. Radiopacity is achieved by including barium sulphate, silver–tin alloy or silver–glass cermet with the glass powder, but these methods produce an opaque material. Strontium or lanthanum may replace calcium in the glass for aesthetic materials requiring translucency. Strontium may also increase the cariostatic effect of the cements.

Opacity

Early cements were too opaque but newer versions have opacity values near those of composite resins.

Strength

The compressive strength is comparable with that of silicates (around 200 MPa) but the flexural strength (10–40 MPa), even though tripled in later materials, is low and renders the materials unsuitable for Class IV or large Class II restorations in adults.

The compressive strength at one year may double that at 24 h.

Cariostatic effect

A fluoride flux is used in the manufacture of glass-ionomer cements and fluoride is released into enamel, dentine and cementum. The solubility of enamel in contact with glass-ionomer cement decreased by 52% and, after 4–5 years, 84 cervical erosion restorations showed no secondary caries.

Storage

The shelf-life is similar to that of composite resins. Glass-ionomer cements should not be refrigerated because:

1. In the powder/liquid forms the polymeric acids may crystallize.
2. In the powder/water forms, condensation on opening the cold bottle can cause partial polymerization of the freeze-dried acid, which will retard setting and reduce the physical properties of the set cement.

Water loss or gain

Dehydration causes crazing and cracking and produces an opaque restoration with increased susceptibility to staining and microleakage.

Susceptibility to dehydration decreases with time but may persist for 1–15 days according to the material.

Water absorption can cause swelling and surface disruption and protection is required for 10–30 min after placement. Rubber dam may protect unset cement from moisture but can cause desiccation of unprotected cement with resultant shrinkage and crazing.

INDICATIONS

Restorative materials

1. Erosion/abrasion lesions without cavity preparation
2. Class V carious lesions
3. Class III carious lesions
4. Deciduous teeth
5. Sealing and filling occlusal pits and fissures
6. Repair of defective margins in restoration
7. Minimal cavity preparations (tunnel preparations)
8. Core build-up of posterior teeth
9. Sealing root surfaces for overdentures

Fast-setting lining cement and bases

1. Lining cavities where biological seal and cariostatic action are required
2. For the laminate or sandwich technique
3. Sealing and filling occlusal fissures with early caries

Luting cements

Particularly in patients with high caries rate (fluoride release).

CONTRAINDICATIONS

(Because of low flexural strength, lack of translucency.)

1. Class IV restorations
2. Large areas of labial enamel where appearance is of major importance
3. Conventional Class II cavity preparations
4. Replacement of lost cusps

USING GLASS-IONOMER CEMENTS

Mixing

1. Use a plastic, agate or cobalt–chromium spatula to avoid discoloration of glass particles.
2. Use the powder/liquid ratios and proportioning devices recommended by the manufacturer.
3. Hold the dropper bottle vertically and allow the drop to form by gravity or squeeze the bottle gently.
4. Agitate the powder bottle before using the measuring scoop, as failure to do so can increase the powder dispensed by 15%.
5. Use a clean, dry, cool (not below the dew-point) glass slab or a fresh sheet from a mixing pad.
6. Mix over a small area to minimize water loss and material waste.
7. With a folding action, incorporate all the powder rapidly and complete the mix in 20–30 s.
8. Do not add liquid to a mix that is too thick — start a new mix.
9. Place the material in the cavity immediately after mixing and within 1.5 min of the start of mixing.
10. Keep the bottle closed. Water gain to the freeze-dried powders will retard the set and reduce the physical properties of the cement.

Clinical placement

1. Select shade.
2. Clean abrasion lesions with pumice and water only or remove caries and create retention if appropriate.
3. Line deep areas of cavities (within about 1.0 mm of pulp) with calcium hydroxide.
4. A surface conditioner may be applied.
5. Dry the cavity but do not dehydrate the dentine.
6. Place the cement and contour with a precontoured soft metal matrix.
7. Allow material to set for manufacturer's recommended time.

8(a). Remove matrix and cover immediately with varnish or light curing bonding resin. (Copal varnish is not effective and petroleum jelly may be removed by the tongue.)

(b). If no gross excess, discharge patient and instruct to remove matrix at end of day.

9. Trim gross excess with hand instruments — avoid rotary instruments at this stage.
10. Re-apply protective coating.
11. Delay finishing for 10–15 min or till next visit.

Fissure sealants

In fissures without apertures, use resins, but in patent fissures, where a sharp tip of probe will enter fissure, glass-ionomer cement may be used as follows.

1. Isolate tooth.
2. Apply polyacrylic acid for 20 s to fissures — wash, dry. Do not use pumice and water as particles may obstruct fissures.
3. Tease low-viscosity mix into fissures with probe tip.
4. Cover with thin occlusal wax.
5. When set, remove wax and protect with varnish.
6. Check occlusion, remove excess with hand instruments or small round bur.
7. Re-apply varnish.

Luting cements

Advantages over conventional cements include:

  (a) cariostatic because of fluoride release;
  (b) low solubility when set;
  (c) high strength;
  (d) good bond to dentine, enamel and amalgam;
  (e) protects pulp from acid-etching procedures.

Disadvantages. For luting, problems may be:

  (a) early cements were radiolucent;
  (b) high solubility if not protected against water loss or gain while setting;

(c) post-cementation sensitivity — attributed to low initial pH, and may be avoided or reduced by:

    (i)   using optimum powder/liquid ratio;
    (ii) calcium hydroxide protection of deep areas;
    (iii) avoiding use in young teeth with large pulps;
    (iv) not removing smear layer with polyacrylic acid conditioner.

NEW CONCEPTS

'Microcavities' can now be prepared as the material bonds to the tooth and leaches fluoride.

For a **tunnel restoration**, a small round bur is used to 'tunnel' under the marginal ridge to remove the caries. Good illumination, usually from a fibre-optic, is required to ensure all the caries has been removed. Some workers advocate staining the cavity with a dye to check complete removal of caries.

Chemical removal of any remaining caries can be performed with an agent containing N-monochloroglycine.

The 'tunnel' is flushed with 20% stannous fluoride followed by copious water rinsing and air-drying. This will help to remineralize any subclinical caries left.

Because of the good bonding to tooth substance, the marginal ridge is supported and should resist fracture.

Laminates and sandwiches

Etching the surface of a glass-ionomer cement with 37% phosphoric acid for 15–20 s produces a rough surface to which composite resin may adhere. This produces a 'composite-ionomer sandwich'.

The glass-ionomer acts as a 'dentine substitute', as its physical properties are similar to those of dentine. The composite is viewed as an 'enamel substitute' in these bonded restorations.

Recent research has shown that treating the glass-ionomer with acid solutions can lead to pulpal damage if the water rinsing is not carried out thoroughly.

Some forms of base-liner cements do not require etching, and the composite resin-bonding agent can be directly applied to the base. These materials set within about 4 min and are radiopaque.

An extension of this technique can be used with the cementation of certain porcelain inlays for posterior teeth.

Light-cured glass-ionomer cements

Light-cured, glass-ionomer base-liner materials retain the advantages of bonding to dentine and enamel and fluoride release with the additional advantages of increased working time and a setting time reduced to a 30 s light-cure. When set the materials are not susceptible to water loss or gain.

The materials have higher early compressive, tensile and flexural strengths than conventional glass-ionomer lining cements. They also exhibit a rapid rise in pH on curing—calcium hydroxide sub-lining of deep cavities is claimed to be unnecessary.

In one formulation the powder is a photosensitive fluoroaluminosilicate glass and the liquid an aqueous solution of polyacrylic acid and HEMA (hydroxyethylmethacrylate) with a photoinitiator.

After mixing the powder and the liquid, a 30-s light-exposure will cure a 2 mm layer of material. Without light-activation the setting time exceeds 10 min.

Refrigeration prolongs shelf-life but the photosensitive powder and liquid must be protected from exposure to light.

Suitable as a lining or base under composite resins, amalgams, porcelain and cast restorations, their instant setting, when light-cured, makes them well suited to the composite 'sandwich' technique.

FURTHER READING

Atkinson A. S., Pearson G. J. (1985). The evolution of glass-ionomer cements. *Br. Dent. J.*, **159**, 335–7.
Council on Dental Materials and Devices (1979). Status report on glass ionomer cements. *J. Am. Dent. Assoc.*, **99**, 221–6.
Knibbs P. J. (1988). Glass-ionomer cement: 10 years of clinical use. *J. Oral Rehabil.*, **15**, 103–5.
Knibbs P. J., Plant G. C. (1986). A clinical assessment of a rapid setting glass-ionomer cement. *Br. Dent. J.*, **161**, 323–6.
Knibbs P. J., Plant G. C., Pearson G. J. (1986). A clinical assessment of an anhydrous glass-ionomer cement. *Br. Dent. J.*, **161**, 99–103.
Knibbs P. J., Plant G. C., Shovelton D. S. (1986). An evaluation of an anhydrous glass-ionomer cement in general dental practice. *Br. Dent. J.*, **160**, 170–3.
McLean J. W., Wilson A. D., Prosser H. J. (1984). Development and use of water-hardening glass-ionomer luting cements. *J. Prosth. Dent.*, **52**, 175–81.
Paterson R. C., Watts A. (1987). Toxicity to the pulp of a glass-ionomer cement. *Br. Dent. J.*, **162**, 110–12.
Walls A. W. G. (1986). Glass polyalkenoate (glass-ionomer) cements: a review. *J. Dent.*, **14**, 231–46.
Wilson A. D., McLean J. W. (1988). *Glass-ionomer Cement*. Chicago: Quintessence.

Chapter 27

Resin-bonded bridges

The use of the acid-etch technique in bridgework for the replacement of missing teeth was first described in 1973. As techniques have proliferated, the bridges have been called by various names, the most popular of which include adhesive bridges, acid-etch bridges, Rochette bridges, Maryland bridges and resin-bonded bridges. The techniques all use composite resin to bond the pontic to the etched enamel of the adjacent abutment teeth and have the major advantage over conventional bridges of requiring little or no reduction of sound tooth substance.

TYPES OF BONDED BRIDGE

Resin-bonded bridges may be of two distinct types:

1. A pontic tooth, consisting of an acrylic denture tooth, a natural crown or a composite pontic is bonded directly to the etched enamel of abutment teeth using composite resin.

2. A cast metal framework carrying an acrylic or porcelain pontic is constructed and this is bonded to the abutment teeth.

Resin pontics

The pontic may be an acrylic denture tooth or fabricated from composite resin using a cellulose acetate crown-form. They may be made at the chairside or in the laboratory on a plaster cast and should incorporate three essential design features:

1. The pontic must fit the abutment closely to minimize the thickness of composite resin in the joints.

2. The pontic should slightly 'wrap around' the abutment teeth to locate it positively.

3. Mechanical retention grooves must be cut in the proximal surfaces of acrylic pontics as composite resin does not bond well to acrylic.

To improve the success of these bridges dovetail cavities or threaded pins have been used in the adjacent teeth but these procedures are not reversible and should be avoided. Pontics have been modified by the incorporation of orthodontic wire, stainless-steel mesh, orthodontic pads and perforated, heat-cured acrylic retaining flanges.

Resin pontic bridges survive well when replacing missing lower incisors, but should generally be considered as provisional replacements for upper anterior teeth. They may not require occlusal clearance for retaining flanges, may be completed in one visit, and have the advantage of low cost. They may replace a partial denture while a denture stomatitis resolves or a socket heals and resorbs before placing a conventional bridge.

Natural crown pontic

This uses the crown of a patient's natural tooth which has been extracted or severely traumatized. The crown is sectioned from the root to produce a pontic of appropriate length, and the pulp chamber is then thoroughly cleaned, dried and filled with resin. The enamel of the proximal surfaces of the abutment teeth and the pontic is etched, and the clinical crown is bonded back into its original position in the arch.

METAL FRAMEWORK BRIDGES

These are the most widely used of the resin-bonded bridges. The pontic may be heat-cured acrylic but porcelain is preferred. Retainers or flanges may be perforated or non-perforated.

Perforated retainers

Used in Rochette bridges (1973), these rely on macromechanical retention. The retainer may be 0.5 mm thick and perforations, about 1 mm in diameter, should taper towards the fit surface and have rounded edges to reduce stress concentrations. Few large or many small perforations seem to perform equally well.

Advantages
  1. The perforations can be made without special laboratory equipment.
  2. Specialized composite resins are not required for bonding.
  3. No additional visit is necessary for try-in.
  4. The bridge can be simply removed by drilling the resin out of the perforations, and subsequently rebonded.

Disadvantages
  1. The perforations weaken the metal retainers which have to be increased in thickness to compensate for this.
  2. The exposed composite is prone to wear, plaque accumulation, water absorption and leakage.
  3. The resin protrusions seem to be the site of clinical failure.

Non-perforated retainers

Non-perforated retainers avoid some of the problems of perforated retainers and use various methods for bonding the resin to the metal.
Electrolytic etching is used in Maryland bridges: it differentially dissolves the metal surface to create microporosities which allow micromechanical retention of the resin.

Advantages

1. The retaining flanges are thinner and smoother than perforated flanges and produce less interference with the occlusion.
2. The composite resin is covered so there is no wear or plaque accumulation on the surface.

Disadvantages

1. The metal etching procedure is technique-sensitive.
2. Only some non-precious alloys can be used.
3. Alloys (not available in the UK) containing toxic beryllium etch best.
4. Different alloys require specific acids, current density and etching times.
5. It is difficult to check that the etch pattern is retentive.
6. Mechanical damage or saliva contamination of etched surface reduce the bond, but may be avoided by applying unfilled resin to the etched surface before try-in, or trying-in the bridge before etching.

Chemical etching achieves effective etching without expensive electrical etching equipment but necessitates the use of highly corrosive mixtures, e.g. nitric and hydrochloric acids and methanol.

To avoid the handling of acids and because of inconsistencies with etching, other methods of bonding the resin to the metal are constantly sought and include:

1. Mesh retention. A nylon mesh (Duralingual technique) may be incorporated into the wax pattern of the flange, but adaptation to the tooth surface is difficult and casting requires special care.

2. Bead retention. Resin retention beads have been incorporated into the fit surface of the wax pattern. The presence of bead retention after casting can be easily checked and it is less susceptible to contamination than micromechanical retention systems.

Disadvantages are over-contouring of the flanges, and poor adaptation to the tooth surface, especially into small grooves and rest seats.

3. Salt crystals. Water soluble salt crystals (150 μm), incorporated into the fit surface of the wax pattern, are dissolved to create a pitted surface after casting for retention of the resin. Careful investment and casting techniques are essential.

All alloys may be used with the above three macroretentive devices, which are more easily confirmed than etched surfaces and less affected by contamination during manipulation.

4. Porous coating. A porous coating (20–50 μm thick) of a metallic material (Inzoma) may be fused to alloys by heating in a porcelain furnace. The micromechanical retention is claimed to equal that of etched surfaces.

Chemical bonding to framework

Compared with mechanical retention, frameworks for chemical bonding are simpler to make and use all the fit surface for bonding:

1. Tin plating. A crystalline layer of tin, electrochemically deposited on the metal increases the surface area to aid micromechanical retention. Chemical adhesion with composite resin results when this layer is oxidized electrolytically using an acidified potassium permanganate solution or by heating in air at 1000°C for 2 minutes. Precious and semi-precious alloys may be used but the surface is vulnerable to saliva contamination. In one clinical study of tin-plated retainers with acrylic pontics, over a mean observation period of 22 months, 8.2% of 84 anterior bridges but none of 68 posterior bridges became detached.

2. Silane coating. A silane solution is vapourized in a flame to deposit a 1 μm layer of silicon dioxide on the casting surface. A thin film of silane is painted on the surface and dried before bonding with composite resin.

A special furnace is necessary, only porcelain pontics can be used, and no clinical data are yet available.

Grit-blasted retainers

This is the simplest method of surface preparation of retainers, but requires the use of specialized resins that bond chemically to the metal. One filled resin cement with a phosphate monomer bonds to grit-blasted non-precious alloy retainers, but precious alloys require tin plating. It is self-curing but strongly retarded by oxygen, so cement at margins of flanges must be covered with protective gel to exclude air. Bridges have survived over five years clinically.

A cement based on 4–META and methyl methacrylate bonds to grit-blasted cobalt–chromium and nickel–chromium alloys.

Another uses a composite resin plus a metal primer containing methacrylate-phosphate groups.

The long-term durability in water of the bonds has not been established for all these systems.

INDICATIONS FOR RESIN-BONDED BRIDGES

1. Best suited to single-tooth spans when the abutments are sound or have small carious lesions or restorations. Longer spans may be used if the occlusion is favourable, e.g. anterior open bite or large overjet.
2. When the appearance of the abutment teeth is satisfactory.
3. When adequate occlusal clearance can be achieved for the retainer without exposing dentine on the abutment tooth.
4. When the pontic space is appropriate.
5. Opposing a full denture.
Particularly suited to:
6. Patients with periodontal disease — because the gingival margin problems with conventional bridgework are less likely to occur.
7. Young patients where a conventional bridge is best avoided because of the pulp size or risk of trauma to teeth weakened by conventional preparations.
8. Use as a temporary bridge — because it is reversible.
9. Elderly or medically compromised patients.

CONTRAINDICATIONS FOR RESIN-BONDED BRIDGES

1. Unfavourable occlusion — Angle Class I, division II. It is difficult to create occlusal clearance on the palatal surfaces of the abutment teeth without

penetrating the dentine, and the deep overbite and steep anterior guidance can cause rapid detachment of the bridge.

2. If abutments have inadequate enamel for attachment, e.g. caries, large restorations, eroded enamel, sparse or poor quality enamel, fractured teeth, partially erupted teeth and short clinical crowns.

3. Where full coverage is necessary for aesthetics or realignment, e.g. non-vital abutment teeth, pontic space too wide or too narrow.

4. Marked alveolar ridge loss.
5. High caries rate — poor oral hygiene.
6. Inadequate posterior support — for anterior bridge.
7. Unequal mobility of abutment teeth.
8. Parafunctional habits, e.g. bruxism, nail biting, pencil chewing.
9. Long-span bridges — these place undue stress on abutment teeth.

ADVANTAGES OF RESIN-BONDED BRIDGES

1. No or minimal tooth reduction — confined to enamel.
2. No risk of pulp damage — especially in young patient.
3. No local anaesthetic required.
4. Retainers are supragingival — so excellent periodontal tolerance.
5. Simplified impression technique — no gingival retraction.
6. Cheaper than conventional bridge.
7. Reduced chairside and laboratory time.
8. Clinical procedures are brief and atraumatic.
9. Temporary crowns and bridges not necessary.
10. Reversible if minimal tooth reduction.
11. Fewer potential problems in service with recurrent caries, thermal sensitivity, occlusal interference.
12. Better accepted than partial denture.
13. Can be one visit for resin or natural tooth pontics.

DISADVANTAGES OF RESIN-BONDED BRIDGES

1. Cannot be used if palatal enamel on abutment teeth is missing.
2. The debonding rate is too high in some cases.
3. Cannot compensate for discrepancies in abutment tooth size, shape or colour, or pontic size.
4. No trial period is possible.
5. Flanges may reduce translucency of thin abutment teeth.
6. Increased wear of opposing teeth against metal flanges.
7. Thick flanges of adequate strength may interfere with the occlusion.
8. Composite resin in perforations may wear and encourage plaque accumulation.

DESIGN FEATURES

The design of the framework aims to transfer potential tensile and shear forces into compressive forces at the bonding site. Thus:

1. Create a single path of insertion in an occlusogingival direction by minimal reduction of the abutment teeth.
2. Use the maximum area for bonding with the retainer, terminating about 1 mm supragingivally and proximally on the marginal ridge.
3. If necessary, create 1 mm occlusal clearance for the flanges of an upper anterior bridge.
4. Use occlusal or cingulum rests as vertical stops.
5. Use proximal grooves to increase retention if essential but avoid extensive tooth preparation as the procedure is then no longer reversible.
6. With thin abutment teeth avoid 'greying' of the incisal edge (caused by the metal showing through) by reducing the incisal extension of the retainer.
7. Extend the pontic beyond the distobuccal and mesiobuccal line angles of the abutment teeth.
8. Wrap the casting around the labiofacial line angles.
9. Ensure the casting seats positively with no displacement possible in a labiolingual direction.
10. Cantilevered bridges may be considered where the adjacent tooth has a porcelain crown, insufficient enamel for adequate retention or where it is not practicable to provide adequate clearance for a wing.
11. Hybrid bridges — if one abutment requires crowning a movable attachment should be incorporated between the pontic and the crown. In case of bond failure the retainer can then be rebonded without removing the firmly cemented crown.

TOOTH PREPARATION

Must be confined to enamel.

For upper anterior teeth, preparation may involve:
1. Reduction of proximal areas to produce near-parallel surfaces.
2. A knife-edge finishing line supragingivally.
3. Cingulum rests.
4. Proximal grooves to enhance resistance to lingual displacement.
5. Reduction of the lingual fossa or opposing lower incisal edge to create about 1 mm occlusal clearance.

For posterior teeth preparation may involve —
1. Creation of occlusal rest seats about 1.5 mm diameter and 0.5 mm deep in the enamel of the marginal ridge or the lingual fissure.
2. Reduction of the proximal and lingual surfaces to move the survey line closer to the gingival margin so increasing the area available for bonding.

BONDING TECHNIQUE

1. Clean the abutment teeth with pumice and water in a rubber cup.
2. Try-in the bridge to check the fit, occlusion and appearance. (If the casting is contaminated with saliva return it to the laboratory for etching or grit blasting, or clean with phosphoric acid, rinse and dry.)
3. Isolate the area.

4. Replace existing restorations in the bonding areas of abutment teeth with composite resin.
5. Etch the enamel with 37% phosphoric acid for 60 s.
6. Wash with water for 20 s and dry with oil-free air.
7. Apply the resin to the fitting surfaces of the bridge. (Do not use light-cured resins.)
8. Use opaque resins to avoid the greying effect with thin abutment teeth.
9. Fit the bridge and retain in position with light finger pressure.
10. Remove gross excess which exudes before it sets.
11. Remove excess cured resin with hand scalers or finishing diamonds and points.
12. Check the pontic is clear of the occlusion in all excursions of the mandible with articulating paper or shimstock.
13. Instruct the patient in the use of a floss threader to maintain bridge hygiene.
14. Advise patients to seek advice immediately if they notice a bridge is loose, as caries, although reported rarely under retainers, can progress rapidly to involve the dentine if the bond to enamel fails. If detachment is detected the bridge must be rebonded immediately, unless established that failure is at the resin–metal interface and that the enamel is protected by a layer of composite resin.

Rebonding failed bridges

1. Before rebonding a bridge, seek the cause of failure (especially occlusal interference) and eliminate if possible.
2. Remove resin completely from the enamel of the abutment teeth and the framework.

FAILURE RATES AND CAUSES

Determining the failure rate for resin-bonded bridges from the literature is no less difficult than for conventional bridges. One study of resin-bonded bridges and splints placed by 17 dentists, using different resins, retention systems and retainer designs, found for bridges that 81.5% after 12 months and 73% after 18 months were in place without needing rebonding.

Early failure (e.g. within 2 days) may be caused by contamination of the etched surface (metal or enamel) with blood, saliva or grease, movement of the resin whilst setting, excessive occlusal loads, or poor fit of the casting.

Long-term failure may result from fatigue fracture of the resin; water breakdown of the bond between resin and enamel or resin and metal. Trauma, biting hard objects such as ice, or torquing forces on cantilever bridges may cause failure at any stage.

Failure rates are likely to be higher if abutments with large restorations are used and if patients with marked parafunctional habits are not excluded.

The bond to composite resin that has been in the mouth is half of that to freshly bonded composite so existing restorations are best replaced by composite resin at the visit the bridge is bonded.

Bond failure to the metal occurs more frequently than to the enamel.

CONCLUSIONS

Resin-bonded bridges have not eliminated conventional bridgework but they are being used increasingly as improvements in design and retention increase their success rate and widen their range of applications.

Acrylic or composite pontic bridges are best confined principally to replacement of anterior teeth, but bridges with a cast metal substructure may be used in the posterior part of the mouth.

Their role is increasing significantly as caries rates fall and reluctance grows to undertake the massive reduction of tooth structure required for conventional bridgework when the abutment teeth are perfectly sound.

Resin-bonded bridges should not be considered the 'easy option' to conventional bridges. Many of the clinical and theoretical principles of conventional bridgework apply to resin-bonded bridges and case selection may be even more important for their success. Thus:

1. The patient's oral hygiene and attitude must be appropriate.
2. The patient's expectations of appearance must be achievable.
3. Occlusal relationships must be correct:

    (a) Anteriorly, incisal guidance must be avoided or confined to light contact on the pontic in protrusive movements.

    (b) Posteriorly, contact on the pontic should be restricted to centric function — contact in lateral excursions should be eliminated — or restricted to light group function.

    (c) Adequate posterior support must be present for resin-bonded bridges as with conventional bridges.

4. Stable abutment teeth should be used.
5. Parallelism, adequate length and surface area, and a definite path of insertion are required.

FURTHER READING

Council on Dental Materials (1987). Etched-metal resin-bonded prostheses. *J. Am. Dent. Assoc.*, **115**, 95–7.

Ibsen R. L. (1973). One appointment technic using an adhesive composite. *Dent. Surg.*, **49**, 30–2.

Marinello C. P., Kerschbaum T., Heinenberg B., *et al.* (1987). Experiences with resin-bonded bridges and splints — a retrospective study. *J. Oral Rehabil.*, **14**, 251–60.

Rochette A. L. (1973). Attachment of a splint to enamel of lower anterior teeth. *J. Prosth. Dent.*, **30**, 418–23.

Simonsen R., Thompson V., Barrack G. (1983). *Etched Cast Restorations: Clinical and Laboratory Techniques*. Chicago: Quintessence.

Tay W. M. (1988). Resin-bonded bridges: 1. Methods and materials. *Dent. Update*, **15**, 10–14.

Chapter 28

Advanced tooth wear

MECHANISM

1. *Erosion:* a chemical process involving acid dissolution, or chelation of enamel constituents at a near-neutral pH.
2. *Abrasion:* the physical removal of tooth substance by agents introduced into the mouth, e.g. toothbrushes and toothpastes.
3. *Attrition:* a physical process where tooth substance is removed by the movement of teeth against each other, with or without an abrasive material intervening.

AETIOLOGY

There is no independence for the three modes of tooth tissue loss; differing patterns of wear reflect the relative contribution of each mode, and the principal cause indicates the main line of treatment.
  The main contributing factors are:

  (a) dietary constituents;
  (b) masticatory habit;
  (c) parafunction;
  (d) age;
  (e) general dental state.

CLINICAL PRESENTATION

The condition may present as two populations: a 'younger' group where tissue loss most frequently occurs from the labial or lingual surfaces of the teeth, and an 'older' group where loss is predominantly from the occlusal or incisal surfaces.
  The 'older' group does not represent a progression from the 'younger' group but results from the different mechanisms of loss. Features of both may be present in some cases.

PATIENT EVALUATION

Early diagnosis is important.
  During the history and examination particular attention should be paid to:

1. The patient's perception of the problem.
2. The patient's attitude to possible treatments. Treatment is time-consuming and cooperation is essential. Misgivings regarding this indicate simplicity in treatment planning.
3. The occurrence of gastric reflux: this may be a result of anorexia nervosa or chronic alcoholism. Confirm by reference to medical practitioner rather than by over-persistent interrogation.
4. The following aspects of the dental history:

    (a) onset of awareness of the problem;
    (b) estimated rate of progress of the condition;
    (c) past dental history—relevant to (2) above;
    (d) dietary factors, particularly low pH foods;
    (e) parafunctional habits;
    (f) occupation.

5. The following aspects of the examination:

    (a) teeth present and their status (restoration, angulation, rotation, periodontal condition, mobility);
    (b) prostheses (type, material, condition);
    (c) the occlusion (with natural teeth and prostheses where worn);
    (d) the inter-occlusal clearance ('free-way space');
    (e) the sites and degree of wear;
    (f) radiographic appearance of the teeth (particularly size and position of the pulp chambers);
    (g) vitality testing (caution is required in interpreting results);
    (h) mounted study models;
    (i) the space available for restorations.

TREATMENT PLANNING

There are three options:

1. *No active intervention.* Reassurance and periodic review to check on changes in the pattern or progress of the condition.

2. *Prevention of further wear.* If in early stages, dietary counselling may be all that is required.

Construction of protective appliances, to be worn as necessary. Thin, vacuum-formed polythene mouthguards may be used and may double as a vehicle for the application of fluoride preparations.

If parafunction is suspected, two such guards should be provided, one to be worn at night, the other during the day (excluding meal times). After about 2 weeks these should indicate sites and degrees of wear. Further investigations and occlusal adjustment may be indicated.

If the destructive agent is an essential dietary component, e.g. HCl in achlorhydria, advise use of a straw or of post-consumption mouthwashes.

3. *Restoration.* Firstly, it is essential to assess the space available for restorations. Acrylic appliances resembling record blocks are constructed at the

desired vertical dimension of occlusion. These are adjusted to give even contact around the arch. Worn teeth are overlaid as necessary. After one week's wear the patient's toleration of the appliance is assessed. The appliance is adjusted as necessary, usually by reduction in height. The patient is reassessed at weekly intervals with adjustments as necessary. Once the patient is comfortable and can wear the appliances for extended periods, this is taken to be the vertical dimension of occlusion at which the permanent restorations are constructed.

TREATMENT OPTIONS

(A) Extraction of tooth remnants and provision of conventional partial or complete dentures

Indications
1. Where the patient does not wish to receive more complex alternatives.
2. Where the tooth remains are not readily savable.
3. Where surgical reduction of the alveolus is indicated.

Contraindications
None, but see 'Disadvantages' below.

Advantages
1. Treatment is rapidly completed.
2. Treatment is relatively simple clinically.
3. Immediate denture technique may be used.

Disadvantages
Heavy occlusal forces may result in:
(a) excessive bone loss;
(b) pain under the dentures.

(B) Provision of partial or complete overdentures

Indications
1. Tooth wear has reduced crown height by about two-thirds or more.
2. A small number of teeth is involved.
3. Sufficient space is available.

Contraindications
1. Less than about two-thirds crown reduction.
2. Large numbers of teeth involved.
3. Multiple devitalizations are required to prepare teeth.
4. Patient motivation and cooperation is low.
5. Less than 'good' oral hygiene.

Advantages

1. Good appearance.
2. Less bone loss where roots retained.

Disadvantages

1. Require a high standard of home care.
2. Ideally require regular fluoride application to teeth.
3. Clinically time-consuming.

(C) Restoration using crowns

Porcelain crowns

Usually contraindicated since they:

(a) require excessive tooth preparation;
(b) often fail to withstand the occlusal stresses.

Post crowns

Contraindicated because they:

(a) require excessive tooth reduction;
(b) may cause root fracture.

Porcelain bonded to metal crowns

Indications for these are:

(a) most suitable for 'erosion' type wear;
(b) stabilizing occlusion on buccal/posterior teeth.

Contraindications are short clinical crowns.

Advantages of bonded crowns are that:

(a) less tooth preparation is required;
(b) they will withstand occlusal stresses;
(c) they will withstand wear;
(d) they protect the tooth remnant.

Disadvantages. Such crowns may:

(a) cause excess wear of opposing teeth;
(b) if they fail, produce a result less favourable than before.

As with overdentures, space is critical. If insufficient space is available, one cannot lengthen the tooth by crowning, and therefore cannot improve appearance.

(D) Restoration using composite resin (acid-etch and/or pin retained)

Indications

1. Where sufficient suitably placed enamel is available for etching.
2. Where there is sufficient space to accommodate length of pins.

Contraindications

1. Where only dentine remains.
2. No space for pins.
3. No occlusal support from natural teeth.

Advantages

1. Usually require little or no tooth preparation.
2. Easily replaced in most instances.
3. Require less clinical time than more complex restorations.
4. Independent of laboratory facilities.

Disadvantages

1. Often inferior appearance.
2. May be dislodged if no other occlusal support.
3. May give rise to iatrogenic damage to opposing teeth (abrasive).

THE EFFECTS OF TOOTH WEAR

On individual teeth

1. Laying down of secondary dentine if slow wear.
2. Sensitivity of teeth.
3. Pulpal exposure, with or without abscess formation if rapid wear.

On the vertical dimension of occlusion (VDO)

1. Reduction in VDO if rapid wear, with increased interocclusal clearance.
2. Maintained VDO if slow wear due to compensatory over-eruption; interocclusal clearance unchanged—wear of the teeth should *not* be used as an indicator of VDO status.

On the temporomandibular joint

1. Some evidence associates attrition and joint pathology.
2. Remodelling of the joint (condylar and articular components) is common in both animals and man.

3. Complex factors influence remodelling, including masticatory function.
4. Changes claimed as a result of advanced tooth wear are similar to those from increased pathological change from other causes.

On function

Loss of function is rarely a presenting complaint. There appears no reason to believe that advanced tooth wear per se significantly reduces the functional capacity of the dentition.

POST-TREATMENT PROBLEMS

Increased VDO

Outcome is unclear and evidence is contradictory.

Temporary increases in VDO using 'orthopaedic' interocclusal appliances are highly effective in the treatment of temperomandibular joint and mandibular pain-dysfunction syndromes. Some evidence exists that teeth may be intruded by long-term occlusally directed loads, or at least that histological changes indicating bone and root resorption may occur. The minimum force required to produce these effects is not known with certainty. Restorations may be dislodged. A patient's most likely complaint is likely to be discomfort.

Provision of overdentures

Caries and periodontal disease will rapidly destroy retained teeth unless home care is exemplary.

Chapter 29

Occlusion in restorative dentistry

Dental occlusion is a static, closed relationship between the cusps or masticatory surfaces of the upper teeth and those of the lower teeth. There are many such stationary positions of contact between the maxillary and mandibular teeth but for practical clinical purposes the following positions are referred to:

1. *The intercuspal position*—maximal contact between the cusps and their opposing fossae or marginal ridges. In dentate subjects, the mandible is in its most cranial position and, when the mandible is in a central position, the term centric occlusion is applicable.
2. *The retruded contact position*—contact between opposing teeth when the mandible is retruded. The mandible can, in many subjects, be made to assume a position posterior to intercuspal occlusion as the condylar heads are drawn upwards and backwards, either by the actions of the elevator muscles or by externally applied pressure. The mandible is then said to be in *centric relation* (to the maxilla) and, in this position, opening can take place by rotation of the condyles, resulting in a reproducible arc of movement that allows a separation of the opposing incisor teeth of about 20 mm in adults. The imaginary axis through the condyles is known as the terminal hinge axis.
3. *The protruded position*—this is usually taken to be the edge-to-edge position of the incisors, and occurs when the condyle has moved downwards and forwards in the glenoid fossa.
4. *Left and right lateral occlusion*—a position of contact between the opposing teeth as the mandible moves to the left or the right. This commonly involves contact between opposing canines that have guided the path of movement but other teeth may be involved.

These occlusal positions are, by definition, determined by the number, shape and position of the teeth; as the teeth wear down, are restored or removed, these positions may change. The retruded arc of closure, however, is determined by the muscles and by the bony anatomy and ligaments of the temporomandibular joints. It therefore remains relatively constant and reproducible regardless of changes in the dentition. Opposing teeth, however, are rarely in a static relationship for more than very brief periods. During function and parafunction, the teeth slide over each other and this dynamic relationship is known as *articulation*.

JAW MOVEMENT

The complex three-dimensional nature of jaw movement can most easily be understood if each dimension is considered separately. The outer limits of jaw movement in the sagittal, horizontal and frontal planes are reproducible for a particular subject and each is known as a border movement. The border movements define a space or envelope within which the mandible can move. Because they are reproducible, they can be recorded and the information transferred to an articulator, which will then be capable of simulating, to varying degrees, jaw movement.

Figure 29.1 illustrates the characteristic outer limit of movement in the median sagittal plane of point between the lower incisor teeth in relation to the static maxillary teeth. This is eponymously referred to as Posselt's envelope. In Fig. 29.1, the arc 'a' is produced by rotation of the heads of the condyles when they are in a retruded position in the glenoid fossae. It is known as the terminal hinge axis and is usually about 2 cm in length. The point at which the teeth first meet in this arc (1) is known variously as centric relation, posterior border position, retruded position, or ligamentous position. From this point the mandible can move anteriorly and cranially until the teeth are in maximum intercuspation. This point (2) is known as centric occlusion, intercuspal position, or tooth position.

Further protrusion occurs as the lower incisors slide down the palatal surface of the upper incisors (2–3). This is incisal guidance and in the natural dentition the posterior teeth begin to separate (disclude). The lower incisors can then move over the incisal edges of the uppers (3–4) and into reverse overlap (4–5) until the mandible assumes its most cranial protruded position (6). Opening from this point takes the arc 'b' until maximum opening at point 7 is achieved. At this point the heads of the condyles are rotated and have translated forwards to their limit.

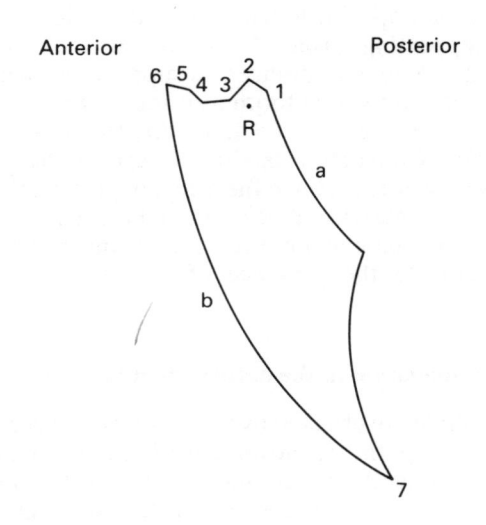

Fig. 29.1 *Posselt's envelope.*

Posterior determinants

Condylar guidance
Sagittal angle
Immediate side shift
Progressive side shift

Angle of orientation of occlusal plane

Anterior determinants

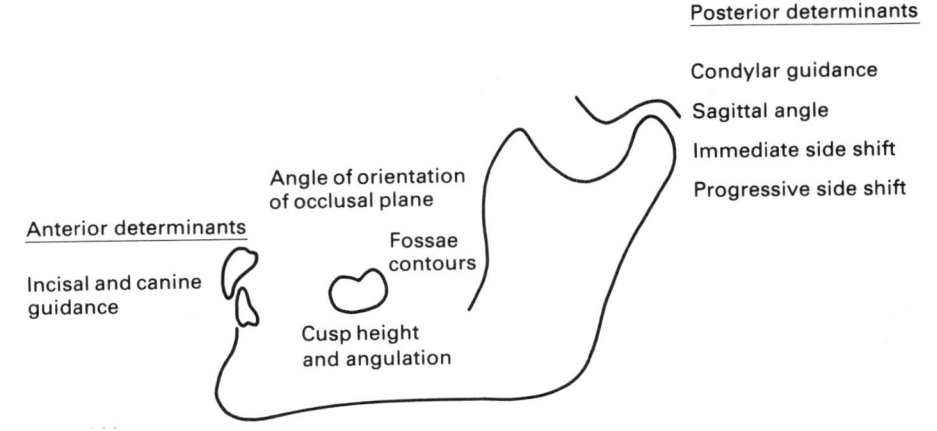

Incisal and canine guidance

Fossae contours

Cusp height and angulation

Fig. 29.2 *Determinants of articulation.*

Points 1 to 6 in Fig. 29.1 are determined by the teeth, and this component of the envelope is lost when all the teeth are extracted. The only point which is reproducible is 1, and then only by deduction of the occluding face height from the rest position (point 'R'). This reproducible position is recorded when jaw relationships are registered for complete dentures.

Occlusion in the natural dentition

The position which the lower jaw assumes, relative to the maxilla, when the teeth are in maximum intercuspation (centric occlusion) is determined (i) by the contact between the *buccal cusps* of the lower teeth and their opposing fossae or marginal ridges, and (ii) also by the contact between the *palatal cusps* of the upper teeth and their opposing fossae or marginal ridges. These cusps are therefore known as **supporting cusps**. Alterations to their shape either by restorations, wear or grinding will modify this supporting function, allowing rotation or eruption of the individual tooth as it seeks to re-establish contact. Alterations to all the supporting cusps could modify the relationship between the lower and upper jaws. Conversely, the buccal cusps of the upper teeth and the lingual cusps of the lower teeth have the effect of guiding the mandible on its path of closure into the intercuspal position and are known as the **guiding cusps**. Alterations to their shape will not result in changes in the relationship between opposing teeth. In the presence of a crossbite, the situation is reversed.

Articulation in the natural dentition

Movements of the mandible are effected by the elevator and depressor muscles but the three-dimensional paths of movement of the lower jaw are guided anteriorly by the anterior teeth and posteriorly by the temporomandibular joints. These determinants of articulation are illustrated in Fig. 29.2. The side towards which the mandible moves is known as the working side and the side away from which it moves is the non-working. In the natural, unworn dentition, canine guidance usually results in early separation of the opposing surfaces of the posterior teeth on lateral movement; the term 'balancing side' to describe the non-working side is therefore inappropriate.

The Bennett movement and Bennett angle

The Bennett movement is the lateral shift of the mandible which occurs during the initial phase of lateral masticatory (and parafunctional) movements (Fig. 29.3; A→B). Further lateral movement of the mandible involves a downwards, forwards and medial movement of the head of the condyle on the non-working side (Fig. 29.3; B→C). The amount of movement varies from one individual to another but is reproducible for the same individual. The angle formed by this movement relative to the sagittal plane is the Bennett angle (average 15°). The curved arc of movement is reproduced as a straight line (A→C) on the Dentatus Articulator. On fully adjustable articulators it is reproduced as immediate side-shift (A→B; range 0–2 mm) and progressive side-shift (B→C; average 6°).

The clinical significance of the immediate side-shift is that it is a tooth contact articulation, that is, it occurs before disclusion becomes effective. The tips of the cusps of the molar and premolar teeth are gliding across the central fossae of the opposing teeth. Thus, when subjects demonstrate a large immediate side-shift, allowance for this must be made in the occlusal contour of restorations if interferences are to be avoided.

The posterior determinants remain constant for any one subject whereas the path of anterior and canine guidance will alter if changes occur in the contours of the upper anterior teeth or the incisal edges of the lower anterior teeth. For example, if the upper anterior teeth are restored with crowns that are constructed with a greater lingual concavity than previously existed, then the anterior guidance angle relative to the horizontal plane will become less steep. One possible consequence of this would be that posterior teeth which previously discluded during protrusion now fail to do so. Similarly, wear of the canine teeth may result in the development of interferences in the opposite

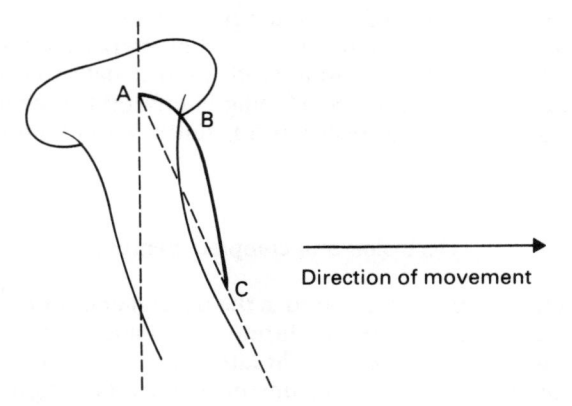

Fig. 29.3 *The Bennett movement and angle.*

(non-working side) quadrant. Thus posterior interferences may develop as a result of changes in the anatomy of the anterior teeth. A healthy, functional articulation, then, depends upon a harmonious inter-relationship between:

(a) the posterior determinants of articulation;
(b) the anterior determinants of articulation;
(c) the cusp height and angle of the posterior teeth;
(d) the angle of orientation of the occlusal plane.

Changes in any of the last three of the above mentioned factors may occur as a result of:

(a) tooth surface loss through attrition, abrasion erosion or trauma;
(b) changes in tooth position either occurring iatrogenically (i.e. orthodontics) or pathologically (e.g. as a result of periodontal breakdown);
(c) changes in crown contour through restorative procedures.

Such changes may result in the development of articulator or occlusal interferences, which in turn may have the following consequences:

1. *Adaptation*—the neuromuscular mechanism has a wide spectrum of adaptability.
2. *Fracture* of a restoration.
3. *Displacement of a crown or bridge*—this may occur when the load produced by the interferences exceed the retentive capacity of the restoration.
4. *Periodontal disease*—there is evidence that trauma from occlusion may act as a cofactor in the location and rate of progression of periodontal disease.
5. *Mandibular pain–dysfunction syndrome*—there is evidence that iatrogenic occlusal interferences result in inceased levels of elevator muscle activity and this could be a primary trigger factor in the aetiology of myofunctional disturbances. Alternatively where high levels of centrally induced muscle activity are present (bruxism), interferences may modify the pattern of psychogenically induced muscle activity causing localization or intensification of symptoms.

An apparent contradiction to this view of the pathogenic role of interferences is the observation that attrition is compatible with periodontal health and is not always associated with temporomandibular joint dysfunction. However, attrition commonly results in a characteristic wear pattern in the dentition which allows the opposing teeth to articulate freely and smoothly over each other and thus occlusal loading is different in character from the damaging oblique forces that occur as a result of cuspal interferences in the unworn natural dentition.

Occlusion and complete dentures

The anterior segment occlusion found in the natural dentition, if reproduced in dentures, results in lack of stability during lateral and protrusive movements. For example, as the teeth meet in right lateral occlusion the denture bases on the left side would tend to tilt away from the denture-bearing area. To counteract this effect, teeth on full dentures are set in *bilateral balanced occlusion*. That is, the teeth on both posterior segments remain in contact in lateral occlusion (the non-working side is now correctly termed the balancing side). Similarly the opposing posterior teeth remain in contact in protrusive occlusion.

Bilateral balanced occlusion can be achieved, on the articulator at least, by setting the teeth so that the following factors are in harmony:

(a) sagittal condyle angle;
(b) incisal guidance angle;
(c) orientation of the occlusal plane;
(d) cusp angle;
(e) curve of occlusal plane.

The cusps form a series of inclined planes which slide over each other as the condyles move downwards and forwards. Towards the back of the mouth the angle of these planes must more nearly approximate the condyle angle (which is approximately 43° to the Frankfort plane or 33° to the occlusal plane) so the teeth are tilted to increase the effective cusp angle. This produces the antero-posterior compensating curve. The flatter the cusp, the greater must be the angle of orientation of the occlusal plane and the greater the compensating curve if balance is to be maintained.

This theoretical concept of balanced occlusion is based on a mechanical interpretation of a complex biological system. In addition, it can be argued that, during mastication, the bolus separates the teeth and balance is irrelevant. However, after deglutition the teeth will contact, not always in the established intercuspal position, and it is desirable that any contact should tend to reseat rather than dislodge the denture bases. Also, as has been stated, most opposing tooth contacts are non-functional.

The objectives for occlusion and articulation in complete dentures are therefore:

(a) maximum intercuspation at a reproducible point on the terminal hinge axis at the correct vertical height;
(b) balanced occlusion in lateral and protrusive positions;
(c) free articulation, i.e. no deflective interferences as the dentures move between these occlusal positions.

This occlusal scheme is also appropriate to maintain the stability of free end-saddle partial dentures. Bounded saddles and fixed bridges should be in harmony with the remaining natural dentition, which will usually be anterior segment occlusion.

Chapter 30

Complaints related to complete dentures

The common complaints (i.e. looseness and pain) relating to complete dentures are usually brought to the dentists' attention either soon after the dentures are fitted or following a period of successful wear when the dentures are perhaps nearing the end of their useful life. In these cases, the complaints can be classified as early post-insertion or late and the time factor may be an important guide to the diagnosis.

There is considerable likelihood that denture faults will cause an overlap of complaints—for example, a loose denture may traumatize the tissues and therefore cause pain. For simplicity, complaints, diagnosis and treatment are presented in tabular form.

LOOSE DENTURES (EARLY POST-INSERTION)

Diagnosis	Treatment
Over-extension	Reduce border
Under-extension	Extend border to full depth/width: (i) chairside technique using rigid lining material (e.g. Peripheral Seal, Total); (ii) laboratory addition after use of greenstick tracing compound and reline impression in clinic
Post-dam absent or ineffective	Add post-dam: (i) chairside technique using rigid lining material; (ii) laboratory procedure after addition of greenstick tracing compound
Inaccurate fit	Rebase/reline Rigid chairside lining material (as above) can be expected to last several months Clinical procedures for laboratory rebase/reline
Teeth or denture base not in neutral zone	Reposition teeth/recontour polished surfaces/remake
Occlusal imbalance or interference	Occlusal correction—small corrections can be achieved at the chairside; however, a remount procedure is recommended to balance the occlusion
Occlusal plane too high	Remake dentures
Posterior teeth encroaching on tongue space	Reduce lingual aspect of teeth. Replace teeth with narrow mould

282

Reduced neuromuscular control (age or neuromuscular disease-related)	Duplicate technique if satisfactory old denture available
Deficient saliva	Determine cause — prescribe saliva substitute

LOOSE DENTURES (LATE)

Diagnosis	Treatment
Inaccurate fit — usually due to alveolar resorption or (rarely) excessive abrasion of impression surface when cleaning	Reline/rebase/remake. Chairside reline (Peripheral Seal, Total) may be possible if condition of dentures is otherwise generally satisfactory

GENERALIZED PAIN UNDER DENTURES

Diagnosis	Treatment
Excessive occlusal vertical dimension (i.e. lack of sufficient freeway space)	Relatively small changes can be made using pre-centric record, mounting on articulator and occlusal grinding If major height change necessary remake one or both dentures
Bruxism	Check — maximum base extension utilized; correct vertical dimension; correct occlusal relationships; consider using permanent soft lining
Atrophic mucosa	As for bruxism but also consider reduction of occlusal loading (use of narrow molar teeth, leave off last molars) Possibly also provide more than the conventional 3 mm freeway space

NB: generalized pain may also be attributed to excessive levels of residual monomer ($>1\%$), denture-induced stomatitis, climacteric, diabetes and certain deficiency states, etc.

LOCALIZED PAIN UNDER DENTURES

Diagnosis	Treatment
Overextension	Reduce border
Occlusal error	Adjust occlusion Discomfort may be related to ridge crest, lingual aspect of lower ridge or occasionally the borders of the denture
Localized pressure	Identify using pressure indicating paste and relieve

Roughness (or imperfections) in acrylic resin	Identify areas and smooth
Prominent mylohyoid ridges	Reduce flange Consider surgical treatment if stability of denture is compromised and discomfort is severe
Superficial mental foramen	Relieve impression surface of the denture. Permanent soft lining may be helpful; only consider surgery to relocate foramen if all else fails
Prominent genial tubercles	Reduce border; surgical reduction may be appropriate if pain is persistent
Sharp (ragged) anterior residual ridge	Relieve impression surface Use permanent soft lining Consider surgical trimming

MISCELLANEOUS COMPLAINTS

Diagnosis	**Treatment**
Pain in muscles of mastication	Correct the excessive or reduced occlusal vertical dimension Check for clenching/bruxism habits
Cheek biting	May occur because teeth are 'new' and therefore not accustomed to them — if so, will correct itself Inadequate soft tissue support — absence of buccal horizontal overlap
Tongue biting	As cheek biting — but consider tongue space available and inclination of molar teeth If appropriate, reduce lingual aspect of lower posterior teeth
Disturbance of speech	With new dentures speech patterns are usually adapted within a few days — if persistent, consider repositioning incisors and/or modifying palatal contour If unsuccessful, copy shape of old dentures
Angular stomatitis	Correct lip support and vertical dimension Improve oral and denture hygiene Since usually related to denture-induced stomatitis, consider use of antifungal agents
Retching	If occurs with new dentures usually reduces with adaptation When it persists, inspect palatal extension, thickness of posterior border and tongue space and correct accordingly; lack of freeway space and loose dentures can also contribute In a minority of cases, when toleration is limited, a palateless denture may be indicated

Excessive saliva	Common complaint in first few days with first-time denture wearers; adaptation rapidly reduces flow to normal
	After cerebrovascular accidents dribbling occurs because saliva is not being swallowed normally
Difficulty keeping dentures clean	Examine dentures for polish and technically well-finished margins around necks of teeth; rough areas or imperfect finish make effective cleaning difficult
	Advise: use acid cleaner if calculus and severe stain present, use alkaline hypochlorite cleaner to remove plaque and to keep denture clean
Denture fracture	Determine cause to prevent recurrence — may have broken when dropped (impact fracture) but midline fracture due to fatigue is common after a period of wear of several years
	Midline fracture usually associated with: median diastema; large fraenal notch, absence of labial flange; inherent weakness following previous repair; wedging action of very worn occlusion
	Laboratory repair is necessary — check relocation of piece(s) and fix together with sticky wax, matchsticks, etc. if doubtful; try in mouth to check location
	Consider an associated rebase to replace old acrylic resin, also add flange, etc. if appropriate

Chapter 31

Impression techniques

COMPLETE DENTURES

Introduction

The retention of complete dentures depends on several factors. These can be summarized as: *muscular forces; physical forces*.

The shape of a denture and the patient's ability to acquire and develop the necessary skills will determine successful muscular control. Impressions will have minimal effect on the design of the polished surface unless used in conjunction with a duplication technique. They will, however, determine the size and shape of the impression surface and therefore play an important role when considering the physical forces, i.e:

1. *Adhesion*—force of attraction between dissimilar molecules in close contact (acrylic resin–saliva–muscosa).
2. *Cohesion*—force of attraction between like molecules (saliva–saliva).

Both are influenced by the nature, quantity and viscosity of saliva as well as the accuracy of fit of the prosthesis. A thin saliva film provides the best retentive force.

It is also important that the flanges of a denture are adequately extended and correctly shaped to produce a facial seal and to provide resistance to the ingress of air, which would otherwise destroy the physical forces. The magnitude of physical retention is also related to the area covered by the denture and it is therefore appropriate to utilize the maximum available.

For optimum retention dentures must be correctly extended and closely adapted to the tissues. This is very difficult to achieve unless the working models are produced from special-tray impressions. Stock trays are manufactured to average sizes and therefore are likely to be less than ideal for any individual. Although modification of stock trays is possible, the resultant impression is still unlikely to be correctly extended. Surveys have shown that relatively few practitioners use special trays and perhaps this is not surprising when NHS fees for denture work are considered.

Preliminary impressions

Preliminary impressions can be taken using either metal stock trays or plastic disposable trays. A high-viscosity, irreversible hydrocolloid (alginate) or impression compound are the materials of choice.

Extent of impressions

1. *Upper:* to the functional depth of the labial and buccal sulci, including the tuberosities and hamular notches, and posteriorly to the junction of the hard and soft palate.
2. *Lower:* to the functional depth of the lingual, labial and buccal sulci and posteriorly covering the retromolar pads.

The aim of the preliminary impressions is to produce correctly extended models on which to make special trays. Accuracy of surface detail need only be limited since this will be an essential component of the working impressions.

Special trays

Self-curing acrylic resin is most commonly used for special-tray construction. It has the advantages of being relatively inexpensive, simple to shape and is rigid in modest thickness. The upper tray should have a small handle placed in the midline of the anterior region, sloping forwards at an angle of 45°. This configuration avoids interference with the lip. On the lower, the handle is vertical and two finger rests are placed, one in each of the second premolar regions. This enables the index fingers to support the tray without interfering with the borders of the impression. Special trays can be divided into two types, spaced and close-fitting.

Spaced special trays

Constructed with a spacer to ensure an even thickness of the elastic impression material for maximum accuracy. Specifically indicated when opposing substantial undercuts exist which could prevent the withdrawal of a close-fitting tray and a non-elastic impression material.

The tray can be constructed with 'built-in' stops, which contact the mucosa, or greenstick tracing compound can be added at the chairside. This should be completed before checking the border extension since the stops will effectively lift the tray away from the tissues and it may then appear underextended. Alginate is the most commonly used impression material (2–3 mm spacer required) — if other elastic materials are favoured (e.g. silicone rubbers) the spacing can be reduced accordingly.

Adhesive specific to the impression material is more efficient than depending solely on holes drilled in the trays for retention.

Close-fitting special trays

As the term implies no spacing is used. Zinc oxide–eugenol paste is the material of choice and is accurate in thin film but requires adequate support — especially at the borders. Correct tray extension is therefore important and can best be achieved by checking that the borders are slightly short (1–2 mm) of the functional depth of the sulci and then using greenstick tracing compound (or other suitable material) to establish the optimum extension. This technique will define not only the depth of the sulcus but also its width. This combination can be used for upper and lower impressions as provided there are no bony undercuts. It has the advantage that it is stable when set and less susceptible to distortion than alginate, a useful adjunct if laboratory services are not available on the premises. No adhesive is necessary for zinc oxide–eugenol but the tray must be clean and dry.

The flabby upper ridge

The combination of complete upper denture opposing lower anterior natural teeth may result in the destruction of the maxillary alveolar ridge opposite the natural teeth and replacement with fibrous tissue. To minimize displacement a low viscosity alginate or plaster of Paris can be used for the impression. An alternative is to take a two stage impression using a zinc oxide–eugenol paste in a close-fitting tray which covers only the firm part and then filling in the anterior region with a fluid mix of plaster of Paris.

Functional impressions

A functional impression material can be defined as 'one which is applied to the fitting surface of a denture for the purpose of securing an impression under functional stresses.' Temporary soft lining materials demonstrate viscoelastic properties, that is they have some plastic flow and some elastic recovery. Although they have an overlap of ideal properties they may still be used as functional impression materials to yield accurate impressions of oral structures.

Since these materials do not harden rapidly, an impression over an extended period is obtained. The muscles and attachments therefore have the maximum opportunity to exert their influence. It is preferable that the denture (plus temporary soft lining material) should remain in the mouth for 4–6 h, bearing in mind that the materials cease to flow and become elastic after a few hours.

The type of case that may benefit from the functional impression technique is one where the old denture has recently become loose because of changes in the denture-bearing tissues. Before applying the functional impression material the border extension of the denture should be checked and corrected. The cast should be poured immediately the denture is removed from the mouth because of the rapid recovery of these materials.

The neutral zone impression

Learning to control the shape of a new denture can be difficult even for the younger person but it is a special problem for the elderly since ageing is characterized by loss of adaptation. This problem can be avoided when there is evidence that an existing denture has been worn satisfactorily. The control of the denture is dependent on habituation (the gradual diminution of responses to continued or repeated stimuli) to proprioceptive signals from the masticatory apparatus, which in turn leads to efficient response by the oral musculature. When a new denture is required it therefore makes sense to construct it to the same overall shape as the original and make most use of the existing habituation. A copy (duplication) technique is recommended in these cases.

However, when no satisfactory denture exists an attempt can be made to provide the technician with information on the potential denture space (neutral zone) where there is least muscular conflict. Provided the artificial teeth and denture base fit into this space the denture should be stabilized by opposing muscle action. Since most problems arise with lower complete dentures, this procedure is most commonly applied to the lower arch.

Procedure

1. A self-curing acrylic resin baseplate is made on the working model to which wire retaining loops are attached, centrally placed.
2. A suitable impression material (e.g. silicone putty using half the normal amount of reactor paste/liquid to allow extra working time, or temporary soft lining material with additional powder in the mix to give it a more viscous body) is placed on the baseplate in the general shape of an occlusal rim.
3. The baseplate is placed in the mouth and the impression material moulded by a range of normal oral muscular movements — swallowing, licking the lips and speaking.
4. When set to a stable form the impression is removed and inspected.
5. In the laboratory, plaster indices are moulded around lingual, labial and buccal aspects and, with the original baseplate removed, molten wax is poured into the space.
6. The artificial teeth are set into the wax by removing only sufficient wax to gain the necessary space — the overall shape of the neutral zone is therefore maintained.
7. The upper teeth are set to the lower and the wax-up is ready for the try-in visit.

PARTIAL DENTURES

Satisfactory partial denture construction is dependent upon a sequence of events being followed:

(a) preliminary impressions;
(b) survey of study casts;
(c) partial denture design;
(d) tooth preparation — rest seats;
(e) working impressions.

This will ensure that adequate thought is given to planning prior to the all-important working impression stage.

Although it is accepted practice to follow this pattern there are occasions when a single-stage impression technique is appropriate. These might include single tooth replacement with a simple acrylic-resin immediate denture.

Preliminary impressions

The presence of natural teeth invariably means that there are undercuts which necessitates the use of an elastic impression material. As with complete dentures, either metal stock trays or plastic disposable trays can be used. The trays might require modification when several teeth are missing. For example, impression compound can be used to adapt extensive edentulous free-end saddle areas prior to the impression being taken in alginate. This ensures that the alginate is used in reasonably even section and hence gives greater accuracy.

Working impressions

The most commonly used impression material for partially edentulous mouths is alginate. It is sufficiently accurate, when supported by an evenly spaced tray, for the construction of cobalt–chromium frameworks. However it does have its limitations:

1. It is likely to tear on removal from severe undercuts.
2. Dimensional stability is poor due to syneresis.
3. The setting reaction is faster at higher temperatures — the material in contact with the tissues therefore sets first, which may give rise to stresses within the material if the tray is moved during setting.

The likelihood of tearing can be reduced by blocking out interproximal areas provided they are not essential to the overall impression. Soft carding wax is a suitable material since it is easy to apply and to remove. If it is necessary to reproduce severe undercuts, then an elastomeric impression material should be chosen, i.e. polyether, silicone or polysulphide. The polyethers are stiffer than other elastomers and may therefore be difficult to withdraw from severe undercuts. All three materials are expensive, relative to alginate, and therefore not frequently used in impressions requiring large quantities of material. They are, however, more dimensionably stable and should be considered when the impression cannot be cast within 30 min of removal from the mouth.

Opinions vary regarding the best impression technique for the lower arch with extensive free-end saddles. The single-stage elastic impression produces a cast which represents the hard and soft tissues at rest (mucostatic). It has been argued that a functional relationship should exist between the various supporting structures. To achieve this and to control the load applied to both teeth and ridges there are two main approaches:

(a) reduce the load;
(b) distribute the load between teeth and residual ridges.

The load can be reduced by leaving a tooth off the saddles and/or by using narrow teeth. Distribution of load is more complex and includes such methods as stress breaking and various combinations of the position of rests and clasps. Mucocompressive impression techniques attempt to distribute the load by reproducing the tissues covering the ridge as they are under load.

Free-end saddle rock (downward movement of the saddle under load) can occur if the denture is constructed using a mucostatic impression when there is displacable mucosa overlying the edentulous ridge. When load is applied to the occlusal surface of the artificial teeth, part of the force is transmitted through the denture base and displaces the underlying mucosa. The degree of movement of the saddle will depend on the load applied and the condition of the tissues underneath it.

Although it is possible to use a dual impression technique comprising a first stage mucocompressive impression of the saddle areas with an overall alginate final impression, this is a cumbersome procedure. An easier, and more effective, way is to construct the metal framework on a cast from a mucostatic impression and then to obtain mucocompressive impressions of the saddle areas in order to modify these areas of the cast. This is known as the altered cast technique.

Procedure for altered cast technique

1. Working impression in alginate taken in evenly spaced special tray.
2. Construction of cobalt–chromium framework with the addition of close-fitting saddles.
3. Clinical trial of the metal framework.
4. Border trimming of the saddles using greenstick tracing compound — or other suitable material.
5. Zinc oxide–eugenol paste (or elastomer or impression wax) impression of the saddle areas ensuring that the metal framework is held firmly in position on the teeth whilst the material sets; no direct load is applied to the saddle areas — this ensures the fit of the framework is not disturbed.
6. In the laboratory the free-end saddles are cut away from the original working cast and the denture then seated in place; the cast is made good by pouring gypsum into the saddle areas.
7. The saddle areas are processed onto the metal framework using the altered working cast.

This technique has the advantage that it should avoid free-end saddle rock occurring with a new denture. However, it requires additional clinical and laboratory stages which, it can be argued, are not always necessary. An alternative approach is to complete construction of the partial denture on the original working cast and to assess the fit in the mouth. If a free-end saddle rock is evident the fitting surface of the free-end saddles will require modification. This can be completed using either a chairside or laboratory reline.

Chairside reline

A chairside reline can be completed using one of the self-curing resins marketed for use in the mouth. Most of these contain polybutyl (methacrylate) monomer to avoid tissue irritation (e.g. Total, Peripheral Seal). The technique is as follows:

1. Having checked for correct extension, the fitting surface of the saddles and the borders are cleaned and dried — they can be roughened if the resin is not 'fresh'.

2. Bonding agent, if supplied, is painted sparingly on the area to be relined.

3. By following the manufacturers' instructions a mix of the resin is applied to the saddle areas and the denture inserted in the mouth.

4. The framework is held firmly in place with no direct load being applied to the saddles.

5. After 2 or 3 min the denture is removed whilst the resin is still rubbery to check that it has not flowed into undercut areas and that there are no imperfections.

6. Excess can be trimmed away with a sharp knife and the denture returned to the mouth for a further period to allow curing.

7. When rigid, the borders are trimmed and polished.

8. A final check is made of the occlusion.

Such a reline should last many months and has the advantage that it is completed with the patient present. A period without the denture is therefore avoided. It is also suitable for domiciliary visits.

Laboratory reline

A laboratory reline requires impressions of the saddles which can be completed using zinc oxide–eugenol paste, elastomers or impression wax. It may be necessary to reduce undercuts to prevent fracture of the stone model when the denture is removed and also to grind a thickness from the fitting surface to make more space available for the impression material. As before, the fitting relationship of the metal framework to the natural teeth must be maintained by ensuring that the occlusal rests are correctly seated throughout the impression. Readjustment of the occlusion must be anticipated.

If a reline at the fit stage of denture construction is a planned procedure, sufficient space to accommodate the impression material can be predetermined by using metal foil 1 mm thick over the saddles prior to adding the acrylic resin in the laboratory.

Chapter 32

Articulators

The articulator is an instrument on which the casts of the maxillary and mandibular dentitions or edentulous ridges are mounted so that their static and dynamic relationships to each other can be reproduced. All articulators consist of an upper and lower arm joined by a hinge or hinges of varying degrees of complexity, and the design of the hinge mechanism is the basis of their classification.

TYPES OF ARTICULATOR

Plain hinge articulators

These instruments have the single function of relating the casts to each other in the intercuspal position only. No movement other than the vertical hinge movement is possible; this path of movement is likely to be inaccurate because the casts are not mounted in the same relationship to the hinge of the articulator as the jaws bear to the hinge axis of the condyle.

Average value articulators

This type of articulator has a double hinge mechanism which allows protrusive movement of the mandibular cast relative to the maxillary cast along a path that guides the hinge axis through an angle based on average values for the condylar path. The angle cannot be adjusted and is usually 30° relative to the horizontal plane. Some average value articulators also have allowance for lateral movement and this usually reproduces the average value for the Bennett movement of 15° relative to the sagittal plane. In addition, the instrument may be designed to allow the use of a face bow to transfer the radius of the arc through which the mandible moves towards the maxilla with the condyle on its retruded axis. Since the condylar angle cannot be adjusted in its relationship to the occlusal plane, it is essential that the casts be mounted with the occlusal plane horizontal and that the orbital pointer is not used with the face bow.

Adjustable articulators

In addition to accepting a face bow transfer record of the radius of the hinge arc of movement, these instruments allow adjustments which may include the following:

1. The condyle angle path in the sagittal plane relative to the Frankfort (horizontal) plane.

2. The condyle path in a medial and medio-protrusive direction (these are known as immediate and progressive side-shift respectively) of the non-working side condyle.

3. The relationship of the angle of the occlusal plane to the Frankfort plane.

4. The intercondylar distance.

5. The angle of guidance of the incisal pin in protrusive and lateral movements — this is anterior guidance.

Arcon and non-arcon articulators

A further subdivision of articulators is based on one aspect of the design of the hinge mechanism. Many types of instrument have the rotating axis element of the hinge fixed to the maxillary arm. This differs from the anatomical situation in which the hinge axis of the condyle bears a fixed relationship to the mandibular teeth since they are part of the same bone, the mandible. The consequence of this is that during protrusion of the natural mandible the axis of movement moves downwards and forwards whereas on this type of articulator (known as the non-arcon) the axis moves upwards and backwards.

In order to achieve a greater degree of accuracy, articulators have been designed with the rotating hinge axis as part of the mandibular arm, thus overcoming the above mentioned problem. Such instruments have become known as arcon articulators (e.g. all Denar models) being *ar*ticulators with *con*dyles.

THE FACE BOW

The face bow is an instrument with two functions:

1. To transfer the distance from the retruded axis of the mandible to the maxillary teeth. In effect this is the radius of the arc of movement of the mandible relative to the maxilla in centric relation.

2. The orientation of the angle of the (upper) occlusal plane relative to the horizontal or Frankfort plane.

Function (1) is carried out by placing the condyle rods centrally over the estimated or arbitrary position of the condyle axes and fixing the bite fork on the upper teeth. Function (2) is achieved by positioning the orbital pointer on the lower border of the orbit; this is the anterior reference point of the Frankfort plane.

Chapter 33

Design of partial dentures

INTRODUCTION

A partial denture is a removable prosthesis provided for a dental arch in which one or more natural teeth remain. Artificial replacement may be necessary if teeth have been lost due to caries, periodontal disease, trauma, planned extractions related to orthodontic treatment, or when some permanent teeth have failed to form (hypodontia).

Although replacement of missing teeth may improve masticatory efficiency and permit better speech patterns, aesthetics is the prime motivating factor for most patients who request a partial denture. Failure to replace missing teeth can lead to a number of consequences which include:

(a) drifting and tilting of adjacent teeth;
(b) over-eruption of unopposed teeth;
(c) disruption of the occlusion;
(d) plaque and debris stagnation areas.

However, the probable advantages of constructing a partial denture should be carefully weighed against the possible sequel of damage to the supporting structures caused by the change in the oral environment. Long-term studies have demonstrated the disastrous effects that can be caused to the teeth over a period of time by poorly maintained partial dentures. It is important that they should be designed and constructed to promote and not endanger the health of the oral tissues. A high standard of oral hygiene is essential.

ORAL HEALTH AND PARTIAL DENTURES

It is well established that plaque is involved in the development of dental caries and gingivitis. The mechanism whereby gingivitis progresses to periodontal disease is less well understood but is probably influenced by variations in the quantity and nature of the plaque. Because the insertion of a foreign body, in the form of a partial denture, into the mouth is likely to affect plaque formation, it is obviously important to design the denture to minimize possible risks. A number of factors can be listed as a result of various scientific studies:

1. Plaque accumulation on a denture is related to the oral hygiene of the individual.
2. Greater amounts of plaque are found in those who wear their dentures day and night.

3. Teeth in contact with a partial denture are likely to accumulate more plaque than those which are not.
4. Wearing a partial denture causes a general increase in plaque levels around the mouth.
5. The areas of the mouth most susceptible to plaque build-up are those underneath or immediately adjacent to the partial denture.
6. The design of the components of the partial denture can influence plaque levels.
7. A partial denture worn in one arch can cause an increase in plaque in the opposing arch.
8. The reaction of the tissues to the damaging effects of plaque, although influenced by its quantity and quality, are dependent more on host tissue response.

PARTIAL DENTURE COMPONENTS

The design of a partial denture and its component parts will influence its ability to attract and retain plaque and food debris. Important principles of design must be followed if a denture is to function successfully and provide an environment that puts the tissues at minimal risk.

Complexity of design

Fussy and overcomplicated designs are not only more likely to collect food debris but are less well tolerated by the patient. Only those components with essential functions should be included; a systematic approach to design will ensure good design concepts are followed. Unnecessary complexity of design will also increase laboratory costs.

Major connectors

Comparative studies of plaque indices with lingual-bar and lingual-plate connectors have shown that plates, which cover both teeth and gingival margins, are likely to be detrimental, causing increased plaque build-up. In the lower arch, it is usually possible to use either a lingual bar or sublingual bar to avoid gingival coverage. In the upper arch a wide variety of plate/strap/bar combinations are possible, however, the concept of avoiding gingival coverage should be followed wherever possible. The Every concept is a 'clean' design allowing maximum palatal coverage but keeping margins free of the gingivae.

Gingival margins

Minor connectors must cover the gingival margins at some point in order to join the component parts to the major connector. In the saddle area, controversy exists as to whether the minor connector should take the form of a close fit against a guide plane contacting the mesial/distal surface of the tooth down to the gingival margin, or a 3 mm open design with a theoretical self-cleansing space. The close-fit, box-shaped option has considerable advantage in terms of retention if the guide planes of the abutment teeth can be made parallel. There is some evidence that the close-fit increases gingival temperatures but differences in plaque levels have not been shown to be significant.

Other research has shown that if gingival margins must be covered by acrylic resin prostheses that they should be as closely adapted as is practicable. If relief is incorporated over gingival margins the evidence suggests that gingival enlargement will occur to fill the space. The larger the relief, the greater the gingival enlargement.

If a plate design is used in the upper arch, every effort should be made to minimize gingival coverage to reduce plaque levels. It is possible to construct mucosa-supported dentures in the upper arch because of the additional large support area of the palate. However, a plate design in the lower arch should take some support from the teeth to avoid trauma to the gingival margins due to the 'gum stripping' downward movement of the denture under occlusal load. A plate designed for the mandible should, therefore, include occlusal rests and cover the greater part of the lingual surfaces of the teeth. It is not practical to maintain gingival clearance with a lower acrylic-resin plate because of the inherent weakness of the material.

Clasps

Clasps will retain plaque against the tissues and should, therefore, be designed to minimize the problem. They should be of simple design on the basis that less metalwork will attract less plaque. There is some evidence that gingivally approaching clasps, because they cross the gingival margin, may be potentially more damaging. However, because of their improved aesthetics and retention capability their use is widespread.

DAMAGE CAUSED BY PARTIAL DENTURES

Poorly designed and/or poorly maintained partial dentures are likely to cause damage to the mouth. An unsatisfactory standard of oral hygiene will aggravate the situation. Possible damage can include:

(a) caries;
(b) periodontal disease;
(c) tooth mobility;
(d) alveolar bone resorption;
(e) wear of teeth;
(f) temporomandibular joint dysfunction.

As already discussed, plaque is the main culprit. A combination of plaque and excessive occlusal loading may result in more rapid destruction of the periodontal supporting tissues. Insufficient tooth support or a rocking framework is likely to overload individual teeth and cause mobility. Similarly, insufficient support and/or saddle under extension may cause excessive loading of saddle areas and alveolar bone resorption. This is commonly seen with lower free-end saddle dentures, which may rock around the distal abutment teeth. Wear of acrylic-resin artificial teeth may place more of the occlusal load onto the natural teeth, leading to progressive wear and possible loss of occlusal vertical dimension. Occasionally, tooth wear and/or poor occlusion of the partial denture may lead to temporomandibular joint dysfunction.

Many of these destructive phases can be reduced or eliminated by regular inspection and maintenance of the dentures, including saddle relines and replacement of worn teeth.

IS A PARTIAL DENTURE NECESSARY?

The decision to make a partial denture will depend on a number of factors which include:

(a) aesthetic considerations;
(b) masticatory function;
(c) stability of the occlusion;
(d) speech;
(e) oral hygiene;
(f) patient motivation.

The loss of anterior teeth with the resultant change in appearance is an obvious argument for tooth replacement (which may of course include bridgework). Masticatory function may not be seriously diminished until a number of posterior teeth are missing, and there is evidence to suggest that many partial dentures do little to improve masticatory function. Bilateral free-end saddle dentures, although the most necessary to improve function, are notoriously difficult to wear and therefore often fail to fulfil expectations.

Single, or small numbers, of missing posterior teeth do not necessarily require replacement. The stability of the occlusion must be assessed and future changes taken into consideration. The time factor is most important. If the teeth have been missing for only a short period of time and there is already evidence of deterioration of the occlusion (e.g. tilting, drifting or over-eruption), then replacement is necessary. Conversely, long-standing tooth loss with little evidence of adverse reaction can be left alone, provided the situation is assessed at regular intervals in the future.

Speech may be affected by the loss of one or more anterior teeth but individuals show remarkable adaptation to the loss of many posterior teeth. Replacement to restore or improve speech should therefore be decided on individual merit.

The standard of oral hygiene may well influence the practitioners' decision to recommend the construction of a partial denture. It is easier for a patient with little motivation to maintain a modest standard of oral hygiene without a denture than with one. If all else is equal it is wiser not to construct a denture.

In many cases, when the decision to replace missing teeth is not clear-cut, it is best left to the patient to suggest partial denture construction. If there is a lack of motivation there is a strong possibility that the prosthesis will fail simply because it is easier not to wear it than to have to persevere. Considerable amounts of money are wasted constructing dentures which are never worn.

INFORMATION REQUIRED FOR PARTIAL DENTURE DESIGN

For satisfactory partial denture design both the patient and the mouth must be assessed. The assessment should include:

(a) patient's response/motivation;
(b) aesthetic considerations;
(c) previous partial denture design and experience;
(d) examination of the mouth;
(e) oral hygiene;
(f) study casts;
(g) radiographs.

It has already been emphasized that patient motivation is of considerable importance and is linked to aesthetics. The dental history should take into account previous denture-wearing experience and the success, or otherwise, of the dentures in relation to their design and materials.

An examination of the mouth should include the teeth and supporting tissues and a measure of the oral hygiene. The mouth should be inspected with and without any existing denture — note being made of its general fit, retention, occlusion and aesthetics.

Impressions of both arches will be necessary for study casts and these can be used for a number of purposes:

(a) surveying;
(b) examination of the occlusion;
(c) trial preparation or alteration of teeth;
(d) partial denture design;
(e) construction of special trays;
(f) explanation of proposed treatment to the patient.

Surveying

Study casts must be surveyed to make the following essential decisions:

(a) path of insertion and removal;
(b) location and depth of undercuts;
(c) need for tooth preparation;
(d) position and material of clasps.

Paths of insertion will be limited by the remaining teeth and tissue undercuts. A suitable path of insertion will provide optimum aesthetics and perhaps utilize existing tissue undercuts for additional retention. An example of this would be when teeth are missing in the upper anterior region and there is a labial bony undercut present; tilting the cast with the heel down may permit close adaptation of the artificial teeth to the natural teeth and more efficient utilization of the labial undercut.

Once the path of insertion is defined the appropriate teeth can be analysed for suitable undercuts and the survey lines marked in pencil. It is generally accepted that a cobalt–chromium clasp should only engage 0.25 mm of undercut (and a wrought wire clasp not more than 0.5 mm), and it is therefore necessary to measure for this depth of undercut and mark its location. If insufficient undercut is available it may be necessary to consider modifying the tooth. If the tooth is sound, the addition of a small bulge of acid etch-bonded composite resin may solve an otherwise difficult problem. When a restoration is required it is possible to alter the shape of the tooth accordingly. Occasionally, crowns may be the only way to provide a satisfactory environment for a retentive partial denture.

SYSTEMATIC DESIGN

A stage-by-stage design plan will ensure that consideration is given to all components, ensuring a logical build-up of the design and a biologically and mechanically correct denture.

It is, of course, possible for a number of designs to fulfil the necessary requirements for the same mouth. Provided certain basic principles are adhered to the prosthesis will function efficiently and will minimize any possible damaging effects. The materials chosen will, of course, influence the design and must be taken into account.

A partial denture must always be considered to form part of an overall restorative treatment plan. Its design should, therefore, be formulated as part of the plan to ensure that restorations are completed so as to optimize the function of the denture and prolong the health of the mouth.

The saddles

A decision must be made on which missing teeth require replacement and the saddles marked accordingly on the design plan.

There are a number of methods of classifying saddles and partially edentulous arches; however, the Kennedy classification is widely accepted. It classifies edentulous areas into four types:

Class I	Bilateral edentulous areas which lie posterior to the remaining teeth
Class II	A single edentulous area which lies posterior to the remaining teeth
Class III	A single edentulous area bounded by teeth anteriorly and posteriorly
Class IV	A single edentulous area which lies anteriorly to the remaining teeth

Modifications are possible to Classes I, II and III but not to Class IV because if teeth other than anteriors are also missing it changes the basic classification to I, II or III.

DESIGN OF PARTIAL DENTURES

Support

Partial denture support can be derived from three sources:

1. *Teeth*. The vertical forces of occlusion and mastication are distributed to the abutment teeth through occlusal, incisal or cingulum rests.
2. *Mucosa*. No support is provided by the natural teeth and the load is transferred through the mucosa to the underlying alveolar bone (and palate in the maxillary arch).
3. *Teeth and mucosa*. Support can be provided by both teeth and mucosa in the edentulous areas in the case of free-end saddle dentures.

The choice of support will depend on the number, location and condition of the remaining teeth. Adequate rests must be provided for tooth-borne dentures and rest seat preparation is usually necessary. Mucosa-borne dentures should be extended to cover as large an area as possible to adequately distribute the load, and for this reason are only suitable in the upper arch.

Retention

Additional resistance to vertical displacement can be provided by retentive units. These comprise a clasp, rest and bracing arm. One of the functions of the rest is to ensure relocation of the clasp into an identical position on the tooth on each insertion of the denture.

There are two basic forms of clasps:

(a) occlusally approaching;
(b) gingivally approaching.

Many variations of these two forms exist but with any clasp only the terminal position of the arm should engage the undercut. The clasp arm is passive in situ until activated when the denture is inserted or removed, i.e. as the retentive portion of the clasp moves towards the survey line. A lateral orthodontic force is produced as the arm moves over the point of maximum bulbosity, and a bracing (reciprocating) component should therefore be included in the design.

Indirect retention

Indirect retention provides resistance to rotational dislodging forces and is necessary in Kennedy Class I, II and IV cases. When the saddles are displaced, rotations can occur around a fulcrum axis, which is an imaginary line drawn through abutment teeth and their retainers. Resistance to displacement of the saddles is provided by placing a rest (indirect retainer) as far as possible from the rotation axis on the opposite side of the arch.

Prevention of horizontal displacement

Anteroposterior displacement of free-end and Kennedy Class IV saddles is possible unless resisted. This can be achieved by placing rests mesially and encircling the teeth with retentive units in the case of free-end saddles. Displacement of Kennedy Class IV saddles can also be resisted by retentive units. Bracing arms and minor connectors play a role in preventing other lateral movements.

Connectors

Major connectors join the components on one side of the arch to the other, and minor connectors are the links between the components and the major connector.

In the upper arch, because of the larger support area of the palate, many variations of major connectors in the form of plates and bars are possible. In the lower arch, there are five main categories:

(a) lingual bar;
(b) sublingual bar;
(c) lingual plate;
(d) dental bar;
(e) buccal bar.

The ideal major connector is rigid, well tolerated by the patient and is sited well away (at least 3 mm) from the gingival margins. The sublingual bar fulfils these requirements for the lower arch. It is placed in the full depth of the lingual sulcus and also utilizes the width of the functional sulcus. Patient toleration is high and, because of the increased bulk, it has maximum rigidity. Although this connector has many advantages its use requires a meticulous impression of the lingual sulcus and its acceptance in general dental practice has been limited.

Choice of materials

Two metals are available for cast metal frameworks — cobalt–chromium and gold. The high modulus of elasticity of cobalt–chromium makes it very suitable for major connectors but greater flexibility is preferable for clasps. Gold has approximately half the modulus of elasticity of cobalt–chromium and is less suitable for major connectors but ideal for clasps. Since cost is obviously an overriding factor the use of gold is limited.

Other materials can be used for simple designs. For example, a lingual bar can be formed from wrought stainless steel; acrylic resin can be suitable for an upper palatal plate. Wrought stainless-steel wire can be incorporated into acrylic resin to form rests or clasps. The choice of materials will depend upon the clinical situation, intricacy of design and cost.

The RPI system

Special mention should be made of the RPI concept which attempts to distribute the masticatory loads between the edentulous saddles and abutment teeth. There is evidence to suggest that if the occlusal rest is placed mesially, more favourable and more evenly distributed loading occurs. A minor connector, the distal plate, joins the rest to the major connector and an I-bar clasp is used with its tip positioned on or anterior to the midpoint of the buccal surface of the tooth. The three parts, rest–plate–I-bar, hold the tooth firmly and no bracing arm is necessary. The distal plate lies on the 3–4 mm long guide plane so that when the denture is fully seated the plate contacts only the lower 1 mm of that surface (the portion over the gingiva is relieved). Thus RPI is:

R — mesial *R*est
P — distal *P*late
I — retentive *I*-bar

Load on the saddle causes the denture to rotate about the occlusal rest. The distal plate and I-bar tend to disengage, preventing further stress being imposed on the abutment tooth.

SUMMARY

Partial denture design should follow four basic guidelines:

(a) simplicity;
(b) support from the teeth;
(c) relief of gingivae;
(d) rigid connectors.

Only those components necessary to serve a definite function should be included in the design, and the smallest number of clasp units compatible with retention and stability should be used. In general, simple designs are better tolerated by patients.

Whenever possible, teeth should be used for support. The additional area of the periodontal fibres reduces the load which would otherwise be taken solely on saddle areas. In the lower arch, with its reduced support area, it is especially important to take advantage of the remaining teeth.

Coverage of gingival margins is likely to increase plaque accumulation, leading to damage of the gingival and eventually the periodontal tissues. If gingival coverage is unavoidable, the denture should be as closely adapted as is practical to avoid tissue growing into the space.

A rigid connector ensures even distribution of forces to all the supporting structures on both sides of the arch. Thin connectors can flex during function and are likely to be easily distorted or fracture through fatigue failure.

Chapter 34

Duplication of full dentures

Duplication has become an increasingly popular method of replacing old and worn full dentures. With this method, one can reproduce the polished surface of the existing dentures, and 'add' a new fitting surface. Aesthetic requirements can also be attended to, and a new denture created, retaining the good features of the old one.

Full dentures are controlled by oral muscles via the polished surfaces. The control is an acquired skill learnt by habituation. This learning process is reduced in elderly patients. Therefore, the duplication of the polished surfaces of the existing dentures for old patients is often the treatment of choice. This can be the case, too, in the replacement of immediate dentures. This may occur some 6 months after the extractions and fitting of the initial dentures, and although resorption of the ridges will have taken place, the teeth on the original denture will be placed in the 'neutral zone' and their position will be of value in the subsequent assessment upon remaking the dentures.

AIM

The aim of duplication, therefore, is to reproduce the features of the existing denture whilst introducing controlled modifications.

METHOD

The methods for duplication are essentially similar, only the materials differ. The object is to encase the denture in a material supported by a rigid tray, remove the denture from the mould, and replace it with a material suitable for use in the mouth as a template for the original. This template must be strong enough to be adjusted in the mouth, and to be worked upon by the technician. For this reason, the template is usually made of cold-cure acrylic as follows.

   1. Using stock plastic trays with alginate to surround the denture — the mould can then be filled with cold-cure.
   2. As above, using heavy-bodied silicone material instead of alginate. This gives a more stable impression, and results in a more accurate template.
   3. Small boxes, such as soap boxes, can be used as a tray system with either material, and wax may be used to replace the cold-cure.

The most accurate of all the above will be the use of silicone material combined with a cold-cure template.

CLINICAL TECHNIQUE

First visit

Treatment plan:

(a) to restore worn teeth and occlusal face height;
(b) to restore the incisal relationship, as this may be in a Class III position due to wear over the years;
(c) to restore the fitting surface.

With the old F/F in the mouth, use a wax wafer to correct the vertical dimension and then to take a registration of the bite. If dramatic changes have to be made, the denture can be built up on the occlusal and incisal surfaces with cold-cure, and the degree of opening which the patient can tolerate assessed over a period of time by adjusting the height of the added acrylic. Centre lines and occlusal planes (anterior and posterior) are marked on the wax wafer. The tooth shade and mould are checked. The duplicates are made by one of the above methods.

In the laboratory the duplicates are aligned on a plane-line articulator using the wax wafer. The teeth are replaced to the marks on the wax wafer.

Second visit

Wax trial of the dentures takes place. If all is well, the impressions can be taken in the acrylic template, using either a zinc oxide–eugenol paste, or one of the light-bodied silicone impression materials. The closed-mouth technique, i.e. taking both impressions at once with the patient's teeth together, is the favoured method. It may be desirable at this stage to border-mould the template with greenstick composition or Peripheral Seal if extension of the original denture was considered inadequate.

Third visit

The dentures are fitted in the usual way, with the customary attention to peripheries and occlusion.

Chapter 35

Problems involving the oral mucosa with particular reference to prosthetics

Such problems can be broadly considered under three headings:
(a) systemic;
(b) dentures;
(c) oral ulceration other than by denture trauma.

SYSTEMIC

Nutritional deficiencies

In the Western world it is rare to see advanced cases of nutritional deficiency. A well-balanced diet consists of adequate intake of protein, fat, carbohydrate, vitamins and mineral salts. Sometimes the intake is adequate but absorption is poor due possibly to gastrointestinal disorder such as Crohn's disease or to the sequlae of jejunal resection or partial gastrectomy.

Inadequate diet is sometimes found in the elderly who do not bother to prepare meals, in the sufferers from gastric ulceration whose treatment involves a restricted diet, and in anorexia due to chronic alcoholism.

Vitamin deficiencies

These are mainly responsible for oral mucosal changes, particularly the B group of vitamins.

B-group deficiencies manifest themselves in the mouth as angular cheilitis, fissuring of the lips and atrophic changes in the tongue. The tongue appears smooth and glazed due to atrophy of the papillae, it is sometimes angry-red and fissured, and often sore. The vitamin deficiencies which produce most changes in the mouth are of riboflavine (B_2), nicotinic acid and pyridoxine (B_6).

Vitamin B_2 is normally absorbed after being acted on by an 'intrinsic factor' produced by the gastric mucosa. In pernicious anaemia this factor is deficient, resulting in inadequate absorption of the vitamin. Folic acid deficiency results in poor development of bone marrow and megaloblastic anaemia.

In dental practice there are very few indications for the prescription of individual members of the vitamin B complex, as a single deficiency of any one is highly unlikely.

The second possible nutritional deficiency is that of iron. It occurs more frequently than the vitamin deficiencies and manifests itself in the form of iron deficiency anaemia. Women are more prone to this than men, particularly in the age group where there is blood loss due to menstruation. In men, iron-deficiency anaemia is rare but does occur when there is occult bleeding from peptic ulcers or blood loss from haemorrhoids.

The oral mucous membrane is pale and there is atrophy of the papillae of the tongue, which also becomes pale. Soreness of the tongue is also a feature. In one study, some 39% of diagnosed anaemic patients complained of soreness of the tongue.

Angular cheilitis is a common condition associated with iron deficiency anaemia.

Xerostomia

Dryness of the mouth is not confined to patients with dentures but when they are present it frequently leads to soreness of the tongue and mucosa.

Xerostomia can be transient, as in acute anxiety — or chronic, when it can be divided into two distinct groups:

1. *Disorders of function*: where the glands are normal but salivary flow is reduced. Common causes are the effects of drugs — tranquillizers, particularly tricyclic antidepressants, antihistamines and hypotensives. Other causes:

    (a) mouth breathing;
    (b) heavy smoking;
    (c) loss of fluid through sweating;
    (d) increased excretion of urine as in diabetes mellitus and insipidus;
    (e) radiotherapy in the region extending from the base of the neck to the base of the skull.

2. *Organic disease of the salivary glands*: Sjögren's syndrome — dry mouth, dry eyes and connective tissue disorder.

The oral tissues are frequently sore, the patient may complain of a burning sensation in the tongue or a metallic taste. There is often superimposed low-grade candidiasis which can result in angular cheilitis and inflamed mucosa.

Tuberculosis

Oral tuberculosis is relatively uncommon today. It usually occurs as secondary to pulmonary tuberculosis. The tuberculous ulcers have an undermined edge. Biopsy or smear culture should be made.

Syphilis

The incidence of syphilis appeared to have been reduced by modern therapy but there is now evidence that the disease is on the increase. Primary chancre is usually on the lips; 'snailtrack' ulcers on the cheeks and tongue (secondary syphilis); and deep 'punched out' ulcers on the palate (tertiary syphilis).

Aphthous ulceration (details in Chapter 43)

The causes of this common condition are still not clear. Onset is around puberty. Typically the ulcers develop in groups of between two to four and take about 14 days to heal without scarring. The first 4–6 days are the most painful. Creams containing local anaesthetic can be used to lessen the pain before meals.

Lichen planus (details in Chapter 45)

The oral lesions frequently precede the skin lesions and tend to give rise to more discomfort. Many appearances have been described: papular, reticular, linear and bullous forms as well as ulceration. Causes are unknown. Trauma should be eliminated, i.e. from hot liquids, smoking, highly spiced foods, denture trauma. Whether it is a premalignant condition is controversial.

Carcinoma (see also Chapters 43, 44, 45)

The commonest cause of malignant oral ulceration is squamous cell carcinoma. The commonest sites are the side of the tongue and floor of the mouth. Any ulcer which has been present for longer than 2 weeks should be biopsied.

DENTURE CAUSES OF ORAL MUCOSA PROBLEMS

Denture induced stomatitis

This occurs most commonly in the upper jaw. The region of the hard palate is often brightly erythematous and sharply delineates the borders of the denture. It is frequently not painful, therefore patients are often unaware of its presence. It occurs more frequently in females, possibly due to endocrine imbalance or vaginal carriage of *Candida*. It can be confined to the palate but frequently there is an associated angular cheilitis (see below). The most common cause is trauma due to the movement of an ill-fitting denture combined with superimposed *Candida* infection. The *Candida* proliferates on the microbial plaque on the fit surface of the denture.

Treatment consists of either leaving the offending denture out (this is undesirable in the elderly) or removing the cause of the trauma by occlusal adjustment and tissue conditioning in conjunction with antifungal treatment.

Inflammatory papillary hyperplasia of the palate

The palatal mucosa acquires the appearance of a mulberry that is raspberry-red in colour. It is believed to be caused by chronic irritation, possibly by long-term movement of a rough denture surface over the palatal mucosa. Treatment involves the removal of the causes of trauma, tissue conditioning and possible surgical removal of the nodules. In severe cases the nodules may remain in reduced form. If new dentures are constructed, the fit surface must be made free from any sharp acrylic spicules by stoning. If a metal palate is required, it should be made of wrought stainless steel not cast chrome.

Angular cheilitis (stomatitis)

This is an erosive, erythematous lesion of the corners of the mouth. It is most commonly seen in denture wearers, where it usually affects both corners of the mouth. If allowed to go untreated for a long period it can result in scarring and, in extreme cases, reduction in the orifice. There is usually superimposed candidal infection and associated denture stomatitis.

Causes
1. Inadequate soft tissue support resulting in creasing of the skin; this in turn results in continued presence of saliva which causes maceration.
2. Overclosure.
3. Iron deficiency anaemia.
4. Nutritional deficiencies, e.g. vitamins B and C, and folic acid.

Treatment consists of elimination of local infection by application of miconazole oral gel together with scrupulous denture scrubbing and disinfection using 0.1% aqueous chlorhexidine.

Denture-induced hyperplasia

Seen in patients who have worn ill-fitting dentures over very long periods. It is most often present as flaps of fibrous tissue at the mucosal reflection in the upper, but more commonly, the lower labial region. There may be single or multiple flaps lying over the other in folds separated by a series of clefts. The cause is chronic alternating ulceration and healing with fibrous reaction to the trauma of an over-extended denture flange.

Treatment

Removal of the cause either by complete removal of the denture or judicious reduction of the flanges. If excessive hyperplastic tissue remains it may have to be surgically removed. A suitable procedure for this is:

(a) impression including the granuloma;
(b) jaw record and wax trial;
(c) before finishing the granuloma is cut from the model;
(d) denture finished with rounded margins;
(e) granuloma surgically removed (see also Chapter 49);
(f) denture inserted without suturing—treat as an immediate denture.

Allergy

Is a state in which tissues become hypersensitive to a substance which is usually harmless. In prosthetics, contact allergy is most suspect. The incidence of allergy to methyl methacrylate polymer is low. Positive skin tests have not generally been obtained in patients thought to have allergy to denture base material; however, a negative result does not necessarily exclude its occurrence on moist oral mucosa.

The patient who complains of allergy is aware of a burning sensation in the mouth. Examination frequently shows an area of redness over the whole of the denture-bearing area.

In view of rarity of proven allergy, possible alternative explanations are:

1. The fit surface reproduces the finest detail of the mucosa, which is irritated by the slightest movement. This is exacerbated by the wearing of the denture at night or by faulty occlusion.
2. Inadequate hygiene of mouth and denture.
3. Denture cleansers often contain chemically irritant components. Failure to remove every trace from the denture before insertion may lead to an apparent 'allergic' response.
4. Free monomer is known to have an irritant affect on mucous membrane. There are occasions where a denture contains much residual monomer due to incorrect processing. The clinical picture is of widespread burning sensation starting very soon after the insertion of new dentures or of one which has been relined. In these cases the mucosa shows extensive inflammation. *Treatment*—subject the denture to further extended processing procedures.

MUCOSAL PROBLEMS CAUSED BY DENTURE TRAUMA

Because some patients have a high pain threshold they are often unaware that there has been damage to the oral tissues. Therefore, even if the patient expresses satisfaction and has no complaints, dentures should be removed and a thorough examination of the mouth should be made. The most common sites of denture trauma are:

(a) in the sulci due to peripheral overextension;
(b) in the region of undercuts on the fit surface of the denture.

The trauma usually takes place during insertion and removal. A common site is the maxillary tuberosity region. Inflammation on the crest of the ridge often arises because of unbalanced occlusion. Other traumatic factors are:

(a) badly designed and too deep a post dam or ante dam;
(b) poorly fitting clasps, which can cause physical trauma;
(c) broken teeth with rough edges, both natural and artificial;
(d) cheek and tongue biting—the common causes are inadequate overjet in molar and premolar regions; dentures not in the neutral zone; possibly incorrect occlusal face height; incorrect occlusal plane.

MUCOSAL PROBLEMS CAUSED BY CHEMICAL OR PHYSICAL TRAUMA

Use of domestic cleaners, e.g. Domestos, for denture cleaning with inadequate rinsing. Ulceration by placing aspirin tablet in the buccal mucosa in an attempt to relieve toothache. Allergic response to some of the earlier topical anaesthetics. Biting of lower lip, tongue or cheeks shortly after inferior block injection.

In all ulcerative lesions diagnosis may be complicated by secondary infection. Microorganisms can gain entry through surface laceration.

INFECTION

Acute ulcerative gingivitis (Chapter 39)

Commonly arises in the presence of pre-existing periodontal disease. Contributory causes can be smoking, emotional stress, nutritional deficiencies — or as complication of a systemic condition such as upper respiratory tract infection. It manifests itself by acute pain, bleeding gums, bad taste and characteristic halitosis. If untreated, ulceration can rapidly spread to the throat and other soft tissues, progressing to severe tissue destruction. In the Third World, where chronic malnutritional states exist, patients can die from cancrum oris as a complication of acute ulcerative gingivitis.

Candidosis

Candidal stomatitis shows as typical white lesions. *Candida albicans* is a commensal of the mouth, throat and vagina. It becomes pathogenic when tissues become debilitated by trauma or disease. The tongue, palate and buccal mucosal are most frequently attacked. In the presence of angular cheilitis the corners of the mouth can be infected. Predisposing factors include old and loose dentures, poor oral hygiene, excessive smoking, nutritional deficiency, diabetes, anaemia and antibiotic therapy. Tetracycline therapy can be followed by sore mouth and candidiasis.

Antifungal agents such as miconazole in conjunction with strict oral hygiene is the treatment. Candidosis is an excellent diagnostic aid in that it may be an early indication of a series of underlying systemic diseases.

Chapter 36

Precision attachments

Precision attachments all consist essentially of two closely fitting components, one incorporated into the natural tooth, the other into a prosthesis; their function is to augment the retention, support and stability of removable prostheses. They may also be used as a joint in fixed/movable bridgework.

Although the design of the many attachments available varies greatly, each consists of a *patrix* and a *matrix*. The patrix usually takes the form of a projecting component or a bar which engages and is enclosed by the matrix. The components may be constructed of wrought or cast precious or non-precious alloys, and may have a nylon or other polymeric resin part. They may be supplied preformed by a manufacturer or cast by a dental technician.

The retentive effect may be achieved either through frictional resistance to movement between closely approximated surfaces of the two components or by the mechanical engagement of undercut areas within the matrix by part of the patrix. These movable minor components of the patrix may take the form of flexible arms and lamellae or spring-loaded plungers.

CLASSIFICATION OF TYPES OF ATTACHMENT

The broad classification is as follows:

1. Stud attachments
2. Bar attachments
3. Extracoronal attachments
4. Intracoronal attachments

These types are now considered in detail.

Stud attachments

These consist essentially of a spherical or cylindrical patrix which engages a matrix which may have two or more flexible alloy lamellae or may include a compressible nylon or PVC insert.

Clinical applications
Stud attachments are principally used for the retention and support of complete overlay dentures. The root-filled abutment teeth are prepared as for a post and core. A casting with a diaphragm is constructed and the patrix

soldered onto the diaphragm. The matrix is then incorporated into the fitting surface of the prosthesis, either at the time of its construction or at a later date using self-polymerizing acrylic in the mouth.

Bar attachments

The patrix of this type of attachment takes the form of a bar which may be pear-shaped, round or rectangular in section. The matrix in the form of a sleeve fits closely against the bar and may be flexible in order to engage the undercut areas of the bar.

Clinical applications

These are used for overdentures and may also be used across saddle areas between abutment teeth to retain a partial denture. The most frequently encountered application for the use of a bar is across two canines when the remainder of the dentition has been lost. Since some rotation of the prosthesis about the bar will take place, the bar must be located at right angles and symmetrically to the median sagittal plane. The root-filled abutment teeth are prepared as for posts with the additional requirement that the two prepared canals must be parallel to allow insertion of the one piece patrix; post and diaphragm component.

Extracoronal attachments

The patrix is soldered onto the prosthetic crown of an abutment tooth and engages the matrix, which is attached to a removable partial denture. The patrix thus projects beyond the crown of the abutment tooth so that the crown preparation will not require any particular modification. However, the patient must be able to achieve adequate levels of oral hygiene to prevent plaque accumulation cervical to the attachment.

Clinical applications

This type of attachment fulfils the roles of the clasp, occlusal rest and guide plane components of a removable partial denture. That is:

(a) retention through the engagement of the patrix in flexible components of the matrix, by frictional resistance and sometimes by the use of spring-loaded plunger mechanisms;

(b) resistance to lateral movement by the approximation of the vertical surfaces of the two major components;

(c) support as the patrix comes to rest under load on the base of matrix.

All of these functions may be achieved more effectively by the use of attachments rather than conventional clasps, at the same time as improving the aesthetics because no clasp arms will be visible. However, the need to prepare abutment teeth for full-coverage crowns must be taken into consideration.

Some vertical rotation of any free-end saddle partial denture must be assumed to take place, so the alignment of attachments on either side of the arch must be parallel to each other and usually to the sagittal plane. Otherwise rotation will be impaired and the resulting transmitted leverage will result in failure of the attachment, the abutment crown, or the support of the abutment tooth.

Intracoronal attachments

The matrix is incorporated within the contours of the crown of the abutment tooth for a removable partial denture. It usually consists of a dovetail-shaped sleeve of precious alloy onto which the metal of the crown is cast. Alternatively, burn-out patterns are available, which form part of the final casting. The patrix is attached to the framework of the prosthesis. The functions are similar to those of the extracoronal attachment but the load is transmitted nearer to the long axis of the abutment tooth and there is no projection to impede plaque control. However, a recess must be cut in the tooth preparation to incorporate the matrix. This type of attachment may also be used as the movable component of a fixed–movable bridge.

GENERAL PRINCIPLES OF ATTACHMENT USE

Many attachments, including most stud and bar attachments, are available in a rigid or resilient configuration, the latter allowing some rotation and vertical movement of the matrix against the patrix. This resilience is usually achieved by the inclusion of a spacer between the two components during their positioning in the laboratory.

The clinician must select the form which is most appropriate. If rigid anchors are used for complete overdentures, the entire load of occlusal function may be transmitted to the attachments and abutment teeth. This may be acceptable only if:

(a) there are more than two abutment teeth;
(b) the denture is constructed using a mucodisplacement impression technique (see Chapter 31) so that some of the load is shared by the mucosa;
(c) relining or rebasing can be undertaken as often as required.

The resilient configuration may therefore often be more appropriate for complete overdentures and for long free-end saddles. Conversely, partial dentures that are essentially tooth-supported should incorporate the rigid form of attachment.

Size of attachment

The vertical and horizontal space available is a severe limiting factor on the size of precision attachments. In general, the use of the largest size of attachment which can be fitted into the space available has the following advantages:

1. The components are stronger and less liable to fracture.
2. There is a greater surface area of contact between the two components, giving better frictional retention and reducing the rate of wear.
3. Greater resistance to lateral loading can be achieved.

Articulated study casts should be prepared preoperatively and an assessment made of the space available before the attachments are selected.

Chapter 37

Implantology

The use of implants to support and retain prostheses replacing missing teeth is becoming an important part of modern dentistry. A wide variety of implant systems are in clinical use and these may be subdivided as follows:

1. *Endosseous* — these include:

    (a) root analogue cylinders having a threaded, unthreaded or basket form;
    (b) cone-shaped implants;
    (c) blade implants.

2. *Subperiosteal* — an open cast-metal framework is placed on the bone surface.

3. *Transosteal* — the transmandibular staple for use only in the anterior region; the implants being united at the lower border.

The successful outcome of any implant procedure is dependent on a combination of the following factors:

(a) biocompatability of the implant material and the effect of its macroscopic and microscopic surface characteristics on the response of hard and soft tissues;
(b) the surgical placement technique;
(c) the status of the recipient tissues;
(d) an absence of loading during the healing phase;
(e) the design and construction of the prosthesis, particularly with regard to loading characteristics and hygiene.

THE BIOLOGICAL RESPONSE TO IMPLANT MATERIALS

Implant materials in current use include:

(a) pure titanium (e.g. Nobelpharma, Straumann) and titanium alloys;
(b) aluminium oxide polycrystalline ceramic (e.g. Tubingen) and aluminium oxide, single crystalline sapphire;
(c) cobalt–chromium–molybdenum alloys (used for cast subperiosteal framework).

The response of bone

Osseointegration is a histological definition meaning a direct contact between living bone and a load-carrying endosseous implant at the light microscopic level. There is a large body of evidence to confirm that such a bone/implant interface, without any intervening fibrous tissue, can become established using correctly inserted titanium and aluminium oxide implants.

The criteria for the development of osseointegration are:

1. A surgical technique for the preparation of the implant bed which controls trauma in order to avoid impaired bone healing. The site must be prepared at very low rotational speeds using copious irrigation, intermittent cutting and sharp instrumentation to prevent temperature rise with the bone.

2. An implant material which is either biologically inert or osseoinductive. The surfaces of many titanium and aluminium oxide implants have micro-irregularities produced either by machining or by plasma-spray coating. These serve to increase the surface area of the interface. The surface should be free of contaminants at the time of insertion.

3. Primary stability should be achieved immediately after insertion. Threaded screw implants are well retained when placed into a precisely prepared bed. Some systems involve a two stage procedure: initially the root analogue is inserted and covered by the mucosal flap or may be left level with the mucosal surface. The implant head is attached during a secondary procedure which may involve re-exposure of the submerged implant. Primary stability may be achieved for systems with a fixed head by the mutual splinting of several implants using caps and a gold bar.

4. An adequate period of healing is required before the implant is loaded. The formation of a woven callus, its lamellar compaction and the ultimate maturation of bone around an implant takes from 16 to 24 weeks.

5. The prosthetic superstructure must be designed so that the functional and parafunctional loading is transmitted evenly to all the implanted fixtures. It should be designed to allow a high level of plaque control by the patient.

The soft tissue interface

There is some evidence that an epithelial attachment analogous to that around a natural tooth can become established at the neck of titanium and aluminium oxide implants. A basal lamina and the formation of hemidesmosomes have been demonstrated. A smooth or polished neck in the transmucosal part of the implant appears to favour this response.

CLINICAL APPLICATIONS OF ENDOSSEOUS IMPLANTS

1. Single tooth replacement.
2. Bridge abutment combined with a retainer on a natural abutment tooth or with implants acting as both bridge abutments.
3. The restoration of the edentulous mandible or maxilla. This may be

achieved either by a fixed prosthesis retained on the implant heads by screws or by a removable prosthesis retained on a bar or other form of attachment linked to the implants.

4. The support of maxillofacial prostheses including artificial eyes and ears.

CRITERIA FOR SUCCESS

1. No mobility of an individual, unattached implant when tested clinically
2. No evidence of peri-implant radiolucency
3. Less than 0.2 mm vertical bone loss annually after insertion
4. An absence of abnormal signs or symptoms such as pain and paraesthesia

In the context of (1) to (4) above, a success rate of not less than 85% after 5 years and not less than 80% after 10 years should be demonstrable. Longitudinal studies have now established that several implant systems are capable of fulfilling the above criteria.

FURTHER READING

Albrekktsson T., *et al.* (1986). The long-term efficacy of currently used dental implants: A review and proposed criteria of success. *Int. J. Oral Maxillofac. Impl.*, **1,** 11–25.

Part Four

Oral Medicine, Pathology and Surgery

Chapter 38

Pharmacology and therapeutics

This chapter covers:

(a) antimicrobial agents;
(b) analgesics;
(c) sedative agents.

It is by no means complete but attempts to cover the drugs most commonly used in dentistry and some new drugs which may find their way into common dental usage.

Dosages given in the text are recommended adult doses unless otherwise stated. Children's doses should ideally be calculated by body weight. As a general guideline children 1–5 years old receive one-quarter of the adult dose; those 6–12 years receive half the adult dose.

Doses for children are stated in the individual drug entries of the *British National Formulary (BNF)*.

WRITING A PRESCRIPTION

The following information should be clearly stated on a prescription form:

(a) full name of patient;
(b) address of patient;
(c) age of patient;
(d) the full name of the drug to be prescribed—it is preferable to use non-proprietary names whenever possible;
(e) dose and frequency, e.g. 250 mg, four times a day;
(f) duration of course in days or quantity to be supplied;
(g) form of medication, e.g. tablet, lozenge, elixir, capsule, etc;
(h) directions—i.e.

    (i) route of administration, e.g. oral, topical;
    (ii) how is medication to be taken; sucked, swallowed, chewed, etc.;
    (iii) timing of doses, e.g. on an empty/full stomach;

(i) special instructions/contraindications/warnings, e.g. metronidazole interaction with alcohol; benzodiazepines and driving.

ANTIMICROBIAL AGENTS

These will be considered in three major groups.
1. Antibiotics
2. Antifungal
3. Antiviral

They may be used for prophylaxis, e.g. the prevention of infective endocarditis, or therapeutically, e.g. the treatment of thrush, herpes or acute ulcerative gingivitis.

ANTIBIOTICS

By definition antibiotics are substances produced by microorganisms which act in minute concentration to kill other organisms (bacteriocidal) or prevent them from proliferating (bacteriostatic). In this text the term antibiotic will be used to include both naturally occurring (true antibiotics) and synthetic antimicrobial agents. The antibiotics described are those which are more commonly used in the treatment of orofacial conditions and in prophylaxis during dental treatment. It is far from complete and further information can be obtained from the references given at the end of the text.

Penicillin

When used unqualified penicillin refers to benzyl penicillin (pen G), the first natural penicillin to be discovered. Since the isolation of the penicillin nucleus several different types of penicillins have been synthesized; they may be broadly divided into the following four groups:

1. *Injectable/long-acting penicillins*
   e.g. benzyl
        procaine   } Triplopen
        benethamine
2. *Phenoxymethylpenicillin* (pen V)
3. *Broad-spectrum penicillins*
   e.g. ampicillin
        amoxycillin
4. *Penicillinase-resistant penicillins*
   e.g. cloxacillin
        flucloxacillin

The use of penicillin as an antibiotic in man was first reported in 1941. Penicillins have since proved to be the most generally useful and safest antibiotic available. All penicillins act by interfering with bacterial cell wall synthesis, making them bacteriocidal. They are active against Gram-positive organisms and Gram-negative cocci.

One major concern with penicillin is that of hypersensitivity, which may manifest a number of symptoms ranging from transient skin rash to fatal anaphylaxis. It is therefore important to specifically ask a patient whether they

PHARMACOLOGY AND THERAPEUTICS

have experienced any allergic reactions to penicillin in the past. Patients with a history of atopy, e.g. hay fever, asthma, eczema, are more prone to react to penicillin.

The penicillins used most commonly by dental surgeons are phenoxymethylpenicillin and amoxycillin.

Phenoxymethylpenicillin (pen V)

Dental uses. Antibiotic of choice for majority of dental infections with the exception of acute ulcerative gingivitis (see metronidazole). Also used prophylactically following oral surgery.

Dosage. Standard dose: 250 mg, four times daily (q.d.s.) on an empty stomach for 5 days. A loading dose of 500 mg may be given to decrease the time taken to reach peak plasma levels.

Excretion. Via the kidney.

Spectrum of activity. Narrow spectrum — may be augmented with metronidazole for the treatment of pericoronitis or osteitis.

Side-effects/contraindications. Hypersensitivity; renal failure — care on dosage.

Amoxycillin

Dental uses. Prophylaxis of infective endocarditis; treatment of sinusitis.

Dosage. Prophylaxis for endocarditis: 3 g orally 1 h prior to procedure. Other uses — 250 mg orally three times a day (t.d.s) for 5 days. Well-absorbed even on a full stomach.

Augmentin

Amoxycillin + calvulanic acid (β-lactamase inhibitor). Extends the spectrum of activity of amoxycillin by inhibiting β-lactamases. Useful for penicillin-resistant staphylococci, gonococci and strains of *Escherichia coli*.

Has been used dentally to treat oral infections in immunocompromised patients.

Cephalosporins

The cephalosporins have a similar structure and mode of action to penicillins. They are active against a broad spectrum of organisms and are resistant to penicillinase. Although advocated initially as being safe to give to individuals allergic to penicillin, they are no longer regarded as suitable alternatives as cross-sensitivity can occur. There is no real indication for the use of cephalosporins for the treatment of oral infections, unless recommended by the microbiologist after culture and sensitivity tests.

Erythromycin

Erythromycin belongs to the macrolide family of antibiotics, so named because they contain a macrocytic lactose ring. Erythromycin was isolated in 1952 and remains the antibiotic of choice for penicillin allergic individuals.

Dental uses. (a) As for phenoxymethylpenicillin in penicillin allergic patients; (b) when penicillin resistance has been detected; (c) prophylaxis against infective endocarditis in penicillin allergic patients who fall into the low-risk endocarditis category.

Dosage. 250 mg q.d.s. orally for 5 days. As with penicillin a loading dose of 500 mg may be given. The estolate is more reliably absorbed but should only be used for courses of less than 7 days.

Prophylaxis for endocarditis—1.5 g erythromycin stearate 1 h prior to procedure; 500 mg 6 h later.

Excretion. Via the liver.

Spectrum of activity. Bacteriocidal—narrow spectrum; Gram-positive organisms and spirochaetes.

Side-effects/contraindications. Estolate—hepatotoxic after about 10 days, leading to jaundice, pain, fever. If drug stopped, complete recovery.

Stearate—gastrointestinal upset in high dose.

Drug interactions. With digoxin; warfarin; carbamazepine—decreased reduction of rate of excretion leading to potentiation of their effects.

Clindamycin

The Endocarditis Working Party of the British Society for Antimicrobial Chemotherapy has recently (January 1990) recommended the use of single dose Clindamycin (600 mg orally 1 hour prior to treatment) as an alternative to erythromycin for antibiotic cover.

Vancomycin (macrolide family)

Dental use. Prophylaxis against infective endocarditis in penicillin allergic high-risk patients, e.g. patients with prosthetic heart valves.

Dosage. 1 g vancomycin as an infusion over 1 h.

Spectrum of activity. Bacteriocidal against Gram-positive bacteria only. Very narrow spectrum.

Side-effects. Intensely irritant when injected—thrombophlebitis; red man syndrome—generalized erythematous rash and fever following infusion. Tinnitus—prolonged use may lead to deafness.

Metronidazole

Metronidazole is a synthetic antimicrobial agent. It was initially introduced for the treatment of trichomoniasis. It acts by inhibiting bacterial nucleic acid synthesis.

Dental uses. Drug of choice for acute ulcerative gingivitis. May be used with or without pen V for the treatment of pericoronitis; osteitis, periodontal disease.

Dosage. 200 mg t.d.s orally during or after a meal for 3–4 days depending upon the severity of the condition.

Physiology. Metabolized in the liver; Excreted in urine and saliva.
Side-effects. Nausea; metallic taste; transient rashes.
Contraindications. Hypersensitivity; also avoid during pregnancy and lactation—unless essential.
Drug interactions. (a) Alcohol—disulfiram type of reaction; (b) warfarin—potentiation of anticoagulant effect; (c) phenobarbitone—increased metabolism of metronidazole; (d) cimetidine—increased plasma concentration.

Gentamicin

Gentamicin belongs to the aminoglycoside family of antibiotics. It is the most active antibiotic of the group, being highly effective against Gram-positive bacilli and *Staphylococcus aureus*. Its only real use in dentistry routinely is for prophylaxis against infective endocarditis in high-risk patients, in combination with either amoxycillin or vancomycin. As it is not absorbed from the gastrointestinal tract it is given as a stat 120 mg dose either intramuscular, 20 min prior to the procedure or intravenous, immediately before the procedure. In common with other aminoglycosides gentamicin is highly toxic to the VIIIth cranial nerve. However, if given as one dose for prophylaxis, no problems should arise.

Sulphonamides

Sulphonamides are the drug of choice in severe orofacial trauma, if a cerebrospinal fluid leak is suspected, as prophylaxis against meningitis. They are one of the only antibiotics capable of crossing the blood–brain barrier.

Teichoplanin

Teichoplanin is a new glycopeptide antibiotic, as yet unlicensed in the UK, which may prove to be a useful substitute for vancomycin or indeed erythromycin for dental prophylaxis against infective endocarditis in patients allergic to penicillin. Teichoplanin is active against all Gram-positive organisms and is more active than vancomycin against streptococci, including *Streptococcus viridans*. It can be given intravenously immediately prior to the procedure or intramuscularly 2 h before the procedure. Unlike vancomycin, infusion over 60 min is not required as it is far less toxic. The recommended dosage for antibiotic prophylaxis is 400 mg intravenously as a bolus. For high-risk patients, teichoplanin should be used in conjunction with gentamicin for adequate prophylaxis.

ANTIFUNGAL AGENTS

Nystatin

Polyene binds to cytoplasmic membrane of fungal cells making them osmotically unstable.

Active against most oral yeasts; resistance does not occur.
Not absorbed by gastrointestinal tract.

Dosage. 100 000 units q.d.s for at least 2 weeks.

Format. **Pastille**—flavoured for better patient compliance; contraindicated in diabetes (sucrose).

Ointment—inert base, may be used orally.

Suspension—proven use in oral candidosis; adheres to oral mucosa. Treatment of choice for thrush and for young children.

Amphotericin

Polyene (like nystatin) therefore, similar mode of action. Less toxic than nystatin: can be given intravenously if necessary; however, may cause thrombophlebitis, febrile reactions, exfoliative dermatitis, anaemia, renal damage.

Dosage. Orally 10 mg q.d.s for at least 2 weeks.

Format. **Lozenges/suspension**— thrush, acute atrophic candidosis, denture stomatitis, chronic hyperplastic candidosis.

Ointment—angular cheilitis, denture stomatitis, chronic hypoplastic candidosis.

Miconazole

In the imidazole group of antifungal agents: active against yeasts, but unlike nystatin, resistance may occur. Also bacteriostatic against Gram-positive cocci including *Staph. aureus*. Clinically very useful in treatment of angular cheilitis and chronic mucocutaneous candidosis.

Dosage. (i) Tablets—250 mg q.d.s, for 2 weeks; (ii) oral gel (sugar-free) 25 mg/ml—5–10 ml applied to lesion q.d.s.

Ketokonazole

An imidazole antifungal agent—hepatotoxic. Reserved for treatment of otherwise intractable candidal infections which have failed to respond to other less toxic agents, e.g. candidosis in immunocompromised patients.

Dosage. 200 mg once daily with food for 14 days.

ANTIVIRAL AGENTS

Acyclovir

Acyclovir has replaced idoxuridine as the drug of choice in the treatment of oral herpes infections.

Acyclovir, an analogue of deoxyganosine, is the antiviral agent of choice for the treatment of herpes infections. Once inside the virus, acyclovir is converted to acyclovir triphosphate by viral thymidine kinase, which blocks further production of viral DNA by inhibiting viral polymerases, disrupting viral replications. Cellular DNA polymerases are unaffected by an acyclovir triphosphate.

Acyclovir is most effective against herpes simplex types I and II followed by the varicella-zoster and Epstein–Barr virus. Cytomegalovirus is the least sensitive of the herpes group of viruses to acyclovir. Resistance to acyclovir has been detected, however, to date, all mutant viruses have been found to be non-virulent.

For effective treatment of herpes infections it is essential to begin treatment at the earliest possible stage of infection. The main effect of acyclovir is to prevent new lesions forming or progressing. Very early treatment with acyclovir may prevent latency, i.e. herpes labialis and herpes zoster.

Preparations of acyclovir

Tablets 200 mg/400 mg
Suspension 200 mg/5 ml
Cream 5% w/w — only agent in *Dental Formulary*
Ointment 3% w/w

A freeze-dried preparation of acyclovir is available for intravenous use.

Recommended treatment of oral herpes with acyclovir

Primary herpetic stomatitis. 200 mg tablet or suspension, 5 times a day, 4-hourly omitting the night dose, for 5 days. Infants under 2 years, half dose.
Prophylaxis of immunocompromised: 200 mg q.d.s.
Herpes labialis. Acyclovir cream applied to lesion five times a day for 5 days. If healing not complete apply for further 5 days. Therapy should begin in the prodromal phase.
Contraindications. Hypersensitivity to acyclovir or propylene glycol in case of cream.
Precautions. In systemic use — beware renal impairment; pregnancy; the elderly.

ANALGESICS

Analgesics may be divided into three main groups:

(a) peripherally acting;
(b) centrally acting;
(c) combination analgesics.

PERIPHERALLY ACTING ANALGESICS

1. Salicylates, e.g. aspirin; diflusinal
2. Anilines, e.g. paracetamol
3. Pyrazoles, e.g. phenylbutazone — no dental use
4. Non-steroidal anti-inflammatory agents, e.g. mefenamic acid, ibuprofen

Those agents prescribed for the treatment of pain by the dental surgeon will be further discussed.

Aspirin

Properties. Analgesic; antipyretic; anti-inflammatory; uriosuric.
Actions. Peripheral action:
↓ vascular permeability
↓ kinin production
↓ prostaglandin synthesis
↓ platelet adhesiveness
↑ bleeding time
Central action on hypothalamus:
↓ body temp
Dosage. 300–900 mg, 4–6 hourly, not exceeding 4 g a day.
(Lethal dose 25–30 g.)

Peak plasma levels are achieved 2 h after absorbtion and aspirin has a half-life of 2–8 h. It is metabolized in the liver and excreted by the kidney. Aspirin blocks pain mediators, e.g. prostaglandin E_2. It is most effective given prior to the onset of pain, while the local anaesthetic is still effective.

Contraindications and toxic effect

1. Children under 12 years — *Reye's syndrome* (rare acute encephalopathy and fatty change of the liver)
2. Anticoagulant therapy — bleeding time
3. Peptic ulceration — 70% patients suffer gastrointestinal irritation
4. Allergy
5. Blood dyscrasias
6. Tinnitus — first sign of overdose

Despite the enormous number of aspirin consumed usually in the UK (2000 tons = 6 billion tablets), adverse reactions are rare.

Paracetamol

Properties. Analgesic; antipyretic — less so than aspirin; anti-inflammatory — very mild.
Dosage. 500–1000 mg, 4–6 hourly.

Metabolism. Well absorbed, 25% plasma bound; metabolized in liver, excreted by kidney.

Contraindications and toxic effects

Contraindicated in: hepatic impairment; alcoholism; and with anticoagulants.

Overdose. Apparent recovery followed by liver failure: 15 mg cause irreversible liver damage; 25 mg — fatal.

Advantages of paracetamol over aspirin

1. No haemostatic interference
2. No gastric irritation

Diflunisal

Member of aspirin family with similar properties to aspirin; however, less hypersensitivity reported. No increase in bleeding time; less gastric irritation.

Dosage. 250–500 mg b.d.s. (Note: aspirin is prescribed q.d.s.)

Metabolism. Rapidly absorbed, peak plasma levels within 2 h; half-life, 7–11 h.

Contraindications/toxicity

(See aspirin.) Diflunisal has been reported to increase the incidence of dry socket.

Non-steroidal anti-inflammatory drugs (NSAIDs)

NSAIDs, if given as a single dose, have an analgesic activity similar to that of paracetamol.

In full, regular dosage, NSAIDs have both lasting analgesic and anti-inflammatory effects.

Caution in use of NSAIDs

Care in prescription of these drugs is necessary in:

(a) elderly;
(b) peptic ulceration;
(c) allergic disorders;
(d) pregnancy;
(e) renal/hepatic impairment;
(f) those taking anticoagulants.

Toxic effects

Side-effects are very variable and may include:

(a) gastrointestinal discomfort;
(b) nausea;

(c) diarrhoea;
(d) hypersensitivity — angio-oedema, asthma, rashes;
(e) vertigo;
(f) tinnitus;
(g) fluid retention;
(h) blood disorders.

Two NSAIDs are commonly prescribed for dental pain:

1. *Mefenamic acid* (Ponstan) 500 mg t.d.s.
2. *Ibuprofen* (Neurofen, Brufen), 200–400 mg, 6–8 hourly.

Care should be taken when prescribing as to the cautions and toxic effects associated with these drugs and patients should be advised to take tablets with a meal to minimize gastrointestinal upset.

CENTRALLY ACTING ANALGESICS (major analgesics)

All cause respiratory depression and addiction; relevant examples are:

(a) morphine
(b) methadone
(c) pethidine
(d) pentazocine
(e) nalbuphine
(f) dextrapropoxyphene
(g) codeine
(h) dihyrocodeine

They are not good oral analgesics; by mouth, peripherally acting compounds act as satisfactorily as centrally acting ones and are much safer.

Nalbuphine (Nubain)

Nalbuphine (Nubain) will be the only centrally acting analgesic to be described in further detail as it is the only major analgesic which may be used in dental practice. Nubain is a new analgesic, equipotent with morphine; however, it has fewer side-effects than morphine and less abuse potential. As with all narcotics respiratory depression does occur with Nubain. Its effects may be reversed with naloxone. Nubain as a stat. intravenous dose of 10 mg has been used to improve analgesia and allow a significant reduction in the mean dosage of midazolam (see below) required to produce satisfactory sedation for minor oral surgery.

NB. Careful monitoring of a patient is necessary if any central nervous system (CNS) depressants are used in combination with benzodiazepines for sedation techniques.

Distalgesic (NO DENTAL USE)

Distalgesic is a combination analgesic containing:

dextropropoxyphene, 32 mg (central action) + paracetamol, 325 mg (peripheral action)

Dosage. 2 tablets 6–8 hourly; less than 8 tablets a day.
Side-effects. Addiction; respiratory depression; hepatotoxicity.
Overdose—20–30 tabs.

Codeine

Codeine is a natural alkaloid, one-twelfth the strength of morphine. It produces little sedation or euphoria so decreases risk of addiction.

Uses

1. For moderate pain — particularly useful combination analgesic
2. Cough suppression
3. Diarrhoea

Combination analgesics containing codeine

Aspirin (400 mg) + codeine (8 mg)
Aspirin (250 mg) + paracetamol (250 mg) + codeine (6.8 mg)
Paracetamol (500 mg) + codeine (8 mg)

Dosage. 1–2 tablets, 4–6 hourly.
Useful analgesics for dental pain.

LOCAL ANALGESICS (see also Chapter 42)

Without doubt the most frequently used drugs in dentistry. They usually contain analgesic agent, vasoconstrictor, preservative, anti-oxidant and modified Ringer's solution.

Lignocaine + adrenaline

A very effective and safe local analgesic agent; available as 2% lignocaine hydrochloride + 1:80 000 or 1:100 000 adrenaline, 2 ml sol.

Toxic effects

Systemic. These toxic effects are:
(a) **lignocaine:** cerebral depression — high dose needed; excitation of myocardium; hypersensitivity — very rare;
(b) **adrenaline:** palpitations — intravascular injection; disturbance in cardiac rhythm and fibrillation.

Maximum recommended dose
1. 10 ml (5 cartridges) in a healthy adult
2. less than 6 ml — in patients with cardiac disease

Drug interactions
1. Monoamine oxidase inhibitors — no real evidence that adrenaline is potentiated as it is broken down by catechol-O-methyl transferase
2. Tricyclic antidepressants — no clinical evidence to support drug interaction as used in dental procedures.

Precautions
Patients with history of cardiac disease: recommended dosage, less than 6 ml lignocaine + adrenaline.

Prilocaine + felypressin

Available as 3% prilocaine hydrochloride with 0.03 unit/ml felypressin; 2 ml self-aspiration cartridge.

Toxic effects. For **prilocaine,** these are:
(a) cyanosis due to methaemoglobinaemia;
(b) hypersensitivity — very rare.

Felypressin has no known adverse systemic effects or drug interactions. It is only available with prilocaine.

Mepivicaine

Available 3% plain (without vasoconstrictor); short duration — 30 min.
2% mepivicaine with 1:100 000 adrenaline — duration 60 min.
May be useful in children or the handicapped, particularly for inferior dental blocks as self-injury less likely due to short duration.

SEDATION (see also Chapter 41)

Low risk compared to general anaesthetics in competent hands.
Agents of choice — **benzodiazepines**

Properties
(a) minor tranquillizers
(b) sedative/hypnotic
(c) anxiolytic
(d) muscle relaxant

Toxic effects
(a) CNS depression
(b) ↓ blood pressure

(c) drowsiness
(d) lethargy
(e) muscle weakness

Benzodiazepines are potentiated by other CNS depressants, e.g. alcohol, nubain, major tranquillizers.

The most commonly used benzodiazepines in dentistry are midazolam, diazepam and temazepam. The first two agents are compared in Table 38.1 (see Chapter 41 — intravenous sedation).

Table 38.1
Comparison of two commonly used benzodiazepines

Midazolam	Diazepam
Water-soluble	Lipid-soluble
Non-irritant to vessel wall	Highly irritant to vessel wall
Potency 2× diazepam	Potency ½× midazolam
Max recommended dose i.v., 10 mg	Max recommended dose i.v., 20 mg
Requires slow infusion	Requires slow infusion
Signs of sedation appear slowly	More obvious signs of sedation
Matabolites — non-active	Active metabolites give second peak effect
Good amnesia	Poor amnesia
Half-life 2 h	Half-life 4 h

Cimetidine (H_2-blocker) delays clearance of benzodiazepines.

Midazolam has now superseded diazepam as the agent of choice for intravenous sedation for dental procedures.

Temazepam

A minor metabolite of diazepam, commonly used for the treatment of insomnia. It has short half-life (approx 4 h) and causes little hangover effect. Temazepam elixir (30 mg) has recently been found to be an excellent oral sedation agent for use in dentistry. Peak plasma levels with a maximal sedative effect occur some 45–60 min after administration, the patient recovering sufficiently to be escorted home some 45–60 min after administration.

Flumanezil (Anexate)

Anexate, an imidazobenzodiazepine, is a specific benzodiazepine antagonist that allows rapid reversal of conscious sedation with benzodiazepines by specific competitive inhibition for benzodiazepine receptors. It is considered in detail in Chapter 41.

REFERENCE

Working Party of the British Society for Antimicrobial Chemotherapy (1990). Antibiotic prophylaxis of infective endocarditis. *Lancet*, **335**, 88–9.

FURTHER READING

Cawson R. A., Spector R. G. (1989). *Clinical Pharmacology in Dentistry* 5th edn. Edinburgh: Churchill Livingstone.
Cawson R. A. (1986). Update on antiviral chemotherapy: the advent of acyclovir. *Br. Dent. J.*, **161**, 245–51.
Maskell, J. P., *et al.* (1986). Teicoplanin as a prophylactic antibiotic for dental bacteraemia. *J. Antimicro. Chemother.*, **17**, 651–9.
Rosenbaum, N. L. (1988). Flumazenil—the first benzodiazepine antagonist. *Dent. Update*, **15**, 278–83.

Chapter 39

The periodontium: diseases and treatment

THE PERIODONTIUM IN HEALTH

The human periodontium is composed of four interdependent structures:

(a) gum (gingiva);
(b) alveolar bone;
(c) cementum;
(d) periodontal membrane.

Gingiva

The gingiva include three types of specialized epithelia and their underlying connective tissues by which they are organized. The types of epithelia are:

(a) stratified squamous *outer epithelium*;
(b) *sulcular* (or *crevicular*) *epithelium*;
(c) *junctional epithelium* (formerly called the attached epithelial cuff).

Outer epithelium

This extends from the gingival margin to the mucogingival junction (Fig. 39.1). In health it has the following histological features:

(a) rete ridges;
(b) four layers of cells;
(c) keratinized or parakeratinized outer layer.

The outer epithelium is often called *attached gingiva,* but for reasons which will be explained later, this may not always be correct.

In health the outer epithelium is pale pink or pigmented, firm, and with a finely stippled surface. Its width varies round the mouth, being widest labially to the maxillary incisors and narrowest buccally to the mandibular canines and third molars. Its normal width may be modified by a prominent or instanding tooth, by the eruptive position of a tooth, and by the presence of frena and mucosal bands.

It is regarded as part of the masticatory mucosa of the oral cavity. Its most apical boundary, except in the palate, is the mucogingival junction, a fixed boundary identifiable histologically by the fact that alveolar mucosa has a non-keratinized epithelium and its connective tissue has elastic fibres and fewer collagen fibres, unlike the outer epithelium.

Sulcular epithelium

This lines the gingival sulcus or crevice. It may be regarded as a transitional epithelium, being bounded at the gingival margin by the outer epithelium and at the base of the sulcus by junctional epithelium (see below). Its histological structure is characterized by:

(a) short rete ridges;
(b) basal and spinous layers only;
(c) absence of keratinization.

Junctional epithelium

This extends apically from the base of the histological sulcus (where it meets sulcular epithelium) to the cemento–enamel junction. A specialized epithelium, it has the following features in health:

(a) no rete ridges (any epithelial downgrowths are pathological);
(b) basal layer and spinous layer only;
(c) non-keratinized;
(d) 1–30 cells thick (much thinner than outer epithelium);
(e) rapid turnover (2–4 days), cells being shed into the sulcus;
(f) highly permeable (to cells, fluids, and bacterial products);
(g) derived from reduced enamel epithelium.

Junctional epithelium is attached throughout its length in health to enamel via basement laminae and hemidesmosomes. Thus it conforms to Gottlieb's

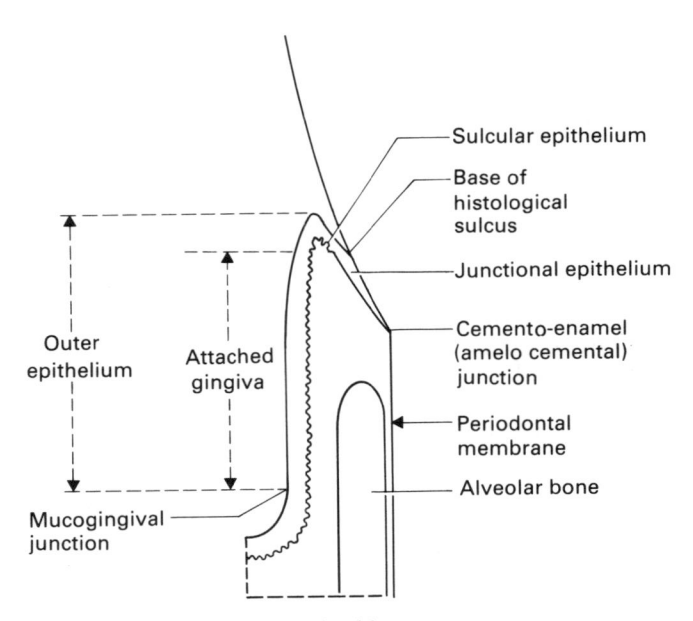

Fig. 39.1 *The human periodontium in health.*

concept of 'Epithelansatz' (epithelial attachment), and not to Black's concept of a deep crevice extending between the gingival margin and the cemento–enamel junction. However, such an attachment cannot be rigid, but must allow for the movements of eruption. There is also evidence that, in health, junctional epithelial cells have a shifting, dynamic adherence to the crown of the tooth, a property which they lose only when plaque-related pathological changes occur.

The position of the healthy gingival margin is related to the eruptive position of the tooth. As the tooth begins to emerge into the mouth the gingival margin may recoil apically, or its level may change only slightly as the tooth moves past. At times the gingival margin may stay at a high level on the crown for an extended period, and may then become liable to trauma and plaque accumulation, which in turn may contribute to pericoronal inflammation and false pocket formation.

Estimations of the depth of the sulcus (crevice) are liable to error because a measuring probe may inadvertently penetrate the delicate wall of the sulcular or junctional epithelium. Such a value is now called the 'clinical sulcus' in order to differentiate it from the 'histological sulcus' which is the depth determined under the microscope. The latter value is usually 0.5–2.0 mm in the fully erupted tooth. Probing the healthy sulcus should not cause bleeding.

The gingiva in health is firmly bound down via its connective tissues to the periosteum of the underlying alveolar bone. The gingiva is also attached to the tooth itself via connective tissue fibres radiating from the supracrestal cementum and also via the junctional epithelium. Thus *attached gingiva* may be defined as that portion of the outer epithelium which is attached to the bone and tooth as just described; its most coronal limit corresponds to the base of the

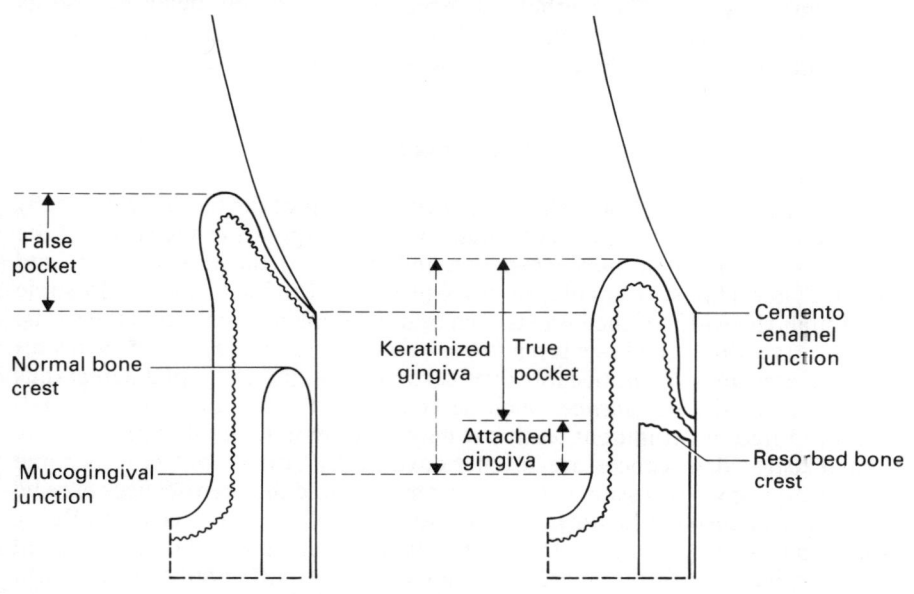

Fig. 39.2 *The classic types of periodontal pocket: (left) a false pocket; (right) a true pocket.*

sulcus, and its apical limit is the mucogingival junction (Fig. 39.1). Where true pockets develop the amount of actual 'attached gingiva' will be correspondingly reduced although the width of keratinized gingiva may be unaltered (Fig. 39.2).

The shape of the *interdental papilla* conforms to the curvature and width of the crowns which bound the interdental area below the contact areas. Between the molars, with their broad contact areas, the gingiva linking the buccal and lingual papillae dip to form a col-like area. Between the incisors, which have a narrower contact point, a col is usually absent. Between other teeth of intermediate size the interdental gingiva has a correspondingly modified form, and variations may occur wherever teeth are not in normal alignment. The shape of the papillae and interdental gingiva may also be a reflection of underlying osseous morphology. The interdental gingiva is particularly susceptible to the effects of plaque accumulating apical to the contact zones.

Gingival connective tissue

This consists of cells and a matrix together with blood vessels, nerves and lymphatics. The cellular component includes fibroblasts, lymphocytes, macrophages, plasma cells, mast cells and polymorphonuclear leukocytes. The matrix has both collagenous and non-collagenous components. Components of ground substances include mucosubstances, mucine, mucoprotein, acid mucopolysaccharides and glycosaminoglycans.

Where the gingiva is very thin, so that the basement membranes of the outer epithelium, sulcular epithelium and junctional epithelium are very close, the width of connective tissue is correspondingly reduced and in time may be inadequate to sustain the epithelium, which may gradually begin to lose its vitality. This possibility has been advanced as part of the explanation for the development of gingival recession in otherwise clinically healthy gingiva.

Alveolar bone

The morphology of the bone which supports the roots of the teeth is genetically determined. In general its buccolingual width corresponds to the width of the roots it supports. It is hence broader and flatter in the molar areas, and narrower and almost triangular in cross-section in the incisor areas. In some individuals the width of the bone is such that it completely embraces the roots; in other individuals the bone is narrower or even incomplete, and in such sites the bone crest may dip noticeably over certain roots; the U-shaped defect thus created is called a *dehiscence*. Such defects are probably more common adjacent to tilted or prominent teeth but may occur in individuals with properly aligned teeth; dehiscences are usually covered by gingiva but may become evident as gingival recession occurs. It seems possible that dehiscences may be a principal underlying factor in the development of gingival recession. Being usually buccal or lingual to the roots, dehiscences (and related O-shaped defects called fenestrations) are often not visible on radiographs of the teeth. Even where dehiscences occur, more than enough bone usually remains to support the teeth.

The basic histology of alveolar bone will be familiar to readers. The different densities in the structure of the bone are responsible for the variety of patterns seen on radiographs, and these patterns themselves may appear to vary according to the angulation (vertical or horizontal) of the X-ray tube. Bone defects which do not involve loss of cortical bone may not show up on X-ray films. However, the tapering crests between some mandibular incisors in health may produce on radiographs an appearance of disease. As is well known, the normal distance between the cemento–enamel junction and the healthy bone crest is not more than 2 mm, so that any value greater than this suggests disease, but any value less than this in a fully erupted tooth may suggest incorrect angulation of the X-ray tube. Also, where teeth are tilted, or where the cemento–enamel of adjacent teeth are at different levels, the healthy bone crest often slopes accordingly, which may resemble features of disease.

Cementum and periodontal membrane

Cementum has an inorganic component of 46% which increases when cementum is exposed to oral fluids; there is no clear evidence that periodontally involved cementum is 'softer' than uninvolved cementum.

Primary (acellular) cementum forms in conjunction with root dentine in the presence of the epithelial sheath of Hertwig. Sharpey's fibres make up much of its structure. Secondary (cellular) cementum forms in response to functional demands and is laid down over acellular cementum. Both forms are laid down by cementoblasts, some of which become incorporated into cementoid and thereafter into cementum and are then called cementocytes. Channels that link the lacunae in which cementocytes reside permit the transportation of nutrients and maintain the vitality of cementum. The periodontal membrane is the source of these nutrients, and furnishes pluripotential cells from which cementoblasts differentiate; thus the periodontal membrane acts as both a pericementum and periosteum. If periodontal membrane is destroyed (as in disease) cementum loses its nutrition.

Towards the apex of the tooth the thickness of cementum is 150–200 μm, but becomes much thinner (16–60 μm) near to the cementum–enamel junction where, presumably, much of it may soon be removed by subsequent scaling procedures. Undisturbed cementum may treble in thickness during adult life.

Maintenance of health

Defence of the periodontium is a function of the following mechanisms:

(a) rapid turnover and shedding of junctional epithelial cells into the sulcus;
(b) the epithelial barrier within the sulcus which prevents bacteria entering the underlying connective tissue;
(c) repair potential of the junctional epithelium;
(d) gingival fluid;
(e) neutrophils entering the sulcus by transmigration through the junctional epithelium;
(f) saliva.

The passage of an exudate (gingival fluid) through the junctional epithelium and into the sulcus is a feature of health and disease. Much attention is currently focused on the increased flow and altered cellular and biochemical constituents of crevicular fluid as a marker, and possibly prognostic indicator, of disease.

THE DISEASED PERIODONTIUM

Chronic gingivitis

The studies of Löe and his colleagues in the mid-1960s showed a relationship between plaque accumulation and the development of gingivitis.

After being thoroughly cleaned, a tooth surface rapidly becomes covered with a structureless film of salivary glycoproteins—the acquired pellicle. Within a few hours this begins to be colonized by aerobic, Gram-positive coccoid bacteria; these are mainly streptococci but other organisms are also found in small numbers. This adherent film of bacteria accumulates on the tooth surface both supragingivally and in the sulcus.

At a histological level, changes in the gingival tissues may be evident within 2–4 days of the onset of plaque accumulation. These changes, regarded as the initial response to bacterial products diffusing into the tissues, include:

(a) vasculitis of vessels subjacent to the junctional epithelium;
(b) chemotactic movement of increased numbers of granulocytes (mainly neutrophils) through the junctional epithelium from the subjacent vessels to the sulcus;
(c) increased production of gingival fluid;
(d) alteration of perivascular connective tissue;
(e) possible early changes in the junctional epithelial cells nearest to the sulcus.

Neutrophils form the first line of defence, therefore any defects in their numbers or functions may predispose the host to an escalation of the disease process.

The first-formed, Streptococcus-dominated, plaque, if left undisturbed, will be supplanted within days by an anaerobic Actinomyces-dominated plaque. Within the tissues the features of the initial response are enhanced and, within 4–7 days, T-lymphocytes begin to infiltrate the connective tissue, marking the onset of a phase called the 'early lesion'. Other features of this phase include:

(a) early proliferation of the basal cells of the junctional epithelium;
(b) further loss of collagen from the marginal connective tissue;
(c) fibroblasts undergo cytopathic changes.

The immune response in the tissues continues with the appearance of plasma cells in the inflammatory infiltrate which they, and B-lymphocytes, may eventually dominate. This phase is called the 'established lesion' which, according to some studies, develops within 3 weeks of undisturbed plaque accumulation. However, in some instances, the early lesion may have a longer duration than was previously reported. Other changes also become more evident. The gingival margin swells because of increased amounts of tissue fluid. By its imperceptible detachment from the enamel surface and continued proliferation of its basal layer to form rete ridges, junctional epithelium becomes converted to pocket epithelium. Macrophages and large numbers of neutrophils accumulate in the pocket wall. Further collagen breakdown occurs.

In Löe's studies, clinical signs of gingival inflammation did not appear until the tenth day of undisturbed plaque accumulation in a few individuals; such changes appeared later in the other subjects. Thus, in some instances, the established lesion may have been reached by the time clinical changes are evident. Clearly, as histological changes precede clinical changes by several days, and are themselves preceded by biochemical changes, an appearance of gingival health is no guarantee of normality within the tissues.

As is well known, the clinical features of gingivitis are:

(a) redness of the papillae and possibly gingival margin;
(b) loss of stippling;
(c) shiny or glassy appearance of the involved tissues;
(d) swelling or blunting of the inflamed tissues;
(e) false pocket formation (Fig. 39.2);
(f) bleeding on toothbrushing or gentle probing (such bleeding is *never* normal).

Amongst the participants in Löe's study, such features resolved within a week after toothbrushing was resumed, although it is reasonable to suppose that resolution at a histological level took longer.

Although with undisturbed plaque accumulation under experimental conditions there is a transition from an aerobic coccal flora to an anaerobic flora, characterized firstly by filamentous forms and slender rods, and later by spirochaetes and vibrios, the associated clinical changes are probably related more to the quality of organisms than to the presence of specific types (the so-called non-specific plaque hypothesis). In patients routinely practising inadequate plaque removal, long-standing gingivitis is commonplace, but it is difficult to interpret such clinical features in the light of experimental gingivitis studies over a known period and based on prior normality. For example, some specimens of severe gingivitis have shown a dominancy of lymphocytes (both B and T forms) over plasma cells. Two studies have shown that, over a 21-day period of experimental gingivitis beginning from health, changes were either typical of an early lesion or an initial lesion, the latter suggesting that only after 6 months of neglected oral hygiene would plasma cells dominate the inflammatory infiltrate.

It is also well known that young children may have less gingivitis than adolescents with the same plaque levels, indicating that gingival reactivity increases gradually from early childhood to adulthood. In later adolescence, gingival inflammation changes from being an indicator of poor oral hygiene to being a sign of initial periodontal disease. In older patients, age may be of little importance in the observed response of the tissues to experimental plaque accumulation if there has been no prior evidence of susceptibility to periodontitis. However, people who have shown a prior susceptibility to periodontal disease may develop gingivitis more readily in experimental studies than non-susceptible individuals; younger patients in the former group may show greater tendency to bleeding on probing than older subjects. Older patients may have an altered host response to plaque microorganisms, developing gingivitis more readily than younger subjects.

Chronic periodontitis

A fourth phase of periodontal disease, called the 'advanced lesion', has been described. This refers to the extension of the lesion into the alveolar bone and periodontal membrane and its subsequent progression to produce significant loss of alveolar support with formation of true pockets. Loss of collagen continues to occur subjacent to the pocket epithelium, but fibrosis may occur at more superficial sites. The cellular infiltrate is dominated by plasma cells. Osteoclasts are present at the crest of the resorbing bone (which is in advance of the pocket base), their presence and activity being governed by various host and bacterial factors.

The factors which initiate the shift from gingivitis to periodontitis are being intensively investigated. As yet, however, there is no apparently sure way of predicting which sites may progress and when. The issue is complicated by the realization that some sites may not progress from gingivitis to periodontitis at all, and also that sites where periodontitis has developed may progress only intermittently. Thus a practitioner recording a patient's periodontal status for the first time has no sure way of knowing the history of the lesions seen, and has to be aware that potentially the condition could suddenly deteriorate. Nevertheless, relating the extent of periodontal destruction to the patient's age may help to assess the patient's predisposition to disease; thus we can categorize patients in broad terms into high- or low-risk groups, and target treatment appropriately. Application of this same principle may help in the treatment of specific sites, as no two sites in the same mouth may behave identically.

Sites which undergo rapid deterioration may stabilize and repair, sometimes without treatment, but this favourable response is unpredictable and perhaps uncommon. Assessment of probing depth is not a reliable indicator of present disease activity. Bleeding on probing indicates plaque-induced inflammation at the base of the pocket (the probe having disrupted thin or ulcerated pocket epithelium there) and hence is an indicator of disease activity but not necessarily of progression. The production of pus on probing is a similar indicator.

An extensive range of microbes has been implicated in periodontitis. In general, as disease activity increases, the number of motile organisms and spirochaetes increase, and coccoid forms decrease. Gram-negative rods are commoner in active sites than non-active sites. Organisms regularly found in active sites include *Bacteroides intermedius, Actinobacillus actinomycetemcomitans*, and *Wolinella recta*; organisms sometimes found in active sites include *Fusobacterium nucleatum, Capnocytophaga gingivalis*, and *Eikenella corrodens*. 'Active sites', in this context, refers to rapid loss of connective tissue attachment including alveolar bone. There is some evidence that sites of active periodontitis may have raised levels of B-lymphocytes and abnormal immune regulatory mechanisms possibly involving T-helper cell subsets. Also *A. acti-*

nomycetemcomitans and *B. gingivalis* may activate human peripheral monocytes to produce interleukin-1 and tumour necrosis factor. There is still some uncertainty about how extensively microbes may invade pocket walls in periodontitis, although trauma (e.g. from injudicious scaling) may enhance this tendency.

Much interest is presently focused on the possible relationship between certain types of periodontal disease and the predominating subgingival microflora. Thus many investigators currently identify at least three types of periodontitis, generally known as juvenile periodontitis, rapidly progressive periodontitis, and slowly progressive periodontitis — the last perhaps being the same as or similar to adult chronic periodontitis. The different terms in popular usage highlight the problem of defining disease activity either by reference to the age of the subject or to the currently perceived amount of attachment loss, and there is no definite way of estimating what microorganisms may be particularly implicated in a clinically determined level of periodontal disease. Thus treatment often begins at an empirical level. A form of periodontitis which remains unresponsive to conventional non-surgical or surgical therapy has currently attracted the label of 'refractory periodontitis', a term to be used with caution since it implies that all basic treatment has been completed.

In a patient with 'periodontitis', any one or more of the following features may be present:

(a) loss of supporting bone;
(b) true pockets (Fig. 39.2);
(c) gingival enlargement;
(d) gingival redness;
(e) gingival fibrosis;
(f) blunting of papillae;
(g) gingival destruction;
(h) ulceration;
(i) gingival recession exposing root;
(j) sensitivity of exposed roots;
(k) root caries;
(l) bleeding on probing/with toothbrushes/with hard foods/spontaneously;
(m) increased exudate;
(n) pus;
(o) abscesses;
(p) combined 'perio–endo' lesions;
(q) mobility of teeth;
(r) drifting/tilting of teeth;
(s) tooth extruded from socket;
(t) plunger cusps;
(u) food wedging;
(v) soreness/itching/pain;
(w) bad breath;
(x) bad taste in mouth.

Surprisingly, some patients with periodontitis may be unaware of any significant symptoms.

Bone loss varies in its pattern and extent. In slowly progressive adult chronic periodontitis, the average rate of loss has been estimated as 1.0 mm for each decade of life. If this is so, patients may be expected to have lost about half the alveolar support of certain teeth by their seventh decade of life, notably of the first permanent molars, which are the first teeth to be involved in periodontal disease in the mid-teens. It is unlikely that such bone loss progresses at the steady rate which such an estimate may suggest and, as is well known, variations are commonplace as proposed in what have been called the 'random burst' and 'asynchronous multiple burst' models of disease progression. In general, multi-rooted teeth are more vulnerable to advancing periodontal disease because plaque accumulates in inaccessible inter-radicular sites, and maxillary molars are more prone than others to progressive disease because two furcation entrances are on interstitial surfaces where plaque most readily accumulates and where tooth cleaning by the patient is most difficult. In addition, vertical bone loss is regarded as an indicator of more rapid destruction than horizontal bone loss. However such variations may also be related to bone morphology. Thus vertical bone loss is more likely to occur adjacent to posterior teeth because cancellous bone immediately under the broad contact zone is likely to be resorbed more rapidly than the cortical bone. Anteriorly, the narrow crestal bone, which may be entirely cortical in nature, is likely to be resorbed evenly, creating the appearance of horizontal bone loss. Convenient though such differentiation may seem, many variations occur, and, for example, widespread but moderate horizontal bone loss may be found in older patients with slowly progressive periodontitis, and widespread severe horizontal bone loss may occur in rapidly progressive periodontitis. Localized vertical bone loss may be associated with teeth undergoing occlusal trauma, but vertical defects involving the mesial roots of all first permanent molars and the roots of central incisors in an adolescent may denote juvenile periodontitis.

Radiographs often give an inadequate appraisal of bone defects. The bone loss is often more advanced than X-ray films indicate. What on X-ray films is seen as a 'vertical defect' may represent an osseous defect having one, two or three walls, depending on the integrity of any cortical walls that may or may not have cast a shadow on radiograph. Radiographs may not indicate the presence of enlarged crestal margins ('lips' or 'buttresses'), and defects buccal or lingual to roots (such as dehiscences) will usually not be seen.

It is, of course, impossible to know how long an osseous defect seen on a single radiograph has been present or whether it is progressing. Progression can be determined only by taking comparable radiographs, identical in angulation and exposure time, at a later date. Two years is a reasonable interval for this type of assessment in most patients, using vertical bitewing films if a long-cone technique and standardizing device are unavailable. Orthopantomographs are not usually detailed enough for periodontal assessment.

It may seem unnecessary to state that adequate radiographs should be part of a practitioner's assessment of any patient's dentition (whether periodontal disease is suspected or not), were it not for the fact that some still embark on even extensive work without them.

The majority of patients with periodontal disease will have a slowly progressive or chronic form, although certain sites may show more extensive involvement than others. Before reviewing acute disorders of the periodontium, and different aspects of treatment, the features of juvenile periodontitis and rapidly progressive periodontitis will be reviewed. Both these conditions are uncommon, compared with adult chronic periodontitis, but are difficult and time-consuming to manage adequately, making realistic appraisal at the onset essential.

Juvenile periodontitis

The following clinical features characterize this disorder:

1. There are vertical defects involving the mesial roots of the first permanent molars and upper central incisors.
2. Opposite sides of the jaw commonly have identical defects.
3. Deep true pockets correspond to the defects.
4. Involved teeth may drift and/or become mobile.
5. Oral hygiene is often good.
6. There are no known contributory systemic factors.

The condition is usually detected in the second decade of life, and the incidence is about 0.1% of potential subjects. Previous reports have indicated that females may be more susceptible than males (ratio 3:1), with Asians and Afro-Caribbeans most likely to be involved.

This disorder typifies the so-called specific plaque hypothesis. *A. actinomycetemcomitans* and *E. corrodens* are the predominating microorganisms in progressing sites, whereas the former organism may be found alone in non-progressing sites. All subjects show raised levels of IgG chiefly to *A. actinomycetemcomitans*, and to *E. corrodens*, *B. gingivalis*, and *B. intermedius*. *A. actinomycetemcomitans* blocks the cell surface receptors of neutrophils, and there is evidence in susceptible individuals that neutrophils have deficient chemotactic responses.

Treatment is directed at abolishing the active subgingival microflora. This may nowadays be best accomplished by tetracycline given systemically for two weeks or longer which concentrates in the pocket. Flap surgery may also be indicated. With adequate treatment the disorder may be arrested; if not treated, other teeth may later become involved.

Juvenile periodontitis is rarely found in the primary dentition.

Rapidly progressive periodontitis

This uncommon disorder is classically found in Caucasian female patients before the age of 35 years. Oral hygiene is invariably good. The clinical features include:

(a) horizontal or irregular bone loss which is severe and may involve the entire dentition;
(b) extensive deep true pockets;
(c) involved teeth may become mobile and/or drift;
(d) brisk bleeding on probing from all pockets;
(e) overlying gingival tissues often noticeably inflamed in active phases, but less so in quiescent phases;
(f) purulent exudate from active pockets;
(g) unpleasant taste and bad breath.

There is no noticeable deficiency of neutrophil function, but a higher frequency of human leukocyte antigen (HLA) A9 has been reported. Levels of IgG, IgM, and IgA are raised. B-lymphocytes may be in their normal range but T3 cells may be reduced and T4 cells may be markedly reduced. Predominant micro-organisms include *B. gingivalis* and *W. recta*.

There are often no obvious systemic contributory factors, but the disorder is perhaps more common in 'intense' or 'stressed' individuals. The onset of noticeable changes in many subjects seems to be preceded by some crisis (e.g. family bereavement, breakdown of marriage, losing one's job).

Because the disorder has often reached an advanced stage when first detected, prognosis for many teeth may be poor and treatment choices are limited. However, multiple extractions may constitute another crisis for such individuals, and there is some value in trying to keep as many teeth as possible for as long as possible. Initially, intensive antimicrobial therapy may be effective in reducing microbial activity, followed by subgingival debridement perhaps via the judicious use of flap surgery. In time the most involved teeth may be removed as necessary—perhaps singly at intervals. Splinting may be of little value, but occlusal loading on remaining teeth needs to be assessed carefully.

Although juvenile periodontitis and rapidly progressive periodontitis develop in individuals who apparently lack any contributory systemic disorders, practitioners should consider requesting routine systemic investigations (especially for diabetes mellitus, neutropenia and leukaemia) in seemingly healthy subjects who rapidly develop extensive periodontal disease in the absence of obvious local irritants.

Other advanced forms of periodontitis are uncommon but not unknown (e.g. prepubertal periodontitis). As yet the precise aetiology of such disorders is uncertain.

Acute periodontal disorders

This section will be chiefly concerned with acute necrotizing gingivitis (Vincent's disease) and lateral periodontal abscesses. Acute inflammation of the gingival margin of an erupting tooth (percoronitis), especially involving a mandibular third molar tooth, and acute herpetic gingivostomatitis, are dealt with elsewhere in this book.

Acute necrotizing (ulcerative) gingivitis (Vincent's disease)

This well-recognized and sometimes dramatic disorder is commonest in young adults, often being superimposed on a pre-existing plaque-related chronic gingivitis or chronic periodontitis of which the patient may be unaware.

The onset is usually characterized by:

(a) painful gingiva;
(b) spontaneous gingival bleeding;

(c) foul taste;
(d) bad breath.

Clinically, the tips of one or more papillae become blunted and necrotic, each ulcerated site being covered with a yellowish-grey pseudomembrane, and bounded by an intensely inflamed zone. Such changes may spread laterally along the intervening gingival margins or in an apical direction involving the attached gingiva. The necrosis of the tissues is the cause of the spontaneous bleeding. Occasionally the alveolar crestal bone may be exposed—a feature otherwise rare in periodontal disorders.

Factors predisposing to this order are:

(a) poor oral hygiene;
(b) cigarette smoking (which *increases* blood flow through the gingival margins);
(c) 'stress';
(d) possible seasonal variations;
(e) possible viral infections (e.g. of respiratory tract).

It is perhaps significant that this disorder is commonest at a time of life when individuals for the first time may be under particular stress (e.g. leaving home, taking crucial examinations, entering employment or being unemployed after leaving school, courting and/or getting married!).

Despite the intense fusospirochaetal infiltrate which characterizes the ulcerated tissue, the exact role of these and other bacteria, particularly *B. gingivalis*, remains unclear. Nevertheless, this disorder also supports the specific plaque hypothesis.

Treatment centres on achieving rapid relief of symptoms and thorough debridement of involved tooth surfaces. Opinion is divided over the desirability of scaling the teeth at the time of initial diagnosis, which can be very painful. An ultrasonic scaler may be less uncomfortable than conventional scalers, but creates the risk of a highly contaminated aerosol. Conversely, patients who are started off only on systemic antimicrobial therapy may fail to attend review appointments because their symptoms have resolved. Clearly there is no sure answer to this dilemma and the management of each patient has to be decided on the basis of clinical judgement and other considerations.

Metronidazole, 200 mg tablets, given for 5 days at the rate of three per day, is the antimicrobial drug of choice. Patients should be warned against taking alcohol with this drug. It is wise not to prescribe it for pregnant patients for whom penicillin may be an acceptable alternative. For a pregnant patient who is allergic to penicillin, erythromycin may be used, but it is probably wiser to resort to mouthwashes such as buffered sodium perborate (Bocasan®) or chlorhexidine, although neither achieve as complete or as rapid a response as systemic antimicrobials. Tetracycline is not a suitable drug with which to treat Vincent's disease.

Vincent's ulceration may occasionally be superimposed on chronic periodontitis in older patients or in sites with pericoronitis. Its appearance in mouths which otherwise appear healthy is uncommon enough to raise the possibility that such a patient may be immunocompromised in some way (e.g. leukaemia, AIDS).

Acute lateral periodontal abscesses

Such abscesses, which usually arise within the soft tissue wall of true pockets and are hence superimposed on chronic periodontitis, often represent a crisis in the life of a tooth. Dentist and patient may opt for early extraction, in the belief that the prognosis of such teeth is too poor to warrant extensive treatment. However, with brisk but careful management, the prognosis may often be better than imagined.

The symptoms are usually swelling of the gum and pain, but not always together, and often not of the severity associated with periapical abscesses arising as a sequel to pulpitis. Discomfort is not increased by hot, cold, or tapping, and such teeth are not usually 'raised in the bite'. Regional lymphadenitis, pyrexia, and other evidence of systemic involvement, are usually absent. Involved teeth are vital.

Either the abscess may be 'pointing' or its site may be marked by diffuse redness and swelling; the location is invariably between the gingival margin and mucogingival junction, and most arise adjacent to interstitial areas.

Abscesses tend to involve molar teeth slightly more often than non-molars, but are equally dispersed between maxillary and mandibular molars. Sites exhibiting abscess formation tend to have greater probing depths than contralateral non-abscessed sites. Patients seem to be most at risk from periodontal abscess formation during their third and fourth decades of life; the lower incidence of such abscesses later in life may however be related to the earlier loss of the most susceptible teeth.

The development of such abscesses may be related to such factors as:

(a) prevention of drainage from the pocket (e.g. by calculus);
(b) subgingival flora becoming more pathogenic;
(c) trauma to the pocket wall (e.g. by scaling);
(d) bacteria penetrating the tissues;
(e) alteration of neutrophil activity;
(f) systemic modifying factors.

The fact that a fair proportion of abscesses may follow a scaling procedure must not be interpreted as implying that scaling predisposes to abscess formation; the number of scaling procedures far outstrips the number of reported abscesses.

Any of the following reasons may justify an attempt to retain an abscessed tooth:

(a) first abscess at the site;
(b) no major bone loss;
(c) no excessive mobility;
(d) site amenable to further treatment;
(e) good periodontal status of the remaining dentition;
(f) an important tooth (e.g. bridge abutment; aesthetics);
(g) an intact dental arch;
(h) loss of the tooth may lead to problematic over-eruption of the opposing tooth;
(i) teeth distal to the tooth in question may tilt mesially;
(j) a keen patient with good oral hygiene.

A decision on trying to retain the tooth has to be followed by effective therapy to reduce the acute phase:
1. Incise the abscess.
2. Prescribe effective antimicrobial therapy.
3. Arrange prompt and appropriate follow-up treatment which may be non-surgical or surgical; if one root of a molar is involved, the tooth can sometimes be retained by removing the root in question preferably *after* endodontic therapy of the remaining root(s).

Because the microorganisms most likely to be implicated in abscess formation are Gram-negative anaerobic forms, the antimicrobial drug of first choice is metronidazole 200 mg at approximately 8-hourly intervals for 5 days. Penicillin and erythromycin may be less effective and less rapid in effect. Tetracycline is *not* recommended for suspected or proved periodontal abscesses.

If there is inadequate response to antimicrobial therapy the attempt to save the tooth may have to be reconsidered. Other reasons for removing a tooth involved in abscess formation, either immediately or preferably after the acute phase has subsided, are:
(a) recurrent abscess;
(b) advanced bone loss;
(c) marked mobility;
(d) generalized advanced periodontal disease;
(e) several teeth already absent;
(f) disinterested patient with poor plaque control.

Patients who begin to develop abscesses frequently or in multiple should be assessed for underlying systemic disease.

Occasionally abscesses follow such trauma as direct damage to the soft tissue from food impaction or contact from an opposing tooth, or from a 'high filling'. Such abscesses usually respond well to corrective therapy.

TREATMENT OF PERIODONTAL DISEASES

Periodontal disease often responds favourably to simple treatment provided it is done completely and thoroughly. A scheme of treatment is:
(a) note any relevant medical history;
(b) control any acute disease;
(c) control chronic disease — this progresses through three phases:
  (i) oral hygiene phase;
  (ii) corrective non-surgical or surgical phase;
  (iii) maintenance phase.

Acute disorders

Acute periodontal diseases are controlled, as outlined earlier, by:
(a) release of any pus;
(b) antimicrobial therapy;

(c) relief of pain;
(d) other relevant measures, e.g.
- (i) endodontic therapy;
- (ii) extraction;
- (iii) supportive therapy.

Chronic periodontal diseases

These are controlled by means of:
(a) effective plaque control by the patient;
(b) removal of all hard and soft microbial deposits;
(c) elimination or correction, as far as possible, of any modifying factors;
(d) additional therapy as necessary.

Oral hygiene phase

Stimulating patients to adopt proper home-care measures for effective plaque control is important, time-consuming, and often frustrating for dental personnel. Ingrained attitudes are hard to change and, even if patients appear to be persuaded to alter tooth-cleaning methods, the majority still may not adopt lasting changes. General advice on tooth cleaning is rarely enough; precise advice applied to the patient's problem, and frequently reinforced, is needed.

Practitioners are often able to tailor their approach to the patient's situation. A young adult with a relatively clean mouth but with advanced disease has different requirements when compared with an older patient with inadequate oral hygiene but minimal periodontal destruction. In one mouth different sites may require different levels of management, and time needs to be apportioned accordingly. Adequate documentation and other relevant investigations (e.g. radiographs) are essential. Photographs and study casts may be helpful.

It cannot be assumed that patients have an adequate knowledge about plaque and its role in causing disease in their own mouths. Disclosants may be helpful in highlighting plaque which was missed by the toothbrush. There are several simple reasons why patients leave plaque undisturbed when brushing—for example:

1. They do not brush close enough to the gum margin.
2. Their technique is faulty.
3. They spend insufficient time.
4. Their method is haphazard.
5. Their access is limited (various reasons).
6. Their brush needs replacing.

Sometimes spending more time, using an orderly technique, is all that is required to improve matters. The Bass method, however, has the benefit of providing some intrasulcular cleansing.

THE PERIODONTIUM: DISEASES AND TREATMENT   351

There are various hindrances to effective cleansing:

(a) small mouth opening;
(b) brushing creates a retching sensation;
(c) Handicap (congenital or acquired), e.g. —

    (i) blindness and/or deafness;
    (ii) lack of finger(s), hand, arm;
    (iii) arthritis of fingers and/or hands, etc.;
    (iv) neuromuscular dysfunctions (e.g. strokes, multiple sclerosis);
    (v) educational subnormality.

(d) inaccessible sites —

    (i) position of the tooth in the mouth,
    (ii) misplaced teeth,
    (iii) deep pockets;

(e) sensitivity of exposed roots;
(f) sore mouth;
(g) debilitating disease;
(h) extremes of age.

A different size or style of toothbrush, or modifications to the handle of an existing brush, may prove helpful.

Some patients, even if they are able to master an altered technique of toothbrushing, may find interstitial cleansing beyond them. Flossing requires patience and perseverance; occasionally a floss holder proves helpful. Unwaxed floss is generally more effective at cleaning than waxed floss. 'Superfloss' is sometimes useful where spaces exist between the teeth, or between gum and tooth. If larger spaces are present, spiral-wound brushes may be better, since they are more efficient than floss or woodsticks at cleaning the interstitial concavities of some molar roots.

Clearly, very few tooth-cleaning measures adopted by patients will cleanse subgingivally. Nevertheless, after a full programme of treatment for periodontal disease, patients who allow their supragingival plaque control to lapse, or who do not comply with a maintenance care programme, are more likely to deteriorate than those who cooperate fully.

Although many patients set great store by them, mouthwashes are in general of little benefit because they usually fail to gain access to the subgingival plaque front. If conventional cleaning is precluded, such as by soreness of the oral mucosa, an antibacterial mouthwash (e.g. chlorhexidine) may be helpful. Some patients speak favourably of water irrigation devices. Patients may need to be reminded that, whereas food particles may be dislodged by rinsing, etc., plaque is adherent and less readily removed.

Non-surgical phase

Removal of deposits

Removal of all calculus and subgingival plaque is clearly the responsibility of the dentist and hygienist. There are several reasons for removing calculus:

1. Its surface is always covered with a layer of vital plaque;
2. It retains vital plaque in close proximity to the soft tissues;
3. It may prevent the proper outflow of pocket fluids;
4. It may, by retaining plaque at given sites, promote the development of more virulent forms in time;
5. Supragingival calculus may prevent saliva from exerting antibacterial activity at the pocket entrance;
6. Supragingival calculus prevents the patient's oral hygiene measures from being fully effective.

Gross supragingival deposits may be removed with either conventional or ultrasonic scalers. The latter have the benefit of speed and may be less traumatic to inflamed tissues, but they lack the benefit of tactile sensation. This tactile difficulty has led some to the belief that ultrasonic scalers may be less effective than conventional scalers for removing subgingival deposits, and also their size may prevent them from fully entering deep or narrow pockets. However, both methods may be equally effective, although neither may be able to remove subgingival deposits completely. Sonic scalers may be as effective as ultrasonic scalers.

Subgingival scaling procedures result in a reduction in numbers of spirochaetes and motile organisms and an increase in coccoid forms. Thus the pocket microflora reverts to a form more associated with health. Both methods of scaling also reduce probing depths and bleeding scores, by reducing inflammation of the gingival margin and at the base of the pocket. The pocket microflora takes several weeks to return to pre-scaling proportions. The supposed benefit of post-scaling irrigation with chlorhexidine has been questioned of late.

The effectiveness of non-surgical access to pockets is limited by:

(a) pocket depth;
(b) position of the tooth in the mouth;
(c) furcation involvement;
(d) minor surface irregularities;
(e) tolerance of patient;
(f) operator's skill;
(g) choice of instruments.

Interest has also been focused on the possibility that lipopolysaccharide endotoxins from Gram-negative bacteria might be adsorbed into the cementum lining the pocket. The technique of root planing has hence been advocated to remove involved layers of cementum and create a biologically acceptable surface. This particular concept has been questioned of late, although there seems little doubt that the cemental surface in some way is able to harbour microbial forms.

The raising of surgical flaps may give better access for the thorough debridement of root surfaces, particularly for deeper pockets. Nevertheless, thorough non-surgical measures may in the long term prove as effective as surgical measures, even in deep pockets, in retarding or arresting periodontal disease.

THE PERIODONTIUM: DISEASES AND TREATMENT

Modifying factors

As well as factors already mentioned, various other factors may enhance plaque accumulation, hinder its proper removal, or modify the response of the tissues to plaque accumulation.

Local modifying factors. These include:

(a) open lip posture;
(b) shallow buccal vestibule or sulcus;
(c) prominent fraena and/or mucosal bands;
(d) rough enamel surfaces;
(e) reduced buccolingual width of alveolar housing;
(f) imbrication;
(g) close apposition of roots;
(h) partial eruption;
(i) over-eruption;
(j) occlusal factors;
(k) exposed roots (rough, sensitive);
(l) carious cavities adjacent to gingival margins;
(m) calculus;
(n) restorations;
(o) appliances;
(p) partial dentures.

A few comments are pertinent to the above list. When the width of the alveolar bone is narrow, anatomical deficiencies of the crestal bone (dehiscences) may be present (see p. 338). Such deficiencies are also likely to occur where teeth are prominent, as at sites of imbrication. Initially the gingiva covers such sites but may later break down to allow the formation of a Stillman's cleft. Such areas of gingival recession may alarm patients, but they can usually be reassured that they are unlikely to lose the tooth. However, the exposed root is often difficult to clean, both because of sensitivity and access, and gingivitis of the surrounding tissue may ensue; this problem is compounded wherever the vestibule is already shallow or where frena are implicated.

Not all patients have problems in cleaning imbricated teeth. However, where teeth are crowded, roots may not only be prominent (leading potentially to problems already mentioned) but also in close contact, which could theoretically dispose such a site to more rapid downgrowth of plaque and periodontal breakdown, as well as inhibiting instrumentation. Similar problems may occur where teeth are partially erupted or over-erupted.

The presence of wear facets and/or attrition should always prompt questions about bruxism. Mobility and/or movement of a maxillary lateral incisor may be a consequence of occlusion with a prominent mandibular canine. Maxillary premolars, especially those with prominent cusps and deep fossae, should be checked for mobility in lateral movements. A polythene occlusal cover sometimes helps to overcome the effect of occlusal overloading, in conjunction with the above measures. Nevertheless, where there is a combined problem of occlusal stress and periodontitis, current evidence shows that the first need is to remove all microbial irritants from the involved site.

Not all restorations are plaque retentive, but problems may arise if their margins are:

(a) subgingival;
(b) rough;
(c) overhanging;
(d) overbuilt (compressing the gingival papilla);
(e) deficient.

Deficient contact areas may encourage food packing. Placement of matrix bands and/or wedges may damage the gingival tissues, but failure to adapt bands to the concavities of certain roots may permit some restorative material to 'escape' beyond the cavity margin.

Orthodontic appliances, intermaxillary fixation and partial dentures are all potential sources of plaque accumulation. If function and aesthetics are not compromised by the absence of certain teeth, partial dentures may be avoidable, or simple bridges may be a suitable alternative.

Systemic modifying factors. These may include:

(a) puberty;
(b) neutropenia;
(c) leukaemia;
(d) diabetes mellitus;
(e) dietary insufficiency and/or malabsorption;
(f) pregnancy;
(g) drug therapy: —
  (i) oral contraceptives,
  (ii) nifedipine and diltiazem,
  (iii) phenytoin,
  (iv) cyclosporin;
(h) immunocompromising disease or treatment.

Particularly where plaque control is good any of the following features should arouse suspicion of underlying systemic disease:

(a) generalized gingival redness;
(b) generalized gingival enlargement;
(c) tendency to spontaneous bleeding;
(d) soreness of gingiva and/or oral mucosa;
(e) frequent or multiple abscess formation;
(f) unexpected change in the level or severity of disease;
(g) failure to respond adequately to local measures.

Investigations may necessitate referring the patient to a specialized unit without delay.

Clearly the extent to which different patients manifest systemic changes within the mouth varies widely, and it is not possible within the scope of this chapter to provide more detail. Treatment can often be satisfactorily arranged in liaison with the patient's physician or specialist. Occasionally drug therapy can be changed to reduce gingival enlargement. Oral hygiene measures may be supplemented with an antibacterial mouthwash, e.g. chlorhexidine, to control 'pregnancy gingivitis'. Since the hormonal changes exaggerate the local response to plaque, pregnancy gingivitis is to be regarded as an indicator of pre-existing chronic gingivitis which will need thorough treatment after parturition. For patients with a reduced host response, antimicrobial therapy may be indicated more often than would be necessary in a healthy subject.

To the problems which may limit the patient's ability to exercise effective plaque control may be added such difficulties as:

(a) caring for infants or infirm relatives at home;
(b) bereavement;
(c) domestic pressures;
(d) extensive travel;
(e) demands and stress of work (e.g. shift work).

The wise practitioner will seek to be informed of all such 'social factors' which may play a crucial role in the patient's response to dental care.

Additional therapy

Apart from dealing with any plaque-retentive restorations and modifying or replacing certain partial dentures, further therapy may include:

(a) antimicrobial therapy;
(b) orthodontic re-alignment of drifting or crowded teeth;
(c) removal of impacted teeth or those with a poor prognosis;
(d) hemisections or root amputations;
(e) splinting;
(f) frenectomy;
(g) gingival grafts;
(h) corrective surgery for periodontal pockets.

Several of these topics are discussed in the next section.

Antimicrobial therapy

Apart from their use in treating acute periodontal disorders, antibiotics are not an alternative to thorough subgingival debridement. However, antibiotics may be used effectively under one or more of the following circumstances:

(a) widespread bleeding on probing;
(b) pus exuding from a number of pockets;
(c) marked vascularity of the gingival tissues;
(d) scaling procedures limited by profuse bleeding.

As mentioned earlier, such features may also denote underlying systemic disorders, so that ideally systemic investigations should precede the giving of antibiotics.

Various antibiotics have been used in an attempt to halt periodontal destruction, given either systemically or by local delivery systems. At present three drugs remain in general use and are usually given systemically:

(a) tetracyclines;
(b) metronidazole;
(c) amoxycillin.

Tetracyclines. These antimicrobials are active against Gram-positive and Gram-negative cocci and bacilli and spirochaetes, by interfering with protein synthesis. They also inhibit collagenase activity. The recommended dose for juvenile periodontitis, rapidly progressive periodontitis, refractory periodontitis, and sometimes active phases of adult chronic periodontitis, is 1000 mg daily in four equally divided doses for 2 or 3 weeks. Capsules should be taken half an hour before meals and not taken with milk. Tetracyclines may reduce the efficacy of orally administered contraceptive drugs, and should be avoided in patients with renal disease. The addition of nystatin may prevent opportunistic candidal infection.

Metronidazole. This is an antimicrobial drug effective against Gram-negative obligate anaerobes and spirochaetes, and therefore may be ineffective against facultative aerobic organisms. The recommended dosage for treating acute necrotizing ulcerative gingivitis and acute abscesses is 600 mg daily in three equally divided doses for 5 days. Its interaction with alcohol is well known, and is a serious disadvantage for some patients!

Amoxycillin. This is a broad-spectrum penicillin active against Gram-positive cocci and Gram-negative bacilli. Apart from being contraindicated where a history of allergy to penicillin exists, amoxycillin is perhaps less effective than metronidazole in treating acute periodontal disorders and less effective than tetracycline in treating juvenile periodontitis, rapidly progressive periodontitis, and active phases of adult chronic periodontitis. There have been some promising results when amoxycillin has been combined with clavulanic acid (Augmentin®) in the treatment of established refractory periodontitis, but as it is such a valuable drug in other situations, its use in periodontal disorders has to be considered very carefully.

Splinting

Splinting is not a panacea for all mobile teeth, but may be of benefit where:

1. Mobility of a tooth, or a few teeth, is of a temporary nature (e.g. following surgery or trauma).
2. Where teeth have undergone occlusal adjustment for mobility and are expected to become firmer.
3. Where underlying periodontitis is being treated and the involved teeth are expected to become firmer.
4. After orthodontic correction of teeth which had moved as a result of periodontal disease and where, without splinting, relapse could occur.

Splinting may give rise to the following problems:

1. Oral hygiene measures are hampered, usually because interstitial cleaning aids cannot be used.
2. Plaque accumulation may promote further disease.
3. The true status of the involved tooth (or teeth) may cease to be evident.

Before temporary or permanent splints are applied, all supragingival and subgingival deposits need to be meticulously removed and good plaque control by the patient needs to be established. Any adverse occlusal stresses on the involved teeth need to be treated. Where mobility is a feature of untreated chronic periodontitis, removal of all irritants often results in reduced mobility, often to the extent that splints are no longer necessary. Patients need to understand that, because periodontal disease is primarily plaque-related, the wearing of splints may not retard the disease. Polythene occlusal covers may be better than splinting when mobility is the result of bruxism.

Chapter 40

Periodontal surgery

The goal of periodontal therapy is to maintain the health and function of the natural dentition whilst preserving satisfactory aesthetics. As previously discussed, periodontal therapy may progress through three phases:

(a) the oral hygiene phase;
(b) the corrective non-surgical or surgical phase;
(c) the maintenance phase.

Generally, the procedures which may be adopted for periodontal surgery are subject to considerable variability due to prevailing opinion, and this makes the rationale for, and the selection of, suitable and relevant surgical techniques complex. However, it is generally the case that the surgical procedures which most concern general dental practitioners fall into three categories:

(a) gingivectomy techniques;
(b) flap surgery;
(c) mucogingival surgery.

The basic principles underlying the use of these three broad categories of techniques should be understood. This chapter aims to present a rationale for periodontal surgery whilst restricting the description of named techniques to a minimum. It should be appreciated that there is no wholly satisfactory classification of surgical procedures and, frequently, experienced operators adopt an approach which may combine more than one technique.

INDICATIONS FOR SURGERY

1. The persistence of bleeding on probing from the base of pockets following the oral hygiene phase
2. The presence of true pockets with active disease in excess of 5 mm depth
3. An unfavourable contour of the marginal gingival tissues which prevents the patient from being able to maintain an adequate standard of oral hygiene
4. The inability of the operator to remove deposits by subgingival scaling and root planing by non-surgical means
5. To facilitate conservation or prosthodontic treatment
6. To restore function
7. To restore aesthetics
8. The presence of (1) to (6) in combination with good patient cooperation and a high standard of personal plaque control

CONTRAINDICATIONS TO SURGERY

1. Inadequate standard of oral hygiene — it is essential that hygiene therapy has been successful before contemplating surgery, as otherwise the periodontal condition may be worsened as a result of the surgical intervention
2. Doubtful patient cooperation
3. Little bony support remaining and tooth loss inevitable
4. Elderly patient and tooth prognosis adequate if left untreated
5. Medically compromised patient, e.g. immunosuppressed, recent myocardial infarction, leukaemia

Patients who are insulin-dependent diabetics, or who give a history of adrenal incompetence, steroid therapy, rheumatic fever, warfarin therapy, or who have had a renal transplant, should only receive periodontal surgery after consultation with the appropriate medical practitioner

Systemic investigations should be considered for patients who have not responded as anticipated to non-surgical phases of treatment

6. Presence of an acute gingival condition, e.g. pericoronitis or acute necrotizing ulcerative gingivitis
7. Inadequate clinical expertise or facilities

AIMS OF SURGERY

1. To arrest the disease process
2. To restore the health of the tissues
3. To enable the patient to establish a good standard of oral hygiene
4. To increase the bony support and create a new connective tissue attachment
5. To restore function
6. To improve aesthetics

A surgical procedure may not achieve all of these aims.

SURGICAL TECHNIQUES

Very many surgical techniques have been described and it is best to consider them in terms of the following three basic principles:

(a) resection;
(b) reattachment;
(c) repositioning;

Resection

Resection techniques involve the complete removal of both the inner pocket epithelium and the outer soft tissue pocket wall. Examples of such techniques are the conventional gingivectomy and Zamet's replaced flap.

There are a number of methods and instruments available for performing a conventional gingivectomy, and these may include the use of scalpels, handpieces with diamond impregnated stones, periodontal nippers, or electrosurgery.

Electrosurgery has the advantage that it renders the operative field relatively bloodless, which enhances operator visibility, but care must be taken not to remove too much tissue or expose the bone crest, as there is then a danger of necrosis. Additionally, it is claimed that healing after electrosurgery takes longer and that patients dislike the technique.

Use of a water- or saline-cooled diamond stone in a handpiece to remove other than localized areas of tissue is best avoided, since there is a lack of fine control over the amount of gingiva removed.

A scalpel is generally recommended as the preferred method for performing a gingivectomy incision. A variety of knives may be used including a Bard–Parker scalpel with Swann–Morton No. 15 or 12 blades, or a Blake knife with a No. 11 blade.

Operative procedure for the conventional gingivectomy

1. The depths of the pockets to be treated are measured with a periodontal probe and these measurements marked on the outer surface of the attached gingiva using the tip of the probe. Alternatively, this may be done using Crane–Kaplan pocket-marking forceps, but the beaks of these are rather bulky and may not reach the depths of pockets, thereby impairing accuracy.

2. An incision is made at 45° to the long axis of the tooth with the tip of the blade pointing coronally. The angle and position of the incision may be modified according to the desired final contour of the gingiva. The incision should be made apical to the bleeding points which denote the bases of the pockets and should be aimed to excise the full depth of each pocket.

The bone crest must not be exposed and the incision should therefore be approximately 2 mm above the bone crest. The incision should commence at a papilla and should be made from the back of the mouth towards the midline to assist the operator's visibility and control.

It is essential that a sharp scalpel blade is used and more than one blade may be needed to complete a single procedure.

3. The tissue that has been excised is removed using curettes or other suitable instruments. Tissue tags that remain should also be removed.

The exposed tooth surfaces are scaled free of any deposits. Exposed root surfaces are planed and superficial contaminated cementum is removed.

The junction between the incision and the intact gingival tissue may need additional contouring and this may be achieved using a water-cooled diamond impregnated wheel; recontouring with a scalpel is difficult.

4. The wound is covered with a periodontal dressing for up to 1 week.

Disadvantages of the conventional gingivectomy

The conventional, or, as it was formerly named, open-wound gingivectomy is not now generally recommended for the surgical correction of true pockets, since there are a number of disadvantages. These are:

1. Bleeding during the procedure can be problematic and postoperative haemorrhage can occur.
2. Healing of the wound is by secondary intention, and therefore slow.
3. The wound may be painful.
4. A periodontal dressing is required for the initial stages of wound healing.
5. There is a danger of secondary infection developing, even beneath a periodontal dressing.
6. The aesthetic result arising from the excision of gingival tissue may be undesirable.
7. A resection technique may not be used to treat infrabony defects since the bone crest is not visualized.
8. A resection technique may not be used if pocketing has extended apical to the mucogingival junction, or if the surgery will compromise its integrity.
9. If a resection technique is used in the treatment of suprabony true pockets, the exposure of the root surfaces caused by the operation may lead to dentine sensitivity, root caries, furcation exposure, difficulties in oral hygiene maintenance and poor aesthetics.

Advantages of the conventional gingivectomy

1. Restorations that were subgingival prior to surgery may become supragingival after surgery, and therefore accessible to oral hygiene measures.
2. The wound heals with a dento-epithelial junction of normal dimensions.
3. Interproximal spaces are enlarged and this may facilitate plaque control.
4. In areas of the mouth where access may be very difficult, both for the patient and the operator (particularly around the posterior molar teeth), pocket elimination may be the treatment of choice.

Indications for conventional gingivectomy

Because of the many disadvantages of resection techniques, their use tends to be restricted to gingivoplasty, which is:

(a) the surgical removal of hyperplastic gingival tissue that has formed false pockets, e.g. phenytoin hyperplasia;

(b) the correction of gingival contour which has resulted from chronic gingivitis, or from episodes of acute necrotizing ulcerative gingivitis;

(c) a crown lengthening procedure to assist restorative treatment;

(d) the deliberate exposure of furcations when it is considered that this will facilitate oral hygiene measures (rarely).

Gingivoplasty produces very satisfactory aesthetic results when the technique has been correctly applied and performed.

Re-attachment procedures

The periodontal attachment apparatus consists of alveolar bone, cementum, periodontal ligament and junctional epithelium. Ideally, periodontal therapy should not only arrest the disease process, but should also restore lost periodontal attachment and therefore health.

Unfortunately, this is seldom achieved using re-attachment procedures because, on healing, epithelial cells derived from the oral epithelium and from remnants of the pocket epithelium migrate down the surgically exposed and cleaned root surface, forming a long junctional epithelium. This migration of epithelial cells occurs at a much faster rate than connective tissue cells are able to differentiate and form a new and conventional connective tissue attachment.

All the re-attachment procedures, such as the modified Widman flap and subgingival curettage, heal via a long junctional epithelium. This structure is as strongly attached to the tooth as the junctional epithelium in health, but its potential for breakdown in the absence of immaculate plaque control is greater and, therefore, a long epithelial attachment to the tooth is not a wholly acceptable substitute for a new connective tissue attachment.

Purposes of raising a flap

1. To establish a clinical situation where open curettage of periodontal defects can be undertaken
2. To visualize the bone crest and evaluate the extent of bony defects
3. To scale and plane root surfaces and furcations to remove deposits and superficial contaminated cementum
4. To eliminate bulky, overhanging, or ragged osseous margins of bony defects
5. To eliminate overhanging restorations if this has not been achieved preoperatively
6. To stabilize the gingiva by the method of flap replacement
7. To achieve healing where possible by primary intention

Advantages of flap surgery

1. Good access to roots and bony support
2. Scaling and root planing by direct vision
3. Healing by primary intention
4. Low incidence of postoperative pain, infection and bleeding
5. No intentional exposure of roots of the teeth
6. Conservation of attached gingiva

Disadvantages of flap surgery

1. The operative procedure may cause an unpredictable amount of gingival recession
2. The recession which results may cause poor aesthetics and also dentine hypersensitivity, which can be resistant to treatment
3. Exposure of roots and furcations may result in root caries and difficulties in plaque control
4. Flap surgery for shallow pockets may cause loss of attachment

Operative procedure for simple flap surgery

1. It is essential that, at the time of surgery, the operator has an up to date and adequate set of radiographs of the teeth, in order to assist planning of the surgical procedure.

2. It is advantageous to use an adrenalin-containing local anaesthetic solution for periodontal surgery, since this diminishes bleeding and thereby assists vision of the operative field. Infiltrations into the sulcus, as well as into the gingival papillae on both sides of the teeth should be sufficient to achieve anaesthesia.

When possible, a lingual nerve block injection should be avoided, since the patient will lose effective control of the tongue and the operator's access lingually will be more difficult.

3. An inverse or reverse bevel incision is made at a 10–15° angle directed apically to the long axis of the teeth. Swann–Morton blades Nos. 15 or 11 are recommended.

The incision should be made 1–2 mm away from the gingival margin, and should extend down to the bone crest.

The distance that the incision is placed from the gingival margin varies according to the health of the tissues at the time of surgery. If no pocketing is present, e.g. over the root face, there may be no need to excise any gingival tissue and an intracrevicular incision may be made.

It is the opinion of some operators that, even in the presence of pocketing, it is not necessary routinely to excise pocket epithelium and an intracrevicular incision for periodontal flap surgery is preferred.

The incision should commence at a papilla and should have a scalloped outline so as to conform to a desirable gingival contour, and to allow for interproximal coverage when the flap is replaced at the end of the procedure. The scalloping may be exaggerated to increase the likelihood of interproximal coverage, but this may be undesirable if, in order to achieve this, tissue has to be sacrificed in areas which are not periodontally involved.

The palatal incision may be complex particularly if the vault of the palate is shallow, the tissue is hyperplastic, or the pockets are deep. In such cases, it is often necessary to make the palatal incision in two stages. The first incision should be followed by an additional incision to thin the tissue and allow for better flap adaptation.

4. The flap should be elevated using a periosteal elevator or a flat plastic so as to expose the bone crest and allow visualization of bony defects. Each time bone is surgically exposed, some resorption will take place. It is, therefore, important to keep exposure of bone to a minimum and not to disturb the periosteum.

5. Once the flap has been raised, the gingival cuff of tissue that has been excised is removed using curettes. Granulation tissue within bony defects is also removed in the same way.

An ultrasonic scaler may prove useful to loosen any particularly adherent granulation tissue and to commence scaling the root surfaces free from deposits. Amalgam overhangs may also be reduced using an ultrasonic scaler.

As inflamed granulation tissue is removed, bleeding diminishes and visibility for scaling and root planing the teeth, using hoes and curettes, is improved.

6. When the teeth are free from deposits and the bony defects have been cleaned of granulation tissue, the flap may be replaced. Wherever possible, flaps should meet interproximally and if this is achieved (without tension), a periodontal dressing need not be applied.

If, however, flap apposition is not possible interdentally, then a periodontal dressing is essential to protect the blood clot from breakdown and to allow the initial phases of healing to take place undisturbed. The periodontal dressing should be in place for up to 1 week, after which time both the pack and the sutures are removed.

Repositioning procedures

Apical repositioning of a surgical flap has been out of vogue. The purpose of apical repositioning is to preserve or increase the width of the attached gingiva, or to increase sulcus depth. However, the importance of the presence of an adequate width of attached gingiva for health is not so great as was formerly considered to be the case, and it is now more common to use the free gingival graft procedure to gain sulcus depth.

If periodontal pockets are of such a depth that their bases extend below the mucogingival junction, then replacement of a flap apically during surgery onto sound bone will assist stability of the gingiva postoperatively and will maintain or increase the width of the attached gingiva.

Operative procedure for apical repositioning

1. An inverse bevel incision is used to outline the flap (as previously described for re-attachment surgery), and the tissue is reflected beyond, i.e. apical to the mucogingival junction. Depending on the length of the flap being raised, relieving incisions may or may not be necessary.

2. Tissue cannot be apically repositioned on the palate and is repositioned with some difficulty lingual on the lower arch. Particular care is required lingual to the lower molars.

3. A partial- or split-thickness flap is raised, i.e. the periosteum remains in situ. The risk of bone resorption and postoperative discomfort is thus reduced.

4. The periodontal defects are cleaned as described for re-attachment surgery.

5. Often a flap requires to be apically repositioned on one side of an arch only, in which case a sling or continuous suturing technique is indicated. Sutures should not be tied under tension and a periodontal pack is used to help stabilize the flap and maintain it in position. Additional sutures through the periosteum in the sulcus may be required to hold the flap in its new position.

Apical repositioning leads to all the disadvantages associated with exposure of the roots of the teeth, and some operators use a combination of re-attachment with repositioning techniques to keep root and, particularly, furcation exposure to a minimum.

Repositioning does, however, have the advantage that a normal dento-gingival relationship is created, and a number of operators consider that oral hygiene is, in fact, facilitated for the patient by exposing interdental areas, which become wider and easier to clean.

The role of osseous recontouring during surgery

1. No attempt should be made to re-establish physiological bony contour during surgery. Such an approach destroys supporting bone and lessens the chances of bony infill during healing.
2. Supportive bone should never be removed.
3. Bone removal should be kept to a minimum and should be restricted to the reduction of reverse architecture, lipping, and bulky or ragged osseous margins, in order to facilitate flap adaptation. Such removal of unsupporting bone is called **osteoplasty**.

Extractions

Extraction may be considered for:
   (a)   non-functional teeth;
   (b)   excessive bone loss and mobility;
   (c)   partially erupted wisdom teeth which the patient cannot clean;
   (d)   recurrent lateral periodontal abscesses;
   (e)   persistent discomfort;
   (f)   narrow width of bony septa between teeth, when the periodontal disease process affecting one tooth is compromising an adjacent tooth or teeth.

Subgingival curettage

Subgingival curettage is the removal of pocket epithelium as well as a portion of subjacent inflamed connective tissue, using either curettes or a scalpel. The use of a scalpel to remove pocket epithelium without raising a flap is the basis of the excisional new attachment procedure (ENAP).

The ideal aim of subgingival curettage or ENAP is to promote a new attachment of connective tissue and/or epithelium to the cleaned root surface. However, as inflammation subsides, any reduction in probing depth will invariably be due to tissue shrinkage.

In general terms, curettage is seldom used because of the disadvantages inherent in the technique. If, however, the removal of pocket epithelium only is indicated, then it is preferable to achieve this by using a scalpel.

Advantages of subgingival curettage

1. The procedure is relatively non-invasive and does not involve disturbing periosteum or raising a flap.

2. When used to treat a suprabony pocket involving a single tooth, the procedure need not disturb the gingival tissues of neighbouring teeth which may not be periodontally involved.

3. Suturing or the use of a periodontal pack may not be necessary.

Disadvantages of subgingival curettage

1. For true infrabony pocketing, the technique is not suitable since the bone crest is not visualized and infrabony defects cannot therefore be satisfactorily assessed or treated.

2. The procedure is technically difficult and time-consuming.

3. Instrumentation takes place under indirect vision and relies on tactile sense. It is not, therefore, possible to be certain that all the pocket epithelium has been removed.

4. The procedure may be traumatic and involve the removal of more tissue than the operator intended.

Mucogingival surgery

For many years, great emphasis has been placed by periodontologists on the necessity of preserving an adequate zone of attached gingiva to maintain periodontal health. Many surgical procedures have been adopted to increase sulcus depth and/or create wider zones of attached gingiva.

However, it has now been established that a complete absence of attached gingiva can be compatible with periodontal health, provided that oral hygiene can be maintained. Generally, however, a small amount of attached gingiva (as little as 1 or 2 mm), is thought to be advantageous to maintain health.

Both the variety and volume of mucogingival surgery being performed is now less and is focused on the technique of free gingival grafting, for which case selection is very important.

Free gingival graft

There are many causes of gingival recession, which is defined as the migration of the gingival margin apical to the cementum–enamel junction. The first sign of recession may be the formation of a small groove in the gingiva, the so-called Stillman's cleft. The aetiology of gingival recession is unclear, but the principal causes are thought to be as follows:

(a) faulty toothbrushing;
(b) malalignment of teeth;
(c) iatrogenic causes arising from periodontal and orthodontic treatment;
(d) inflammation and chronic periodontal disease;
(e) cervical restorations;
(f) prosthodontic and other appliances;
(g) traumatic occlusion;
(h) ageing;
(i) fraenal attachment;
(j) narrow width or absence of attached gingiva.

The free gingival graft is not designed to be able to treat all of these causes of recession and the main indications are:

1. To increase sulcus depth so that adequate oral hygiene measures may be effectively adopted.
2. To stabilize the attached gingiva in the presence of developing recession.
3. To create some attached gingiva, where previously no attached gingiva was present.
4. To eliminate fraena where these are associated with persistent inflammation, with or without an adequate width of attached gingiva.

Care must be taken that the presence of developing recession is not confused with eruption of the teeth to their full clinical crown length. In young children and adolescents, eruption of the lower incisor teeth may occur unevenly and give the illusion that active recession is present on one tooth relative to another. With growth, this situation usually rectifies itself and the child should be carefully monitored to ensure that good oral hygiene is maintained and no recession develops. Study models may be helpful to monitor the level of the gingival margin. Only where true recession is developing should surgery be considered for a child and, if the necessity for a graft is unavoidable in a young child, a general anaesthetic may be needed. An orthodontic opinion may be advisable in the presence of lower anterior crowding, since judicious extraction may be the treatment of choice.

Grafts cannot significantly reduce recession that is already present, particularly if the soft tissue defect over the root is long and wide. However, if the defect over the root is shallow and narrow, some creeping re-attachment may take place after a modest coronal repositioning of the graft. The gain is not, however, likely to be extensive.

The teeth where grafts are most commonly required are the lower incisors, and the premolar and canine teeth in either arch.

Operative procedure for the free gingival graft

The procedure described below is for placing a free gingival graft into the lower incisor region, but the same surgical principles apply for performing the technique at any site in the mouth.

1. *Anaesthesia.* Local anaesthetic solution containing adrenalin should be injected into the sulcus in such a way that the mucosa balloons up. This, in effect, raises a split-thickness flap and facilitates the incision. Local anaesthetic should also be placed in the palatal mucosa distal to the area from which the graft tissue is to be taken.

2. *Preparation of the graft bed.* An incision is made along the mucogingival junction without penetrating the periosteum. The unattached mucosa is reflected apically by blunt dissection using either a periosteal elevator, or the handle of the scalpel. Any existing fraenal and muscle attachments are released. Thus the graft bed, which often has a semilunar outline, has a base of intact periosteum. It should be slightly larger than the size of the graft that is to be placed.

The marginal gingival tissue of the tooth or teeth to be grafted may or may not be retained. It is desirable to try to maintain a band of marginal tissue since this may improve the prognosis of the graft. Any plaque or calculus deposits present on the teeth must be removed.

The lateral borders of the graft bed may be bevelled using periodontal nippers or a scalpel blade, in order to maximize the apposition of the graft tissue to the borders of the graft bed and, therefore, to encourage the establishment of a good blood supply to the graft.

Once the graft bed has been prepared, a damp swab is placed in the area to control haemorrhage whilst the graft tissue is being taken from the palate.

3. *Obtaining the graft tissue.* The size of the graft needed is estimated. The graft should be larger than the final result requires, since there will be some shrinkage on healing. A tin-foil template of the desired size and shape of the graft may be prepared to assist excision of the graft tissue from the palate.

The graft should be taken from a site approximately 3 mm from the gingival margin and distal to the palatal rugae. To avoid damage to the palatine blood vessels, it is essential that the graft is not taken from tissue too high up in the vault of the palate.

The area to be grafted should first be outlined by a shallow incision no greater than 1.5 mm deep. Commencing coronally the graft is dissected free. A number of specialist knives are available to facilitate taking graft tissue, but in the absence of these a No. 15 blade and a Bard–Parker scalpel handle are quite satisfactory.

The graft should be sufficiently thin so as not to incorporate submucosal fat, and any yellow fat lobules on the undersurface of the graft should be removed.

On its removal from the palate, the graft tissue should be placed between gauze soaked in saline to keep it moist prior to transference to the graft bed.

The graft site will be responsible for the majority of the postoperative discomfort experienced by the patient. The site may be dressed using Stomahesive®, an adherent dressing which dissolves or is lost after approximately 24 h.

4. *Transference of the graft tissue to the donor site.* The gauze swab should be removed from the graft bed and haemorrhage should be further controlled by suction and pressure.

The graft tissue should be transferred to the periosteal bed and secured in place by two sutures, one on each lateral border. Either 5/O silk or Ethibond® 5/O braided polyester coated with polybutylate are suitable sutures. The sutures should not be placed under tension. Another method for securing a graft in position is the use of a cyanoacrylate adhesive dressing, such as Histoacryl®.

Pressure must be applied to the graft for 5 min to promote initial fibrin attachment between the graft and its bed as well as to prevent formation of a haematoma. A periodontal dressing should then be placed for 1 week.

Both the periodontal dressing and the sutures should be removed after 1 week and the patient should be advised to begin gentle oral hygiene measures immediately.

Two months following the surgery, the graft site will have healed. The area will always remain pale by comparison with the surrounding gingiva.

Periodontal dressings

The purposes of a periodontal dressing are:

(a) to protect the wound, particularly if there is no epithelial covering to allow healing by primary intention or, if there is exposure of bone;
(b) to maintain adaptation of the flap to the teeth and underlying bone, especially if the flap has been apically repositioned;
(c) to discourage postoperative bleeding, or the formation of excessive granulation tissue;
(d) to protect interproximal areas from food packing;
(e) to discourage the patient from disturbing the surgical site during the initial phases of wound healing.

Disadvantages of periodontal dressings

1. Rinsing with 0.2% chlorhexidine will not prevent plaque accumulation under the pack
2. Risk of postoperative infection
3. Unsightly and uncomfortable
4. If adapted too tightly interdentally, healing may be compromised
5. Hypersensitivity reactions, particularly to eugenol-containing dressings

Ideal properties of a periodontal dressing

1. Setting time should be sufficient for the dressing to be placed
2. Sufficient plasticity to enable handling and placement
3. Sufficient rigidity to resist displacement
4. Smooth surfaces on setting, to prevent soft tissue irritation
5. Bactericidal, to combat plaque formation
6. Eugenol-free, to decrease the risk of sensitivity reactions
7. Absence of interference with the healing process
8. Cohesive and adhesive

Eugenol-free dressings such as Coe-Pak® or Peripac® are generally recommended. However, even eugenol-free packs may cause hypersensitivity reactions.

Cyanoacrylate tissue adhesives may also be used as dressing materials, either in liquid or spray form. However, the indications for their use are rather restricted, and they can be difficult to handle, particularly when dealing with grafts. After applying a tissue adhesive, a conventional periodontal pack may also be used to ensure that no wound displacement occurs.

ANTIMICROBIALS AS ADJUNCTS TO SURGERY

1. Antimicrobials are not generally indicated or required during or after periodontal surgery.
2. If clinically warranted, a course of antimicrobials may be administered either prophylactically, to commence within the 24 h prior to the surgery or to start immediately after surgery has been performed.

3. The antimicrobials of choice are metronidazole, amoxycillin, tetracycline, or rarely, Augmentin®.

POSTOPERATIVE PROBLEMS FOR THE PATIENT

1. Pain
2. Bleeding
3. Infection
4. Recession
5. Sensitivity
6. Staining of the teeth and their appearance
7. Root caries
8. Maintenance of oral hygiene

POSTOPERATIVE INSTRUCTIONS GIVEN BY THE DENTIST

1. The patient should be reassured, should fully understand the nature of the surgery that has been performed and should be given a set of written postoperative instructions. Details of the operative procedure and the postoperative instructions issued should be meticulously entered into the patient's records.

2. The postoperative instructions should explain:

(a) That the patient may experience some postoperative discomfort. The use of a mild analgesic, e.g. two 500 mg paracetamol tablets BP every 4–6 h may be helpful.

Some operators administer an analgesic to the patient before the anaesthetic has fully worn off to help minimize immediate postoperative discomfort.

(b) The function of the periodontal dressing. The patient should be instructed not to eat sharp or sticky foods that will dislodge the dressing. Saline mouthwashes at regular intervals will help to freshen the mouth. The rest of the dentition should be cleaned as normal.

(c) In the event of post-operative bleeding, the patient should apply pressure using a damp gauze or handkerchief for 20 min. The patient should be given a telephone number with which to contact the dentist in the event of either persistent bleeding, or prolonged and severe pain (which may indicate the presence of an infection).

(d) Should the periodontal dressing be displaced and lost, the patient should be instructed either to contact the dentist, or to cleanse the surgical wound using either a 0.2% chlorhexidine mouthwash, or by gentle brushing.

3. After a maximum of 1 week the patient should attend for review. At this appointment, the dentist should remove the periodontal dressing and any sutures.

The surgical area should be gently cleansed and a 0.2% chlorhexidine solution on a cotton-wool bud is suitable. The teeth may be polished using a rubber cup and prophylactic paste.

In addition to normal oral hygiene measures, the patient may be advised to clean the operative site with 0.2% chlorhexidine on a toothbrush twice weekly for a 6-week period postoperatively, to assist healing.

Of greatest importance is the provision of oral hygiene instruction. Most emphasis should be placed on plaque control of the interproximal areas, since recession generally results in increased interdental exposure following surgery.

4. It is essential that the patient is adequately reviewed and the periodontal condition maintained following a course of either non-surgical or surgical work. A patient may initially be reviewed 6 weeks postsurgery to assess the progress and success of healing, as well as the quality of plaque control.

Failure to review patients has been shown to result in the loss of any clinical improvements that might have been gained, or to precipitate a deterioration in the periodontal condition.

HEALING AFTER SURGICAL PROCEDURES

Conventional gingivectomy

Healing after a conventional gingivectomy is by secondary intention. Epithelialization of the gingivectomy wound is usually complete by 7–14 days after surgery. A new dentogingival unit becomes established by coronal growth of tissue from the line of the gingivectomy incision, and healing of the gingivectomy wound is generally complete by 4–5 weeks.

Flap surgery

Ideally, healing after flap surgery should be by achieving a new connective tissue attachment, i.e. by the establishment of new cementum, periodontal ligament and alveolar bone.

However, there are a number of reasons why this may not occur. The differentiation of cells from the progenitor population of the periodontal ligament (particularly cementoblasts) may take a long time — and, before this can occur, epithelial cells may grow down from the gingival margin between the root face and the connective tissue to form a long junctional epithelium. Epithelial cells may also proliferate from remnants of pocket epithelium that have not been removed during surgery.

The long junctional epithelium, if attached to the tooth surface, is theoretically as strong as a normal junctional epithelium in health. However, in the presence of poor plaque control, it is prone to breakdown at a faster rate than a normal periodontal attachment. Further, it is not possible to prove that attachment to the tooth surface has been achieved without histological examination. A reduced probing depth after surgery may be due to tissue loss, recession, resolution of inflammation at the pocket base such that the probe does not penetrate into the underlying connective tissue, or an inability to probe the full depth of the pocket because the gingival cuff is tight.

It should be emphasized that radiology or re-entry procedures cannot establish that a new connective tissue attachment has been achieved. Histology is the only means of proving this.

Apart from conventional non-surgical or surgical techniques, very many procedures have been developed in an attempt to promote new connective tissue attachment. These include bone grafts, synthetic implants such as hydroxyapatite, and root conditioning with chemicals or proteins such as citric acid or fibronectin. However, none of these techniques have satisfactorily demonstrated new attachment formation, and grafts may result in root resorption or ankylosis.

Isolation of the root surface from epithelial tissues during healing has been shown to allow new bone formation and periodontal ligament cells and cementum to become established on the root surface. This is the basis of the guided tissue regeneration technique, by which an artificial, biologically inert membrane protects the root surface from epithelial downgrowth, whilst differentiation of the connective tissue cells becomes established. Results are encouraging, but there are disadvantages in that the technique is complex and difficult to perform and, at present, a re-entry procedure is required to remove the artificial membrane after the initial stages of healing are complete.

Free gingival graft

For the 3 days after surgery, the graft receives nutrients via the fibrinous exudate between the graft and the graft bed. A haematoma beneath the graft may therefore result in graft rejection. Also, during these first days, the epithelial surface of the graft degenerates and becomes desquamated. If a significant proportion of a graft is positioned over an area of recession on a root face, the graft may be lost because insufficient nutrients may be available to maintain viability.

Revascularization of the graft takes place from 2–11 days postsurgery and anastomoses between blood vessels of the graft bed and the grafted tissue become established after as few as 4 days. Re-epithelialization of the graft takes place by proliferation of epithelial cells from the surrounding tissues. If a graft has been placed over a root surface in an attempt to reduce recession, migration of epithelial cells apically along the root surface may result in some pocket formation. Alternatively, some creeping re-attachment of the graft tissue coronally may occur, but this is rarely of a significant amount. Healing of the graft is completed after approximately 6 weeks.

REASONS FOR FAILURE OF PERIODONTAL SURGERY

The reasons for failure of surgery may be summarized as follows:

(a) wrong choice of patient: poor cooperation, inadequate standard of oral hygiene;
(b) wrong choice of operative procedure;
(c) operative procedure not correctly performed;
(d) operative procedure not able to arrest the disease process;
(e) operator not adequately skilled;
(f) inadequate postoperative maintenance;
(g) failure of patient to maintain adequate postoperative plaque control.

CONTENTS OF A PERIODONTAL SURGICAL TRAY

The instruments selected for use in periodontal surgery are obviously influenced by operator preference, but typical items which may be included are as follows:

Mouth mirror
14W periodontal pocket marking probe
2 Bard–Parker scalpel handles No. 3
2 Blake knives with Allan key
Molt periosteal elevator
McIndoe tissue forceps
4L and 4R curettes
Periodontal hoes 210–213
Excavator 127/128
Mitchell's trimmer
Flat plastic No. 6
Mosquito forceps
Needle holders
Iris straight scissors
Suture 4/O silk on 16 mm curved atraumatic cutting needle
Austin's tissue retractor
Ultrasonic tip
Cross-action towel clip
Galley pot
Syringe for irrigation
Stillet
Cannula suction end
2 absorbent hand towels
Dressing towel
0.9% sodium chloride
Swabs
Coe–Pak periodontal dressing
Suction tubing
LA cartridge and syringe
27G short needle

FURTHER READING

Hall W. B. (1981). The current status of mucogingival problems and their therapy. *J. Periodontal.*, **52,** 569–75.
Lindhe J. (1989). *Textbook of Clinical Periodontology*, 2nd edn. Philadelphia: W. B. Saunders Co.
Ramfjord S. P., Nissle R. R. (1974). The modified Widman flap. *J. Periodontal.*, **45,** 601–7.
Strahan J. D., Waite I. M. (1978). *A Colour Atlas of Periodontology*. London: Wolfe Medical.
Waite I. M., Strahan J. D. (1987). *A Colour Atlas of Periodontal Surgery*. London: Wolfe Medical.
Yukna R. A., Lawrence J. J. (1980). Gingival surgery for soft tissue new attachment. *Dent. Clinics N. America*, **24,** 705–18.
Zamet J. S. (1979). Basic periodontal surgery—a re-evaluation. *Dent. Update*, **6,** 49–64.

Chapter 41

Conscious sedation

Most dental patients are satisfactorily treated with local analgesia alone, but some handicapped individuals, nervous children and adults undergoing emergency treatment, and patients undergoing extensive oral surgery, may require general anaesthesia. A remaining small group may be best treated using local analgesia together with conscious sedation.

Conscious sedation techniques include:
(a) oral sedation;
(b) inhalational sedation (relative analgesia or RA);
(c) intravenous sedation (i.v. sedation).

Inhalational sedation is preferred since it is more convenient for both operator and patient, and the agent can be immediately withdrawn if necessary, permitting the patient to recover.

LEGAL ASPECTS OF CONSCIOUS SEDATION

In 1978, the Wylie report stated:

Our definition of a simple sedation technique is one in which the use of a drug or drugs produces a state of depression of the central nervous system enabling treatment to be carried out, but during which verbal contact with the patient is maintained throughout the period of sedation. The drugs and techniques used should carry a margin of safety wide enough to render unintended loss of consciousness unlikely.

In 1989, the General Dental Council recommended in their Notice for the Guidance of Dentists:

1. Where a general anaesthetic is administered, the Council considers that it should be by a person, other than the dentist treating the patient who should remain with the patient throughout the anaesthetic procedure and until the patient's protective reflexes have returned.

2. This second person should be a dental or medical practitioner appropriately trained and experienced in the use of anaesthetic drugs for dental purposes. As part of a programme of training in anaesthesia the general anaesthetic may be administered by a dental or medical practitioner under the direct supervision of the said second person.

3. Where intravenous or inhalational sedation techniques are employed a suitably experienced practitioner may assume the responsibility of sedating the patient, as well as operating, provided that as a minimum requirement a second appropriate person is present through the procedure. Such an appropriate person might be a suitably trained dental surgery assistant or dental auxiliary, whose experience and training enables that person to be an efficient member of the dental team and who is capable of monitoring

the clinical condition of the patient. Should the occasion arise, he or she must also be capable of assisting the dentist in case of emergency.

4. For these purposes, the following definition of simple sedation should be understood to apply: 'A technique in which the use of a drug or drugs produces a state of depression of the central nervous system enabling treatment to be carried out, but during which communication is maintained such that the patient will respond to command throughout the period of sedation. The drugs and techniques used should carry a margin of safety wide enough to render unintended loss of consciousness unlikely'.

5. Neither general anaesthesia nor sedation should be employed unless proper equipment for their administration is used and adequate facilities for the resuscitation of the patient are readily available with both dentist and staff trained in their use. Resuscitation is very much a matter of skill and timing and dentists must ensure that all those assisting them know precisely what is required of them, should an emergency arise, and that they regularly practise their routine in a simulated emergency against the clock. The Council considers it essential that the equipment necessary for basic life support, including suction apparatus to clear the airway, oral airways to maintain it and positive pressure equipment with appropriate attachments to inflate the lungs with oxygen, must be immediately to hand and ready for use in the operating room.

6. A dentist who carried out treatment under general anaesthesia or sedation without fulfilling these conditions would almost certainly be considered to have acted in a manner which constitutes serious professional misconduct.

It is extremely important that the dental surgery assistant involved conforms to this definition of a second appropriate person and that you practise your emergency procedures with that person at regular frequent intervals.

The 'second appropriate person' must be present throughout the treatment and not leave the surgery at any time. Therefore a third person must be present to fetch and carry out administrative duties and answer the phone. Remember always to have a chaperon present.

ORAL SEDATION

Advantages

Simple and relatively safe, and produces some amnesia.

Disadvantages

Variability in absorption for drugs taken by mouth (the patient may become sedated too soon, or too late); compliance of patient; may make some children *hyperexcitable*. The amnesia and sedation may be a disadvantage in the postoperative period.

Drugs used

These include:

1. *Diazepam*. Diazepam can either be taken as a single dose (5–10 mg for an adult) 1 h before treatment, or in divided doses (e.g. 5 mg the night before treatment, a further 5 mg on waking and another 5 mg 1 h before treatment).

Diazepam metabolites may cause rebound sedation three, four or more hours later.

2. *Temazepam*. 30 mg temazepam taken 1 h preoperatively provides about the same sedation as intravenous diazepam in lipid emulsion (Diazemuls). Temazepam, however, has little 'hangover' effect.

OTHER CONSCIOUS SEDATION TECHNIQUES

Consent to sedation. It is essential to:

(a) explain exactly what is to be done — consent *must* be informed;
(b) give written preoperative and postoperative instruction (see below);
(c) get a consent form signed giving permission for a sedation technique to be used together with local analgesia, and for the operative procedure.

Inhalation sedation (relative analgesia)

Nitrous oxide and oxygen are used (Table 41.1): 20% and 35% N_2O in O_2 commonly allow for a state of detached sedation and analgesia without any loss of consciousness or danger of obtunded reflexes. At these levels, patients are aware of operative procedures and are cooperative without being scared.

Table 41.1
Relative analgesia

Drug	Comments
Nitrous oxide	Analgesic, but weak anaesthetic Non-explosive Minimal cardiorespiratory effects

Advantages

1. It is non-invasive.
2. The nitrous oxide level is easily and rapidly able to be altered or discontinued.
3. Protective reflexes are minimally impaired.
4. The drug is administered and excreted through the lungs, virtually total recovery takes place within the first 15 min of cessation of administration. The patient may, therefore, attend and leave the surgery or hospital unaccompanied.
5. No strict fasting is required beforehand.
6. It confers some analgesia (although local analgesia is often still required).

Disadvantages

1. The level of sedation is largely dependent on psychological reassurance/back-up, i.e. hypnotic suggestion.
2. The nitrous oxide must be administered continuously.

3. Nitrous oxide pollutes the surgery atmosphere; this can be reduced by:
   (a) scavenging;
   (b) venting the suction machine outside the building;
   (c) minimizing conversation by the patient;
   (d) testing the equipment weekly for leakage;
   (e) maintaining the equipment;
   (f) ventilating the surgeries, e.g. open window and door fan and open window air-conditioning.
   (g) monitoring, e.g. Barnsley N_2O Monitor which can be obtained from: Dr O'Sullivan, Quality Control Pharmacist, Barnsley District General Hospital, Gamber Road, Barnsley S75 2EP, England;

4. There are physical problems with maintaining the nose-piece in position with a good gas seal while operating on the patient, and preventing dilution by mouth breathing.

Contraindications to relative analgesia

Psychological. Fear or non-acceptance of the nasal mask.
Medical. Relative analgesia is contraindicated in:

(a) temporary (e.g. heavy cold) or permanent nasal obstruction (e.g. deviated nasal septum);
(b) cyanosis at rest due to chronic cardiac (e.g. congenital disease) or respiratory disease (e.g. chronic bronchitis or emphysema);
(c) severe psychiatric disease where cooperation is not possible;
(d) inability to communicate with the patient;
(e) the first trimester of pregnancy;
(f) patients receiving bleomycin therapy, because of the high concentration of oxygen.

Essential advice to the patient

On the day of treatment
DO eat as normal before treatment
DO take routine medicines at the usual times
DO NOT drink alcohol

After treatment
The effects of the sedative gas normally wears off very quickly and you will be fit to go back to work or travel home once we have finished your treatment. (Although recovery is very rapid and patients may be safely discharged without an escort, they should be discouraged from driving, particularly 2-wheeled vehicles, immediately after treatment.)

Procedure for relative analgesia

1. Check relative analgesia machine is ready and working, that extra nitrous oxide and oxygen are available, and that you are completely familiar with the machine.
2. Lie the patient comfortably supine in the chair with legs uncrossed, and the equipment as unobtrusive as possible. Give patient protective eyewear.

3. Explain the procedure to the patient.
4. Allow O_2 to flow (e.g. 5 l/min for a small adult, 7 l/min for a large adult).
5. Close the air entrainment port if present on the nasal mask.
6. Ask the patient to place the mask onto his/her nose. Adjust the mask and tubing to give a good fit.
7. Warn the patient that the O_2 feels cold.
8. Check that the O_2 flow volume is adequate by:

    (a) asking the patient if he/she is receiving the right amount of air;
    (b) watching the patient to see if he/she is mouth-breathing to supplement the flow;
    (c) watching the reservoir bag to see if it is under- or over-inflating (either suggesting the flow is wrong).

Adjust the rate of O_2 flow until a comfortable minute volume is achieved. The correct volume for each patient must be found at each visit.

9. Turn N_2O flow to 10% (90% O_2). Tell the patient he/she may feel warm, heaviness/lightheadedness, tingling of hands and feet, remote, a change in visual and auditory acuity.
10. Look for *signs of adequate inhalation sedation*:

    (a) relaxation;
    (b) warmth;
    (c) tingling or numbness;
    (d) visual or auditory changes;
    (e) slurring of speech;
    (f) slowed responses, e.g. reduced frequency of blinking; delayed response to verbal instructions or questioning.

11. Maintain 10% N_2O for one full minute; continuing verbal reassurance.
12. Increase the N_2O flow with a minute-long increment of 10% N_2O (to a total of 20% N_2O) and then proceed in minute-long increments of 5% N_2O until the patient appears and feels quite relaxed. Dosage is variable but few patients would need more than 50% N_2O.
13. Do not use a prop—**if the normal patient cannot maintain an open mouth then he/she is too deeply sedated.**

A possible exception may be in the case of a handicapped patient unable to maintain an open mouth even without sedation. If a prop is then used, extra-careful observation of the depth of sedation is essential.

14. If, after relaxing, the patient becomes restless or apprehensive, the level of N_2O may be too high and the percentage should be reduced to a more comfortable level. The patient can then be maintained at an appropriate level until the operative procedure (or that part of it that the patient does not normally tolerate) is completed.
15. Give the local analgesic.
16. Monitor the patient's pulse and respiratory rate at frequent intervals. The patient should be conscious and able to respond when directed. Snoring indicates partial airway obstruction and should be corrected immediately.
17. When the sedation is to be terminated, the N_2O flow is shut off so that 100% O_2 is given for two full minutes to counteract possible diffusion hypoxia.

During this time the patient will be receptive to suggestion.

18. Remove the facemask and slowly bring the patient upright over the next few minutes.

19. The patient can leave the surgery when he/she is totally alert and well — usually after about 15 min.

Intravenous sedation

A benzodiazepine, normally midazolam, is the preferred agent for intravenous sedation (Table 41.2).

Table 41.2
Drugs for intravenous sedation*

Drug	Proprietary names	Adult dose	Comments
Midazolam	Hypnovel	0.07 mg/kg (up to 7.5 mg total dose)	Benzodiazepine. Often preferred to diazepam because: (a) Amnesia is more profound, starting 2–5 min after administration and lasting up to 40 min (with no retrograde amnesia); (b) Recovery is more rapid — midazolam is virtually completely eliminated within 5–6 h, without the recurrence of drowsiness that may follow the use of diazepam; (c) incidence of venous thrombosis is less (than with Valium); However, there are no reliable physical signs of sedation and the variable reaction to the means that the drug has to be given slowly so that depth of sedation can be assessed.
Diazepam	Valium	Up to 20 mg	Benzodiazepine: gives sedation with amnesia. Give slowly i.v. in 2.5 mg increments until ptosis begins, i.e. eyelids begin to droop (Verril's sign). (Rapid injection may cause respiratory depression) Disadvantages: (a) may cause pain or thrombophlebitis; (b) drowsiness returns transiently 4–6 h postoperatively (due to metabolism to oxazepam and desmethyldiazepam); (c) may produce mild hypotension and respiratory depression.
	Diazemuls† (diazepam in lipid emulsion)	Up to 20 mg	Preferred to Valium since, although it has most of the actions above, it causes less thrombophlebitis and therefore can be given into veins on dorsum of hand. Do not give intramuscularly

* Particular caution in the elderly, children and those with liver or respiratory disease. Avoid in pregnancy. Do **not** give pentazocine with a benzodiazepine.
† Avoid in egg allergy.

Sedation with benzodiazepines

Intravenous administration of benzodiazepines produces:
(a) acute detachment for 20–30 min;
(b) relaxation for a further hour or so;
(c) some anterograde amnesia for the same period;
(d) minimal cardiovascular depression.

Midazolam (Hypnovel) is soluble in water and available in a 2 ml ampoule in a concentration of 5 mg/ml or in a 5 ml ampoule in a concentration of 2 mg/ml. Both presentations contain 10 mg midazolam in one ampoule.

Diazepam (Diazemuls and Valium) is not water-soluble. It is available in a 2 ml ampoule in a concentration of 5 mg/ml. It cannot be safely diluted.

Midazolam is preferred because it is non-irritant in aqueous solution, has a much shorter half-life than diazepam (in the region of 1–2 h), no significant metabolites (so that recovery is both quicker and smoother) and has more predictable amnesic properties than diazepam (Table 41.2).

Advantages of intravenous sedation

1. Adequate level of sedation is attained pharmacologically rather than with psychological back-up.
2. Amnesia (removes unpleasant memories).
3. The patient may take a light meal up to 2 h before the treatment session.

Disadvantages of intravenous sedation

1. Benzodiazepines produce no analgesia; therefore local analgesia is needed.
2. Once administered i.v., the drug cannot be withdrawn.
3. Direct laryngeal reflexes may be impaired and therefore a mouth sponge/gauze or rubber dam must be used to protect against inhalation of water or debris.
4. *Patient must be accompanied home from surgery by a responsible adult and may not drive or work machinery including domestic appliances, or make important decisions or drink alcohol for 24 h.*

Contraindications to intravenous sedation

1. Other overriding responsibilities, e.g. caring for young children, shift work
2. Inability to bring a suitable escort
3. Children (a considerable variability in reaction to diazepam has been noted in children and RA is the choice in most cases)
4. Previous adverse reaction to a benzodiazepine
5. Pregnancy (and caution during breast feeding)
6. Severe psychiatric disease, mental handicap or neurological disease
7. Alcohol or narcotic dependency or long-term therapy with other benzodiazepines (may render usual doses ineffective)
8. Liver or kidney disease
9. Glaucoma

10. Potential drug interactions — not necessarily *absolute* contraindications to the careful use of benzodiazepines they include:
    (a) cimetidine
    (b) disulfiram
    (c) L-dopa
    (d) drugs which decrease cardiovascular and respiratory function: e.g. anti-hypertensive drugs, antihistamines, narcotic analgesics (with the possible exception of nalbuphine), hypnotics, sedatives, tranquillisers and anti-epileptics.

Preoperative instructions

These should be written.
On the day of treatment
1. Bring a responsible adult with you, who is able to wait to escort you home
2. Have a light meal at least two hours before your appointment
3. Take any routine medicines at the usual times
4. Do not eat fatty foods or drink **any** alcohol
5. Make sure you will not need to work, drive, drink alcohol or make any important decisions within 24 h following the dental treatment

Preoperative checks
1. Patient's name and address (ask patient)
2. Nature, side and site of operation (check also with patient)
3. Medical history — particularly of cardiorespiratory disease or bleeding tendency. Record initial pulse rate and blood pressure
4. Consent has been obtained in writing from patient or, in a person under 16 years of age, from parent/guardian, and that patient adequately understands the nature of operation and its sequelae
5. Necessary investigations, e.g. dental radiographs, are available
6. Patient has had *nothing* by mouth for *at least* the previous 2 h
7. Patient has emptied bladder
8. Patient's dentures have been removed, and note bridges, crowns and loose teeth. Contact lenses should be removed and eye protection provided
9. Necessary premedication (and, where indicated, regular medication such as the contraceptive pill, anticonvulsants or antidepressants) has been given
10. Anaesthetic and suction apparatus are working satisfactorily and correct drugs are available and drugs not expired. Emergency kit available
11. Patient will be escorted by a responsible adult
12. Patient is warned not to drive, operate machinery, drink alcohol or make important decisions for 24 h postoperatively (see below)

Procedure for intravenous sedation with midazolam

Avoid acting as operator–anaesthetist: have third-party present.

1. Ensure drugs and equipment are ready and discreetly placed.
2. Adjust the dental chair to the supine position and ensure the patient is comfortable, with legs uncrossed.

3. Select a suitable site in the antecubital fossa (or dorsum of the hand) for venepuncture. It is best to avoid the dominant arm/hand.

A small bore needle is usually used but an indwelling needle of the butterfly type can be used so that a patent veinway can be maintained throughout the procedure. The arm should be kept straight with a board if the antecubital fossa is used.

4. Occlude the venous return above the elbow with a tourniquet or ask an assistant to squeeze the arm. Alternatively, place the tourniquet above the wrist to use the back of the hand.

5. Cleanse the skin with a suitable antiseptic (e.g. isopropanol 70% or chlorhexidine 0.5%). Select the most readily palpable vein which is remote from the brachial artery.

6. Unless a butterfly needle is used, bend the needle by about 30° so that it can be placed flat on the skin, bevel upwards, without obstruction from the needle hub or syringe barrel. Tap the vein until it becomes reflexly dilated, tense the skin with one hand distal to the chosen puncture site. Place the needle flat on the skin and press downwards. The skin in front of the needle (and the vein) will bulge up. Slide the needle smoothly along the skin and it will pierce the surface and enter the vein easily.

Pressing the shaft of the needle on the skin is not painful yet acts as a distraction or counter-irritant. If the patient is simultaneously spoken to, this is another distraction and often the small additional stimulus of the needle piercing the skin is unnoticed. The point of the needle is always visible and superficial — there is a decreased risk of penetration of a deeper structure such as an artery. Once through the skin, which is the most painful part of the procedure, the needle can be manipulated so that the technique of entering a vein from the side could be used. Advance the needle until two-thirds of its length is within the vein. The appearance of blood within the tubing on aspiration confirms the correct positioning of the needle.

7. Secure the needle or butterfly needle firmly with non-allergenic tape. (e.g. Micropore).

8. Slowly inject the prepared drug, warning the patient of possible cold sensation at the needle site or as the drug tracks up the arm. Provided one is sure that the needle is correctly positioned, the patient should be reassured that this sensation will pass within a short period of time. Stop injecting if pain is felt, e.g. radiating down the forearm, indicating entry into an artery.

9. Inject 3 mg midazolam over 30 s, then pause for a further 90 s. Much smaller doses are needed in older patients. Give further increments of 1 mg every 30 s until sedation is judged to be adequate. Watch for any adverse responses and particularly any respiratory impairment.

The correct dose has been given when there is slurring of speech and the patient exhibits a relaxed demeanour. Ptosis is not a reliable end-point; adequate sedation with midazolam may occur before ptosis is evident.

10. Give local analgesic in the operative area.

11. Operative procedures may be started after a couple of minutes. Approximately 30 min of sedation time is available for the operator. Since there may be considerable muscle relaxation a prop may be needed to maintain the mouth open. *The airway must be protected because the laryngeal reflexes may be obtunded for the first few minutes after the administration of intravenous seda-*

tives, and eye protection must be used. A barrier to prevent accidental inhalation of debris must be used, and this may be rubber dam, butterfly sponge or a gauze square. Some advocate the use of a small dose of either hyoscine or atropine in addition to the benzodiazepines to reduce the risks arising from excessive salivation or bronchial secretion, but the advantages gained are outweighed by the discomfort of a very dry mouth and the potential dangers of using atropinics.

Patients often become more talkative as their inhibitions are released by the depressant action of the drug, analogous to the effect of alcohol, and may sometimes burst into tears. This is a sign of good relaxation and care should be taken not to overdose the patient in the assumption that sedation is not taking place.

12. Monitor the patient frequently by the pulse (pulse oximeter), respiratory rate and skin colour. The patient should remain conscious and able to respond when directed.

13. At the end of the procedure, slowly upright the patient over 5 min. The patient should recover over at least another 15 min under the direct supervision of a member of the dental team or his/her escort.

14. The patient must not be discharged until at least 1 h has elapsed since the last increment of drug was given.

15. The patient should be discharged into the care of his/her escort and instructions repeated that he/she should rest quietly at home for the remainder of the day and refrain from drinking alcohol, driving or operating machinery or making important decisions for 24 h. These instructions together with any pertaining to the dentistry performed should be given to the escort verbally and on a written sheet for the patient to refer to later, as he/she may still be under the influence of the amnesic properties of the midazolam.

Postoperative instructions to patient

These should be written:

1. Travel home with your escort by car if possible
2. Stay resting quietly at home
3. **Do not** — use complex machinery (e.g. cookers, washing machines, power tools)
   — sign important legal or business documents or make important decisions
   — drink any alcohol

Flumazenil (Anexate)

Anexate is an imidazobenzodiazepine and is a specific antagonist to benzodiazepines. It allows rapid reversal of conscious sedation with benzodiazepines by specific competitive inhibition for receptors. However, as the effect of flumazenil subsides, the sedative effect of the benzodiazepine returns until it is completely eliminated from the body.

Dosage. Available as 5 ml ampoules containing 500 µg of anexate. The initial dose is 200 µg (2 ml) i.v. over 15 s. If desired level of consciousness is not obtained within 60 s, give 100 µg at 60-s intervals up to a maximum of 1000 µg. Usual dose required, 300–600 µg (possibly less for the elderly).

Anexate has a short duration of action (half-life approx. 50 min), therefore repeated doses of anexate may be required until all possible central effects of the benzodiazepines have subsided (midazolam — half life of 2–4 h). If drowsiness recurs an infusion of 100–400 µg per hour may be employed.

Contraindications

1. Hypersensitivity
2. Pregnancy
3. Epilepsy
4. Impaired liver function — metabolized in liver
5. Use of psychotropic drugs — e.g. tricyclics

Adverse effects

1. Flushing
2. Nausea/vomiting
3. Anxiety/palpitations/fear
4. Seizures in epileptics

If patients are given Anexate following intravenous sedation procedures they must still follow the normal instructions given after sedation, i.e. no driving, operating machinery, etc.

FURTHER READING

Barker I., Bulchart D. G. M., Gibson J. et al. (1986). IV sedation for conservative dentistry. *Br. J. Anaesth.*, **58**, 371–7.
Dundee J. W. et al. (1980). Midazolam: a water-soluble benzodiazepine. *Anaesthesia*, **35**, 454–8.
Lindsay S. J. E., Yates J. A. (1985). The effectiveness of oral diazepam in anxious child dental patients. *Br. dent. J.*, **159**, 149–53.
McGimpsie J. G. et al. (1983). Midazolam in dentistry. *Br. dent. J.*, **155**, 47–50.
Scully C., Cawson R. A. (1987). *Medical problems in dentistry*, 2nd edn. Bristol: Wright.
Woolgrave J. (1983), Pain, perception and patient management. *Br. dent. J.*, **154**, 243–6.
Wylie Report (1981). *Brit. dent. J.*, **151**, 385–8.

Chapter 42

Dental local analgesia

ANATOMICAL CONSIDERATIONS

Painful sensations from the dental regions travel in trigeminal afferent nerves running from the periphery to the brain. Pain receptors (nociceptors) form part of a sensory nerve plexus which surrounds each dental site. Nerve fibrils from the receptors collect together to form larger nerve fibres which in turn form large nerve bundles identified by name. Each dental situation is served by *three* nerve plexuses — the outer plexus (buccal or labial), the dental plexus (maxillary or mandibular) and the inner plexus (palatal or lingual). Information from these various plexuses travels to the brain in identified nerve trunks according to the diagram (Fig. 42.1).

Effective pain control for dental procedures depends upon accurate deposition of local analgesia solution to block nerve conduction from the appropriate nerve plexuses. The outer and inner plexuses are relatively easy to render analgesic by simple injection of analgesia solution into the region. Dental plexus analgesia is less easy because the afferent nerves carrying information from the operation site are intrabony. However, in the entire maxilla as well as the incisor regions of the mandible, the outer supporting plates of alveolar bone are relatively thin and porous. Deposition of drug solution onto the periosteum of the desired region will not only produce buccal plexus analgesia directly but, by diffusion of solution through the porous bone, the dental plexus will also be reached.

Such infiltration of solution cannot occur in the canine to third molar regions of the mandible as the bone density here is too great. Similarly, in some cases, the bone density over the maxillary first molar region may be too dense for effective infiltration of analgesia solution to the dental plexus, this being due to the thickness of the overlying zygomatic buttress. In these cases, pain control must be blocked by deposition of analgesia solution around the major nerve trunks conveying sensation from the operation site, where these nerves lie outside bone.

In the mandible, solution must be deposited around the inferior dental nerve where it leaves the mandibular foramen and traverses the infratemporal fossa. The regional block produced renders the entire area served by the inferior dental nerve, peripheral to the point of blockade, analgesic. The same injection renders the lingual nerve analgesic due to its close proximity.

In the maxilla, where bone thickness prevents effective infiltration analgesia of the dental plexus, the regional block approach to overcoming this difficulty is more of a problem. The first permanent molar dental plexus classically sends

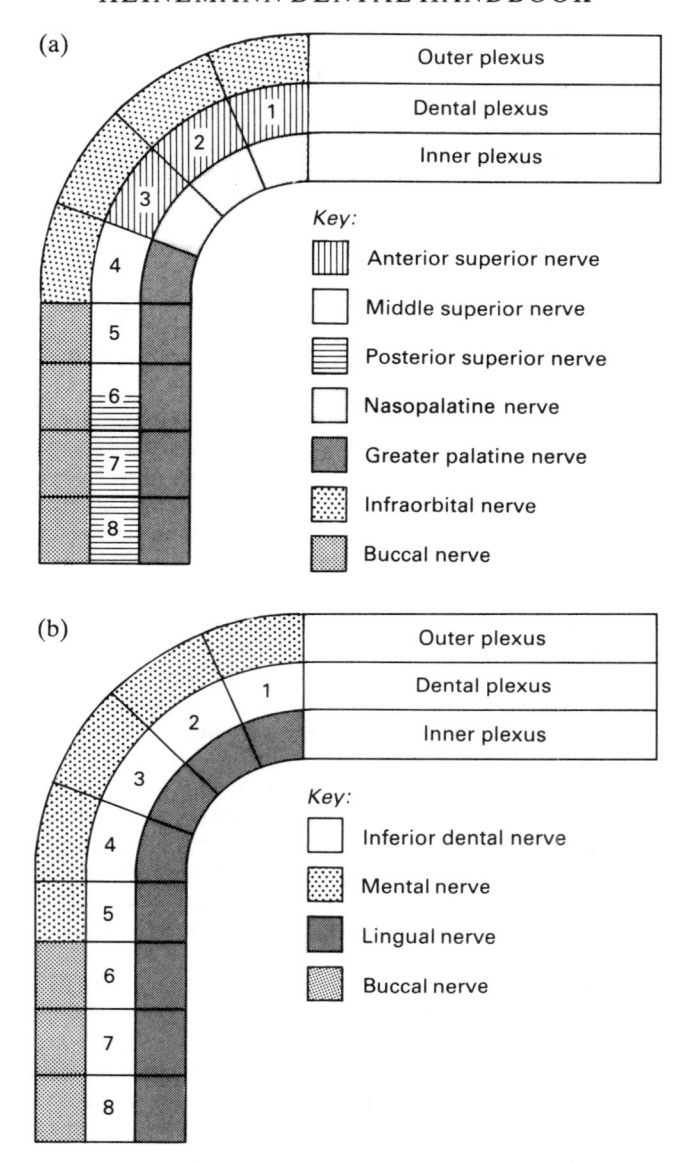

Fig. 42.1 (a) *Nerve supply of maxilla.* (b) *Nerve supply of mandible.*

information to the brain via two pathways: from the mesiobuccal root, information travels in the middle superior alveolar nerves; the remaining dental plexus information travels with posterior superior alveolar nerves. The middle superior dental nerves course towards the infraorbital nerve in its canal, via the lateral wall of the maxillary antrum. Deposition of solution over the lateral wall of the maxillary antrum (effectively over the apex of the second maxillary premolar) will achieve analgesia of these nerves. However, not everyone has middle superior alveolar nerves. Estimates from cadaver dissections reveal that somewhere between 30% and 80% of the population have these nerves missing and afferent information in these cases is assumed to travel with the posterior superior alveolar nerves.

Posterior superior alveolar nerve block is initially a daunting injection to make. The pterygoid venous plexus lies over the infratemporal surface of the maxilla exactly where the posterior superior dental nerves emerge from bone. Needle placement in this region could lead to a dramatic haemorrhage. However, the technique described later (maxillary molar block) achieves effective posterior superior alveolar nerve block without the risk of haemorrhage.

The requirements of local analgesia differ, depending upon the operation to be performed. For conservative procedures, only dental plexus analgesia is required. Inevitably, however, anatomical features mean that there is unwanted soft tissue analgesia whether local infiltration or regional block techniques are employed. For surgical procedures, all three plexuses must be analgesic and cover sufficient area for the operation. Judicious placement of analgesia solution according to the neuroanatomical pathways involved is required. It is worthy of note that the entire palate may be rendered analgesic by only three drops of solution; one drop placed at each greater (anterior) palatine foramen and a third at the nasopalatine foramen beneath the incisive papilla. Further, surgical analgesia in the mandible from the mental foramen to the midline may be obtained by one needle puncture—the inferior dental/lingual nerve block injection. As the mental nerve is analgesic following effective block of these nerves in the infratemporal fossa, all three nerve plexuses in this region of the mandible will be analgesic. Cross-over innervation from the opposite side may affect the analgesia produced in the mid-line, around the mandibular central incisor. It appears that the dental plexus is infrequently (if at all) involved in mid-line cross-innervation. However, the labial and lingual plexuses do have a limited right–left crossover at the central incisor region. Local supplemental infiltration injections resolve this problem.

MODE OF ACTION OF LOCAL ANALGESIA DRUGS

Interaction of a local analgesia drug with a nerve membrane is the basic principle by which all such drugs produce reversible block of nerve conduction. The precise mechanism involved is poorly understood. Details have been given in Chapter 2 and are repeated in brief; the theory is as follows.

In the resting state, a nerve fibre has difference of electrical potential (polarization) between the inner and outer surfaces of its lipoprotein membrane. In the normal resting state this potential difference is maintained by an active 'sodium pump' mechanism at approximately $-70\,mV$. As a stimulus occurs, the intracellular voltage rises, by influx of sodium ions, to $+40-55\,mV$. This is the firing threshold of the nerve fibre and, once reached, depolarization occurs leading to an action potential, which is propagated along the entire nerve length. Immediately after impulse propagation a nerve cannot receive further stimulation; this is the so-called absolute refractory period. During depolarization, sodium ion transfer occurs through ion channels in the

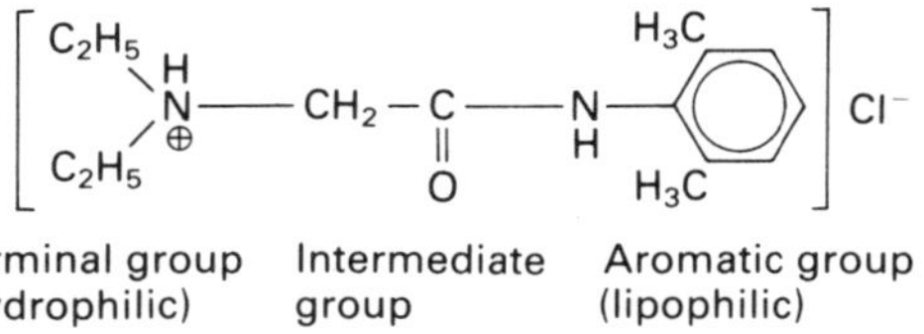

$$\left[\begin{array}{c} C_2H_5 \\ \underset{\oplus}{\overset{H}{N}} \\ C_2H_5 \end{array} \!\!-\!\!CH_2-\underset{\underset{O}{\|}}{C}-\underset{H}{N}\!\!-\!\!\!\left\langle\!\!\!\begin{array}{c}H_3C\\ \\ H_3C\end{array}\!\!\!\right\rangle \right] Cl^-$$

Terminal group (hydrophilic) | Intermediate group | Aromatic group (lipophilic)

Fig. 42.2 *Basic structure of local analgesic compound.*

lipoprotein nerve membrane, which become more permeable. Local analgesia drugs are thought to prevent this permeability of nerve membranes to sodium ions. Common injectable local analgesia drugs of the amide group (lignocaine, mepivicaine, prilocaine) are thought to bind to the sodium channels on the inner surface of the nerve membrane, blocking the passage of ions necessary to produce depolarization and nerve conduction. Normal nerve function resumes when the blocking drug molecules unbind from their receptor sites in the sodium channels.

Local analgesia drugs conform to a common basic structure:

(a) a lipophilic aromatic portion;
(b) an intermediate chain (with an ester or amide linkage);
(c) a hydrophilic portion (Fig. 42.2).

The commonly used base drugs such as lignocaine, prilocaine and mepivicaine have an intermediate chain which contains an amide linkage. The earlier ester types (e.g. procaine) are rapidly metabolized, making working times short, and they were also associated with significant allergy problems. The topical analgesic drugs, benzocaine and amethocaine, are the only agents of the ester type which are sometimes used today. The amides include bupivicaine and etidocaine which are long-acting analgesia drugs but these rarely have a place in dental practice.

Analgesic base drugs are relatively insoluble in water so their soluble hydrochloride salts are used in analgesia solutions. When in aqueous solution the drug exists in both the ionized and un-ionized state. The degree of dissociation between the un-ionized and ionized forms depends upon (a) the drug itself, and (b) the pH of the solution.

For a given pH, a steady-state equilibrium between the two forms is rapidly established. This equilibrium changes as the pH of the solution changes. Each drug has a 'dissociation constant' peculiar to itself—designated the pK_a—which is the pH at which the ionized and un-ionized forms of the chemical compound are present in equal amounts. Effective nerve block results from the action of both forms of the drug. Lipid solubility is dependent upon the un-ionized base drug molecules. To be effective, a drug must enter the lipid-rich nerve membrane to gain access to the sodium channel receptors. However, it is the ionized (dissociated or charged) form of the drug which attaches to these receptors and effects neural blockade. The speed of onset of analgesia reflects the rate of absorption of the chosen drug into the lipoprotein membrane, which is directly related to the amount of un-ionized drug present. Once there, there must be sufficient ionized form of the drug to bind to the receptors and block conduction.

Lignocaine, prilocaine, and mepivicaine have a pK_a of approximately 7.7. When these agents are injected into tissues of pH of 7.4, 65% of the drug exists in the ionized form and only 35% in the un-ionized form. Bupivicaine and amethocaine on the other hand have a pK_a of 8.1 and 8.6 respectively. For these drugs at normal tissue pH, the respective amount of un-ionized drug available is less at 15% and 5% respectively. Consequently, lipid solubility is poor and both bupivicaine and amethocaine have a slower onset of action than the lignocaine types. Very small pH changes greatly affect the balance of ionized to un-ionized forms of a drug. Slight acidic change of tissue pH, which might accompany acute inflammation, has a great affect upon the efficacy of local analgesia drugs. Whilst a lowering of tissue pH favours the formation of the un-ionized form of a drug, and enhances lipid solubility, there is less of the ionized form to occupy the receptor sites and effectively block conduction. Further, biochemical changes in a nerve membrane associated with inflammatory states may extend along the entire course of a nerve and prevent effective local analgesia even when the solution is remote from the infected site.

When an analgesic agent is injected it diffuses radially from the site, becoming diluted as it spreads. Close apposition of drug to nerve is therefore important. The further the diffusion, the fewer molecules there are to effect neural block. Also, dental injections are made into very vascular regions and the concentration of the analgesia solution falls rapidly due to its absorption into the blood circulation. The addition of vasoconstrictors to local analgesia solutions reduces this uptake, enhances the perineural concentration of the base drug and prolongs the analgesic effect. Vasoconstrictors also offset the inherent vasodilator properties of local analgesia drugs, which would further enhance dilution of the injected pool by absorption into the blood circulation.

Adrenaline at a concentration of 1:80 000 is the usual vasoconstrictor added. Where adrenaline is contraindicated, solutions containing the non-adrenergic agent felypressin may be used, though this agent possibly acts less as a vasoconstrictor but rather by enhancing the ability of the base drug to enter the nerve membrane. It is added at a concentration of 0.03 iu/ml which is approximately equivalent to one part in 2 million. Noradrenaline use as a vasoconstrictor is contraindicated as it may produce circulatory failure, even in healthy individuals.

The diffusibility of different agents varies, which also affects analgesic efficacy. For example, lignocaine and prilocaine have very similar pK_a values but in vivo studies suggest that prilocaine is slower in onset than lignocaine. The difference is thought to be related to enhanced ability of lignocaine to diffuse through non-nervous tissues.

Recovery from local analgesia reflects the release of the drug from its nerve-membrane binding sites. The rates at which different drugs are released from these receptors is a measure of their protein-binding ability. Prilocaine and lignocaine have a similar protein-binding ability but that of bupivicaine is much greater, which accounts for its prolonged action. Once released from a binding site, a drug diffuses from the nerve membrane into the surrounding tissue fluid and ultimately enters the circulation. Amide-based drugs are detoxified in the liver and the metabolites are excreted in urine.

The most commonly used local analgesia preparations are:

1. 2% lignocaine with 1:80 000 adrenaline.
2. 3% prilocaine with 0.03 iu/ml felypressin.
3. 3% mepivicaine — this drug is the least potent vasodilator of the commonly used analgesic drugs and produces effective analgesia for short procedures without addition of a vasoconstrictor.

SYSTEMIC EFFECTS AND PRECAUTIONS

Overdosage

All local analgesic drugs are potentially toxic due to their effect upon cell membranes. Undesirable effects occur when there is a sufficiently high blood concentration. It has already been noted that the inherent vasodilatory properties of local analgesic drugs plus the high vascularity of the dental region lead to a rapid rate of drug absorption into the circulation immediately upon injection. The number of injections made, plus the rate of injection, also affects the rate of absorption. The addition of vasoconstrictors to solutions reduces the rate of absorption as well as prolonging the analgesic effect. The circulating level of drug depends upon the rate of absorption, the extent of dilution in the circulation, and the rate of drug elimination. Patients with significantly impaired liver function or who have cardiac failure, where liver perfusion may be greatly reduced, should have the total amount of injected drug carefully regulated. Overdosage is unlikely in a dental patient, but signs to be alert for are a mixture of central excitation and inhibition. These seemingly contradictory effects are due to a common drug effect upon all central nervous system cells, the cells concerned having either excitatory or inhibitory functions. Full resuscitation facilities should always be available. The symptoms suggestive of overdosage are headache, drowsiness, nausea, disorientation, restlessness and uncontrollable muscle twitching. High levels of circulating local analgesia drug cause convulsions and death.

Moderately high blood levels of prilocaine result in methaemoglobinaemia.

Vasoconstrictor effects (see also Chapter 38)

The vasoconstrictor content of local analgesia solutions may have their own deleterious effects.

Adrenaline

Absorption of adrenaline into the circulation is rapid after dental injections, and may cause tachycardia. Further, adrenaline produces a significant fall in plasma potassium concentration within 10 min. This, together with increased endogenous adrenaline release due to fear and anxiety, could precipitate cardiac arrhythmias. This is more likely to occur in patients receiving thiazide diuretic therapy for hypertension, as these drugs not only reduce plasma potassium but potentiate the hypokalaemic effect of adrenaline.

The cardiac-stimulating effects of adrenaline may be particularly hazardous in a patient who has a scarred myocardium resulting from myocardial infarction or who is susceptible to fibrillation, such as a poorly controlled thyrotoxic patient. A system of injection which attempts to avoid inadvertent intravascular injections should always be used. Clearly, intravascular injection would be the most serious event in such patients and would certainly be undesirable in anyone. Rapid transfer of solution away from the intended site would also lead to failure of analgesia. The Astra self-aspirating system is a most appropriate system to attempt to prevent this eventuality.

Felypressin

This vasoconstrictor is an analogue of the pituitary hormone, oxytocin, and produces smooth muscle contraction by a hormonal rather than an adrenergic action. For this reason it has been advocated for patients where adrenaline is contraindicated. It may be preferred to adrenaline where the plasma potassium concern expressed above, for adrenaline, needs to be avoided, as felypressin does not produce hypokalaemia. However, its vasoconstrictor effect upon coronary arteries may present a greater hazard than adrenaline use, though in normal dental dosages this has not been shown to be a problem. Its use in the pregnant female should be restricted, not for the possible abortive effect of the oxytocin-like activity but because it is usually formulated with prilocaine, which more readily crosses the placenta than lignocaine.

Poor blood supply

Inadequate blood supply may be a problem, for example, in patients who have had therapeutic irradiation between the base of skull and clavicles, or who suffer from poorly controlled diabetes. An endarteritis obliterans often exists, and cautious use of adrenaline is often advised, though the reduction of peripheral blood supply after adrenaline use is not as significant as previously thought. However, in such cases, felypressin may be preferred. Certainly, postoperative antibiotics are indicated when surgery is performed. Diabetes per se is *not* a contraindication to local analgesia with solutions containing adrenaline as is sometimes thought. Indeed, adrenaline elevates blood sugar and tends to offset a hypoglycaemic crisis.

Bleeding disorders

Bleeding disorders present a problem to injection analgesia. Any patient with a bleeding tendency, leukaemia, having anticoagulant therapy, treatment to reduce platelet aggregation (e.g. Persantin therapy) or who suffers from severe liver disease (where synthesis of coagulation factors may be impaired) should not receive any sort of dental analgesia injection without the consent of a haematologist. Severe haemorrhage may result.

Allergy

True allergic reactions to modern amide analgesic agents are extremely rare. The usual complaint of 'allergy' surrounds psychosomatic reactions such as fainting or hyperventilation. However, each case must be carefully evaluated, and injections withheld until it is considered safe to proceed. The assistance of an allergy physician may be required. The preservative, methylparabens, formerly added to analgesia solutions, was a common source of allergic reactions, rather than the base drug, and this led to many being diagnosed as 'lignocaine allergic'. Parabens-free solutions should always be used.

Sepsis and cellulitis

Where there is sepsis or cellulitis, local analgesia injections into the site should be avoided. Regional block techniques may resolve the problem. Inferior dental block injections should *not* be given where there is induration of the floor of the mouth as potentially fatal Ludwig's angina may result. Posterior superior alveolar nerve block injections may be given to resolve the problem of sepsis surrounding maxillary premolars and molars. Haemorrhage from puncturing the pterygoid venous plexus may be avoided by adopting the following Adatia technique of 'maxillary molar block'. The needle puncture is made just into the buccal sulcus above the second molar and 1.5–2.0 ml of solution are deposited (after an aspiration test). The needle is removed, and the index finger is placed over the injection site, distal to the zygomatic buttress. The analgesia solution will flow away from the finger pressure to reach high onto the infratemporal surface of the maxilla where the posterior superior alveolar nerves are situated. This will produce effective analgesia as far forward as the maxillary canine in those patients who do not possess middle superior alveolar nerves. In Professor Adatia's, and my own, experience this is successful for 80% of patients.

Epilepsy

Epilepsy is not a contraindication to local analgesia. Although overdosage with local analgesia drugs can produce fits, these are not of the same type as epileptic fits. Indeed, well-controlled epileptics may receive routine dental analgesia without problems though poorly controlled epileptics may be better managed with benzodiazepine sedation plus local analgesia or, if severe, specialist general anaesthesia.

Tricyclic antidepressants and monoamine oxidase inhibitors

Therapy with these drugs is no longer a contraindication to the use of adrenaline-containing analgesia preparations. Noradrenaline, however, *is* contraindicated in patients taking tricyclic antidepressants as potentially fatal hypertension may arise suddenly. It must be remembered that young children may be receiving high doses of tricyclic antidepressants for the management of nocturnal enuresis (bed-wetting). It has already been noted that noradrenaline use is generally contraindicated, even for the healthy.

Overall, there are very few contraindications to careful use of local analgesia in appropriate cases where the length of operation is short and patient tolerance and cooperation are adequate. The safety of modern techniques and preparations has stood the test of time.

FAILURE TO OBTAIN ANALGESIA

Poor localization of drug is the most common cause of failure to obtain analgesia. It is an uncommon problem when infiltration techniques are used. However, regional block failure is usually due to this cause. Large compound nerve bundles, such as the inferior dental nerve, are surrounded by fibrous, adipose and connective tissues which act as a barrier to complete spread of analgesia solution across the entire nerve bundle. The concentric spread of solution from the site of injection dilutes the concentration of drug and makes poor localization even more significant.

The nerve fibres nearest the injected pool may well become analgesic but those furthest from the pool may not acquire sufficient drug to block conduction. Thus, incomplete saturation of the bundle will result, leading to partial analgesia of the field served by the bundle. This is sometimes encountered as failure of pulpal analgesia after inferior dental nerve block, despite the subjective signs of lip analgesia being present. The reverse also holds true; pulpal analgesia is present despite the lack of lip numbness.

The blocked nerves are those saturated with local analgesic drug that are within the effective concentration spread from the injected pool; in the same bundle, the nerves which are still firing have not obtained sufficient drug to block conduction. A supplementary injection may correct this problem, but this is not always so. Solutions containing adrenaline produce profound local vasoconstriction, which when prolonged, such as from repeated injections, may well adversely affect local tissue pH by producing more acidic conditions that then inhibit effective neural block despite effective saturation. A compensating vasodilator injection, such as plain lignocaine, would often reverse this adverse adrenaline effect and supplement the base drug concentration of the area. Sadly, plain lignocaine hydrochloride dental preparations are no longer available.

As an alternative, the potentiating effect of felypressin upon neural absorption of base drug, coupled with its poor vasoconstrictive properties (at the concentration of felypressin used), may rectify the problem of incomplete saturation where the field of analgesia is inadequate. Any beneficial effect from such supplementary injections is *not* due to synergism between the two base drugs, lignocaine and prilocaine.

Anatomical variations, intravascular injections and patient variations will also cause injection failures. These are relatively rare. Intravascular injections should be avoided by use of a self-aspiration injection system.

PSYCHOLOGICAL EFFECTS OF LOCAL ANALGESIA

Most dental patients find dental treatment mentally stressful, particularly when injections into the mouth are anticipated. Consequently, symptoms such as sweating, palpitations and hyperventilation are not uncommon and may be mistaken for adverse reactions to local analgesic drugs. Vasovagal syncope may result from profound fall in blood pressure. Patients should always be instructed to take long deep breaths during injections and, should vasovagal syncope occur, the patient's cerebral circulation must be restored. This is achieved by laying the patient flat with the legs raised. The head should not be below the level of the heart, as cerebral oedema may result and complicate recovery. Folding the patient over such that a head-between-knees position is formed is not recommended. Compression of the abdominal contents against the diaphragm will inhibit recovery by causing breathing difficulty as well as increase the likelihood of gastric emptying.

LOCAL COMPLICATIONS

Pain will result from too rapid a rate of injection or too large a volume of injection. The palate is particularly susceptible to both these eventualities due to the close apposition of the tissues to underlying bone. The action of adrenaline compounds the pressure effect and a large necrotic area results. Injections should *never* be made into the incisive papilla, for the same reason.

Whilst making an inferior dental nerve block injection a patient may feel a sharp pain, likened to an electric shock, in the tongue or lower lip if the lingual or inferior dental nerves are touched by the needle. If these nerves are penetrated by a needle and injection proceeds, then neural damage and prolonged analgesia will result. This is usually transient but may be permanent. Fortunately, such occurrences are very rare. Nerve (and vascular) injuries resulting from dental injections are more likely if needle passage into bony foramina (e.g. the infraorbital or mental foramen) is attempted. Such techniques are not recommended.

Periosteal trauma during injection will result in severe postoperative pain. Care must be taken to make sure such damage is prevented.

Needle-track infections will result from use of contaminated needles or solutions. Analgesia carpules should always be checked for cracks before use. They should *not* be stored in heated containers as such practice reduces the shelf-life of the contained solution. Injection of such degraded solutions may lead to toxic side-effects, swelling and pain. Injection of room temperature solutions has been repeatedly shown to be no more painful than injection of solutions warmed to 37°C.

Re-use of needles and partly used analgesic carpules must *never* be practised as transmission of serious blood-borne diseases from one patient to another will occur. The various forms of viral hepatitis and the human immune-deficiency virus (HIV) are most readily spread in this way.

Haematoma formation will result from perforation of vessels during injection. This rarely presents a problem, however, despite the highly vascular nature of the dental regions. Arterial penetration is very rare indeed as their robust walls resist needle puncture and the vessel tends to roll away from the advancing needle. Veins, on the other hand, are more susceptible to puncture. Bleeding usually stops spontaneously after a short time. Severe bleeding should arouse the suspicion of a bleeding diathesis. Inadvertent intravascular injection will not only fail to produce the required analgesia because the solution is rapidly carried from the desired site in the circulation, but will increase the likelihood of systemic side-effects.

Facial nerve palsy may follow inferior dental block injection, especially when the solution is deposited too far behind the inner surface of the ramus of the mandible. The solution tracks into the parotid gland and blocks nerve conduction in the contained facial nerve. On the affected side, the patient will be unable to frown, move the lips and close the eyelids. The condition resolves as the analgesic effect recovers, though in some cases the condition may persist for a longer period. Eye protection must be prescribed until recovery occurs. Very rarely, analgesic solution spreads into the pterygopalatine fossa, where the ocular nerve supply is then disrupted. This is fortunately an extremely rare occurrence but one which requires urgent reference of the patient to an ophthalmic physician, especially if optic nerve involvement (blindness) has occurred.

Trismus occasionally follows inferior dental nerve block injection, and becomes apparent 2–3 days postinjection. This is thought to be due to local irritation of the medial pterygoid muscle from the injected solution, needle injury to this muscle's fibres or from haemorrhage along the needle track. Infection will compound the effect. The condition usually resolves, but slowly, and may take several weeks to recover completely. Infratemporal fossa infection should be treated with antibiotics. Surgical drainage is required if suppuration occurs.

Lip and soft tissue trauma may result from burning or biting of numb tissues. Specific warnings against these eventualities should always be given, especially in the case of children when the parent should be warned to observe and prevent these problems.

INTRALIGAMENTARY DENTAL ANALGESIA

Recently there has been renewed popularity of this technique, which depends upon deposition of solution directly into the periodontal ligament to effect dental analgesia. Fine-gauge, ultra-short needles are required and instruments specifically designed to produce the high pressures required for injection have become available. Inevitably, the glass carpules frequently shatter during the pressure injection, and these instruments *must* incorporate shielding to contain the glass splinters produced.

The technique is sometimes valuable when failure of analgesia using conventional techniques is a problem, but is contraindicated when local sepsis is present. Routine use is not recommended. The following advantages and disadvantages have been stated.

Advantages

1. Simple to perform.
2. Rapid effect.
3. Absence of unwanted soft tissue analgesia; it has been noted that this is not always so, especially when injections into the molar regions of the mandible are made when lip analgesia can result.
4. Single tooth analgesia; again, this may not be so as the solution can spread to involve adjacent teeth.
5. Very small volume of solution injected; this is not regarded as an advantage by the author. Further, any unused solution in a dental carpule *must* be discarded and *never* used for another patient.
6. Useful for those with bleeding disorders; this 'advantage' must be interpreted with caution. Injections of any sort into such patients should only be made with the specific permission of a specialist haematologist.
7. Useful for children; needle phobia is not overcome, however.

Disadvantages

1. Injection is often painful.
2. Post-injection periodontitis frequently occurs, lasting for 24 h. Frank sepsis can occur, especially when gingival or periodontal health is poor, and these states represent a contraindication to intraligamentary analgesia. Periodontal tissue damage occurs which resolves with scarring after 2–3 weeks. Repeated injections, therefore, may result in permanent damage to the periodontal ligament.
3. Accurate occlusal adjustment of restorations is not possible due to the periodontal dilatation produced by injection.
4. Single, conical rooted teeth (e.g. central incisors or second permanent premolars) may be exfoliated by the pressure of injection.
5. The technique is equivalent to intravenous injection of drug due to its rapid absorption into the blood stream.
6. Unknown, but possible, toxic effects of the injected drug upon developing tooth germs. Injections into the periodontal liagment of deciduous molars flood the developing permanent premolar tooth germs with solution, with the possibility of permanent tooth damage.

Chapter 43

Mouth ulcers

Causes include:

(a) local factors;
(b) aphthae (and Behçet's syndrome);
(c) neoplasia;
(d) drugs;
(e) systemic disorders—
  (i) blood diseases,
  (ii) infections,
  (iii) gastrointestinal disease,
  (iv) skin disease.

Local factors

These include:

(a) trauma (e.g. biting or from an appliance);
(b) heart burn (e.g. pizza palate);
(c) cold burn (e.g. from cryosurgery);
(d) chemical burn (e.g. aspirin);
(e) radiation burn (rare nowadays—but mucositis common);
(f) electric burn (rare).

NB. Sometimes ulcers are self-induced.

Clinical features

1. Any age
2. Usually obvious precipitating factor and history
3. Usually single ulcer of irregular outline
4. Ulcer heals within 2–3 weeks of removal of precipitating factor

Diagnosis

1. History
2. Examination
3. Biopsy *if not healing within 3 weeks*

Management

1. Remove precipitating cause
2. Chlorhexidine 0.2% aqueous mouthwash
3. ± analgesics.

Aphthae (recurrent aphthous stomatitis; RAS)

Caused by unknown factors in most cases but predisposing factors in some include:

(a) familial background (genetic)
(b) trauma
(c) lack, or cessation, of cigarette smoking
(d) luteal phase of menstruation
(e) deficiencies of haematinics (iron, folic acid or vitamin B_{12})
(f) stress
(g) food allergies (possibly)
(h) immune deficiency (e.g. HIV infection)
(i) rarely — Behçet's syndrome (aphthae, eye, genital and other lesions)

Clinical features

1. Usually early onset — child or adolescent (later onset may signify haematinic or immune deficiency)
2. Recurrent multiple ulcers
3. Natural history of spontaneous resolution in third decade in many

Three clinical types of RAS (Table 43.1).

Diagnosis

1. History (exclude Behçet's syndrome, gastrointestinal disease, anaemia, menstrual relationship, etc.)

Table 43.1
Comparison of the three types of recurrent aphthous stomatitis

	Minor	Major	Herpetiform
Frequency	Most common (80% of all)	Uncommon	Very uncommon
Number of ulcers	1–6	1–6	10–100
Size	2–4 mm	5 mm +	Initially pinpoint — later large irregular
Site	Rare on dorsum of tongue, or palate	Any	Any
Healing	5–14 days	1–3 months	Variable — often weeks
Scarring	–	+	±

2. Examination—
    (a) oral
    (b) general (at least skin and eyes)
    (c) haematological (full blood picture, ferritin, folic acid and vitamin B_{12} levels)

Management

1. Treat any identifiable predisposing factor
2. Trial of 0.2% chlorhexidine aqueous mouthwash
3. Topical corticosteroids if above unsuccessful— Adcortyl (triamcinolone paste) or Corlan (hydrocortisone hemisuccinate; 2.5 mg pellets)
4. Refer if intractable ulcers, or suspected systemic disease.

Neoplasia

Many malignant states can cause ulcers but most common causes include:
    (a) oral squamous cell carcinoma (90% or more of all: see below);
    (b) melanoma (usually hyperpigmented lesion in palate);
    (c) Kaposi's sarcoma (usually purple palatal lesion in HIV infection);
    (d) lymphomas (typically in palate/fauces);
    (e) salivary neoplasms (typically in upper lip or palate);
    (f) antral carcinoma (invading palate).

Clinical features, diagnosis and management

Any lump or ulcer persisting for more than 3 weeks should be biopsied or the patient referred immediately.

Oral squamous cell carcinoma (SCC)

Aetiological factors include:

   (a) racial and/or environmental factors (extremely common in SE Asia: see below);
   (b) tobacco habits (especially chewing habits or reverse smoking);
   (c) alcohol;
   (d) others—
       (i)   erythroplasia especially and some leukoplakias (Chapter 45),
       (ii)   iron deficiency in Plummer–Vinson syndrome,
       (iii) erosive lichen planus (about 1% go malignant),
       (iv)   oral submucous fibrosis (in SE Asians mainly),
       (v)   ultraviolet light (lip cancer),
       (vi)   dyskeratosis congenita (rare),
       (vii) discoid lupus erythematosus,
       (viii) infections possibly (syphilis, candidosis, herpes simplex, or human papillomavirus),
       (ix)   immunosuppression (lip cancer).

Clinical features

1. Usually an elderly male
2. Typically a solitary chronic ulcer with raised edges and granular floor
3. ± surrounding leukoplakia or erythroplasia
4. Most common on lateral margin tongue/floor of mouth, or lower lip
5. May also present as lump, fissure, red or white lesion
6. ± pain
7. ± regional cervical lymph node enlargement
8. ± radiographic evidence of bone invasion

Diagnosis

1. History
2. Examination —
    (a) oral (remember cervical lymph nodes)
    (b) radiography
    (c) biopsy essential (choose red area if possible)

Management

Refer for diagnosis if appropriate. Refer for radiotherapy and/or surgery as decided by specialists. Prognosis is still poor for intraoral carcinoma (30% 5-year survival) but good for labial carcinoma (70% 5-year survival).

Drugs causing mouth ulcers

These include:

(a) cytotoxic agents (e.g. methotrexate; which almost invariably causes ulcers);
(b) phenytoin (by inducing folic acid deficiency);
(c) drugs causing chemical burns (e.g. aspirin);
(d) drugs causing lichenoid eruptions or vesiculo-erosive lesions;
(e) many others.

Clinical features, diagnosis and management

1. May be an obvious history
2. Ulcers vary in shape, size, situation and appearance
3. Withdrawal of drug usually leads to resolution
4. Symptomatic care helps (0.2% chlorhexidine aqueous mouthwash)

Blood diseases that may manifest with mouth ulcers

These include:

(a) haematinic deficiencies (see p. 399);

(b) leukaemias (therapy may also precipitate ulcers);
(c) leukopenias (from viral infections including HIV, drugs, irradiation, idiopathic);
(d) leukocyte congenital immune defects (rare).

Clinical features

1. Mouth ulcers in these disorders may resemble RAS, acute necrotizing ulcerative gingivitis, may be non-specific; or may be of herpes simplex virus or other microbial aetiology
2. ± other features in the leukocyte disorders—especially recurrent infections and periodontal disease
3. ± anaemia and/or thrombocytopenia with oral purpura or gingival bleeding (leukaemias or aplastic anaemia).

Diagnosis

1. History
2. Examination—

   (a) oral (remember lymph nodes)
   (b) general examination (especially skin, lymph nodes, liver and spleen)
   (c) haematological (full blood picture, especially white cell count and differential; haematinic assays)

Management

1. Refer to relevant physician
2. Symptomatic treatment of non-specific ulcers with 0.2% aqueous chlorhexidine
3. Treat infections as appropriate.

Infections that can present with mouth ulcers

These include:

(a) *Viruses*
   (i) herpes simplex virus
   (ii) herpes varicella-zoster virus
   (iii) Coxsackie and other enteroviruses
   (iv) Epstein–Barr virus (occasionally)
   (v) human immunodeficiency virus (occasionally)

(b) *Bacteria*
   (i) acute/necrotizing ulcerative gingivitis
   (ii) tuberculosis and atypical mycobacteria (rare)
   (iii) syphilis (rare)
   (iv) others (especially in immunocompromised patients)

(c) *Others*
   (i) rare fungal infections
   (ii) rare protozoal infections
   (especially in immunocompromised patients or travellers outside Europe/N. America)

Only the more common infections, viz. herpes simplex, varicella-zoster and enterovirus infections, are discussed further here.

Oral herpes simplex virus infection

Clinical features

1. *Primary infection*. In young child typically (herpetic stomatitis) — fever, malaise, cervical lymph node enlargement. Diffuse gingivitis, and multiple oral vesicles that ulcerate. Spontaneous recovery in 7–10 days; virus then latent in trigeminal ganglion.
2. *Recurrences*. Typically in adults or the immunocompromised. Precipitated spontaneously, by ultraviolet light, trauma, menstruation or compromised immunity. Lesions on lip usually. Vesicles→pustules→scabs (*herpes labialis*). May be ulcers intraorally especially in immunocompromised patients.

Diagnosis

1. History
2. Examination —
   (a) oral (remember lymph nodes)
   (b) ± full blood picture (if immune defect or blood dyscrasia considered)
3. For primary infection —
   (a) temperature
   (b) ± serology

Management

1. *Primary infection*. Fluids + soft diet; analgesic/antipyretic (e.g. paracetamol); 0.2% aqueous chlorhexidine mouthwash; acyclovir especially in immunocompromised patients.
2. *Herpes labialis*. Acyclovir 5% cream useful.

Herpes varicella-zoster virus infections

Clinical features

1. *Primary infection*. Typically in a child (chickenpox) — fever, malaise, lymph node enlargement; rash mainly on trunk and face (macules→papules→vesicles→pustules→scab).

Non-specific mouth ulcers: usually resemble aphthae.
Spontaneous recovery in 7–14 days: virus then latent, usually in dorsal root ganglia.

2. *Recurrences (zoster or shingles)*. Usually in adult or imunocompromised—if involving the trigeminal nerve, may cause unilateral orofacial pain, rash and mouth ulcers.

Maxillary nerve involved—rash over ipsilateral cheek; ulcers and pain in ipsilateral palate and maxillary teeth.

Mandibular nerve involved—rash and pain over lower ipsilateral face and lip; ulcers and pain in tongue and soft tissues; pain also in mandibular teeth.

Diagnosis

1. History (may be contact history in chickenpox)
2. Examination—
    (a) oral (remember lymph nodes)
    (b) general (skin and rash)
3. For primary infection—
    (a) temperature
    (b) ± serology
4. For zoster—may need to exclude malignancy/immune defect (including HIV)

Management

1. Primary infection—
    (a) fluids + soft diet
    (b) analgesic/antipyretics
    (c) 0.2% aqueous chlorhexidine mouthwash
    (d) Acyclovir in immunocompromised patients
2. Zoster—
    (a) analgesics
    (b) Acyclovir
    (c) 0.2% aqueous chlorhexidine mouthwash

Coxsackie and other enterovirus (usually echovirus) infections

Clinical features

Young child usually. Fever, malaise, lymph node enlargement; mouth ulcers; spontaneous recovery in 5–10 days.
Two main syndromes:
Herpangina. Palatal ulcers but no skin lesions.
Hand, foot and mouth disease. Oral ulcers, and vesicles on hands/feet.

Diagnosis

1. History (may be contact history)
2. Examination—
    (a) oral
    (b) general (at least of hands and feet)
    (c) temperature

Management

1. Fluids + soft diet
2. Analgesic/antipyretic
3. 0.2% aqueous chlorhexidine mouthwash.

Gastrointestinal diseases that may present with mouth ulcers

These include:

(a) coeliac disease (gluten-sensitive enteropathy);
(b) Crohn's disease (regional ileitis);
(c) ulcerative colitis
(d) any disorders that lead to malabsorption or blood loss may predispose to RAS.

Clinical features

Mouth ulcers may resemble RAS (late-onset RAS in particular should raise a suspicion of predisposing factors such as gastrointestinal disease).

Coeliac disease. Ulcers usually like RAS; ± angular stomatitis, glossitis; ± abdominal pain; fatty frequent stool; anaemia; failure to thrive in childhood.

Crohn's disease. Ulcers may be like RAS or also be solitary, persistent and with hyperplastic margins; ± abdominal pain, frequent stool; anaemia; ± angular stomatitis; glossitis; ± facial swelling; mucosal cobblestoning or tags; gingival hyperplasia.

Condition sometimes termed orofacial granulomatosis.

Ulcerative colitis. Ulcers like RAS or irregular chronic ulcers; ± mucosal pustules (pyostomatitis vegetans); ± persistent bloody diarrhoea; anaemia.

Diagnosis

1. History (remember bowel symptoms)
2. Examination—
    (a) oral
    (b) generally (especially for anaemia, weight loss, perianal lesions)
    (c) haematological (full blood picture; ferritin, folic acid, vitamin B_{12} levels)
    (d) ± biopsy

MOUTH ULCERS

Management

Refer to appropriate physician.

Skin diseases that may present with mouth ulcers

These include:

(a) pemphigus (rare but lethal);
(b) pemphigoid (uncommon but may threaten sight);
(c) erythema multiforme (uncommon but incapacitating);
(d) angina bullosa haemorrhagica (ABH; uncommon but worrying to patient);
(e) lichen planus (common but rarely ulcerative; Chapter 45).

Clinical features (Table 43.2)

Table 43.2
Clinical features of skin diseases with oral ulceration

Disease	Age affected	Sex mainly affected	Aetiology	Oral lesions	Other lesions
Pemphigus	Middle +	F	Autoimmune	Erosions Blisters rarely seen but may appear on pressure (Nikolsky sign)	Skin blisters Erosions on other mucosae
Pemphigoid	Middle +	F	Probably autoimmune	Blisters + erosions (± desquamative gingivitis)	± conjunctival erosions and scarring
Erythema multiforme	Young adult	M	? allergic to drugs, micro-organisms	Erosions Blood-stained, crusted swollen lips	± rash (target lesions) ±erosions on other mucosae
Angina bullosa haemorrhagica	Elderly	F/M	? trauma Sometimes steroid inhalers	Blood-filled blisters erosions (especially on palate)	—
Lichen planus	Middle +	F	? immuno-logical Sometimes drugs or dental materials	Erosions (± white lesions) mainly bilaterally in buccal mucosa and/or tongue (± desquamative gingivitis)	± rash (itchy purple, papular on wrists especially) ± lesions on other mucosae, nails, hair loss

Diagnosis

1. History (remember skin, eye and genital lesions)
2. Examination —
    (a) oral
    (b) general (eyes, skin, nails, hair, other mucosae)
    (c) ± serology (autoantibodies to epithelial intercellular cement — pemphigus; or basement membrane — pemphigoid)
    (d) ± haematology (full blood picture and platelets to exclude blood dyscrasia in ABH)
    (e) biopsy: usually also with immunostaining (biopsy not usually needed in ABH or erythema multiforme)

Management

Refer to appropriate physician in most cases.
Pemphigus. Systemic immunosuppressants required.
Pemphigoid. Topical immunosuppressants required.
Erythema multiforme. Systemic or topical immunosuppressants required.
Angina bullosa haemorrhagica. Symptomatic treatment only.
Lichen planus. Topical or intralesional corticosteroids usually.

FURTHER READING

General

Grattan C. E. H., Scully C. (1986): Oral ulceration: a diagnostic problem *Brit. Med. J.* **292**, 1093–4.
Scully C. (1983). An update on mouth ulcers. *Dent. Update*, **10**, 141–52.
Rennie J. R., Reade P. C., Hay K. D., Scully C. (1985). Recurrent aphthous stomatitis. *Brit. Dent. J.*, **159**, 361–7.
Scully C., Cawson R. A. (1988). *Colour Aids to Oral Medicine*. Edinburgh: Churchill Livingstone.
Scully C., Flint S. (1989). *An Atlas of Stomatology*. London: Martin Dunitz.
Scully C., Porter S. R. (1989). Recurrent aphthous stomatitis. *J. Oral Pathol.* **18**, 21–7.
Wray D., Scully C. (1986). The sore mouth. *Med. Int.*, **2**, 1134–7.

Neoplastic ulcers

Henk J. M., Langdon J. D. (1985). *Malignant Tumours of the Oral Cavity*. London: Edward Arnold.
Pindborg J. J. (1980). *Oral Cancer and Precancer*. Bristol: John Wright.
Scully C., Malamos D., Levers B. G. H., Porter S. R., Prime S. S. (1986). Sources and patterns of referrals of oral cancer: the role of general practitioners. *Brit. Med. J.*, **293**, 599–601.

Oral ulcers and drugs

Dreizen S., McCredie K. B., Bodey G. P., Eating M. J. (1986). Quantitative analysis of the oral complications of antileukaemia chemotherapy. *Oral Surg.*, **62**, 650–3.

Scully C., Cawson R. A. (1987). *Medical Problems in Dentistry* 2nd edn. Bristol: John Wright.
Scully C., MacFarlane T. W. (1983). Orofacial manifestations in childhood malignancy: clinical and microbiological findings during remission. *J. Dent. Child.*, **50,** 121–5.

Oral ulcers and systemic diseases

Scully C. (1989). Infectious diseases in oral medicine. In *1988 World Workshop on Oral Medicine* (Millard D., Mason D. K., eds.). Chicago: Year Book Publishers.
Scully C., Cawson R. A. (1987). *Medical Problems in Dentistry* 2nd edn. Bristol: John Wright.
Scully C. (1989) Herpes simplex virus infections. *Oral Surg.*, **68,** 701–10.
Scully C. (1989). Ulcers in association with systemic disease. In *The Mouth in Health and Disease* (Scully C., ed.). Oxford: Heinemann Medical.
Scully C., Porter S. R. (1988). The mouth and skin. In *Relationships in Dermatology* vol. 8 (Verbov J., ed.). Lancaster: MTP Press.
Stephenson P., Lamey P. J., Scully C., Prime S. S. (1987). Angina bullosa haemorrhagica: clinical and laboratory features in 30 patients. *Oral Surg.*, **63,** 560–5.
Van Hale H. M., Rogers R. S., Zone J. J., Greip P. R. (1985). Pyostomatitis vegetans: a reactive mucosal marker for inflammatory diseases of the gut. *Arch. Dermatol.*, **121,** 94–8.
Wiesenfeld D. W., Ferguson M. M., Mitchell D., *et al.* (1985). Orofacial granulomatosis — a clinical and pathological analysis. *Quart. J. Med.*, **54,** 101–13.

Chapter 44

Lumps in the mouth

The many different lesions which may present as lumps or swellings in the mouth may include:

1. *Normal features —*
    (a) pterygoid hamulus
    (b) unerupted teeth
    (c) parotid papillae
    (d) foliate and other lingual papillae

2. *Developmental conditions —*
    (a) maxillary and mandibular tori
    (b) haemangioma
    (c) lymphangioma
    (d) hereditary gingival fibromatosis
    (e) Von Recklinghausen's neurofibromatosis

3. *Inflammatory disorders —*
    (a) abscesses
    (b) pyogenic granulomas
    (c) sarcoidosis and Crohn's disease
    (d) others

4. *Trauma-related disorders —*
    (a) epulides
    (b) fibrous lumps
    (c) denture-induced hyperplasia

5. *Cystic lesions —*
    (a) odontogenic
    (b) non-odontogenic

6. *Hormonally-related lesions*
    (a) pubertal gingivitis
    (b) pregnancy gingivitis/epulis

7. *Neoplastic disorders*
    (a) various benign neoplasms
    (b) primary and secondary carcinomas

LUMPS IN THE MOUTH

  (c) lymphoreticular neoplasms
  (d) other malignant oral lesions

8. *Drug-induced lesions (gingival swelling)*

  (a) phenytoin
  (b) nifedipine
  (c) cyclosporin
  (d) others

9. *Others*

  (a) angio-oedema
  (b) amyloidosis

Some of these conditions are now considered further.

DEVELOPMENTAL

Tori

Clinical features

1. Common, especially in mongoloids
2. Bony hard asymptomatic swellings with normal overlying mucosa
   Maxillary tori — centre of hard palate
   Mandibular tori — lingual to premolars

Diagnosis

1. History (may not be noticed until adult life)
2. Examination

Management

1. Usually — reassurance only
2. If causing difficulties in denture construction — surgery.

Haemangioma (see Chapter 45)

Lymphangioma

Clinical features

1. Congenital asymptomatic lesion often on tongue
2. Variable appearance — often likened to frog-spawn

Diagnosis

1. History
2. Examination

Management

Reassurance.

INFLAMMATORY

Abscesses (dental abscesses)

Clinical features

1. Usually follow caries/trauma
2. Usually preceded or accompanied by pain
3. Swelling usually tender and on buccal aspect of jaw, except with abscesses on upper lateral incisors or palatal roots of upper molars

Diagnosis

1. History (usually there is a preceding pulpitis)
2. Examination (note especially the vitality of associated teeth)
3. Radiography

Management

1. Drain the abscess (through root canal or by incision of fluctuant abscess or by tooth extraction)
2. ± antimicrobials.

Pyogenic granulomas

Clinical features

1. Proliferative, often painless, swelling
2. Typically on lip, tongue or gingiva

Diagnosis

1. History
2. Examination
3. Biopsy

Management

1. *Pregnancy epulis* — conservative management preferred
2. Other pyogenic granulomas — usually excise.

Sarcoidosis

Clinical features

May present orally as lump, xerostomia or salivary gland swelling

Diagnosis

1. History
2. Examination
3. Biopsy of oral lesion (granulomas)
4. Chest radiography (especially to exclude hilar lymph node enlargement)
5. Blood tests — serum levels of angiotensin-converting enzyme and adenosine deaminase are increased
6. Kveim test (usually positive)
7. ± gallium scan (may be positive in lymph nodes and salivary glands)

Management

Refer to physician.

Oral Crohn's disease

Clinical features

Variable combination of:
   (a) cobble-stoning of mucosa;
   (b) mucosal tags;
   (c) labial or facial swelling;
   (d) gingival hyperplasia;
   (e) angular stomatitis;
   (f) mouth ulcers.

Diagnosis

1. History (note especially gastrointestinal symptoms and relation of clinical features to dietary components)
2. Examination (including abdominal)
3. Biopsy of oral lesions (lymphoedema and granulomas)
4. Haematology (full blood picture and assays of iron and folic acid which tend to be reduced)

Management

1. Exclusion diet if there seem to be dietary factors
2. Intralesional corticosteroids may reduce oral swelling
3. Refer to physician.

TRAUMA-RELATED

Fibrous lumps (fibroepithelial polyps)

Clinical features

Gingival fibrous lumps (*epulides*) are typically firm and painless, arising buccally from interdental papillae.

Other fibrous lumps (including *denture-induced*; see Chapter 35) are hyperplastic, firm and painless, usually with normal overlying mucosa.

Diagnosis

1. History
2. Examination
3. Biopsy

Management

Excise.

NEOPLASIA

Any oral lump or lesion that does not regress within 3 weeks of the removal of identifiable predisposing factors should be regarded as sinister and biopsied.

OTHER CAUSES

Angio-oedema

Most angio-oedema is a Type 1 allergic reaction usually in relation to drugs (e.g. penicillin). A minority is due to hereditary deficiency of an inhibitor of complement activation (C1 esterase-inhibitor deficiency). The danger from both types is of facial and lingual swelling, airway obstruction and possible asphyxia.

Clinical features

1. *Allergic angio-oedema* — rapid onset following contact with allergen:

    (a) ± urticaria
    (b) ± anaphylaxis

2. *Hereditary angio-oedema* — rapid onset after trauma (e.g. dental extraction); often a positive family history

Diagnosis

1. History (swelling ± family history)
2. Examination (between attacks shows nothing remarkable)
3. Complement studies (C2, C3, C4 and C1 esterase inhibitor)

Management

1. Dental treatment is best carried out in hospital
2. *Allergic angio-oedema* — avoid allergen, treat attack with intramuscular or subcutaneous adrenaline and intravenous corticosteroids; maintain airway — give oxygen
3. Hereditary angio-oedema — refer to physician; androgenic steroids such as stanozolol reduce attacks.

Amyloidosis

Amyloidosis is a rare condition characterized by protein deposition in tissues including the tongue — a cause of macroglossia. Patients should be referred for specialist care.

FURTHER READING

Lumps in general

Scully C. (1983). Lumps and swellings in the mouth. *Update*, **26**, 1651–7.
Scully C., Flint S. R. (1989). *An Atlas of Stomatology*. London: Martin Dunitz.

Tori

Eggen S., Nátvig B. (1986). Relationship between torus mandibularis and number of present teeth. *Scand. J. Dent. Res.*, **94**, 233–40.
Rezai R. F. (1985). Torus palatinus, an exostosis of unknown aetiology. *Compend. Contin. Educ. Dent.*, **6**, 149–52.

Angiomas

Stal S., *et al.* (1986). Haemangioma, lymphangioma and vascular malformations of the head and neck. *Otolaryngol. Clin. N. Am.*, **19**, 769–96.

Granulomatous conditions

Van Maarsseveen A.C.M.T., *et al.* (1982). Oral involvement in sarcoidosis. *Int. J. Oral Surg.*, **11**, 21–9.

Wiesenfeld D. W., *et al.* (1985). Orofacial granulomatosis — a clinical and pathological analysis. *Quart. J. Med.*, **54,** 101–3.

Epulides

MacLeod R. I., Soames J. W. (1987). Epulides: a clinicopathological study of 200 consecutive lesions. *Brit. Dent. J.,* **163,** 51–3.

Angio-oedema

McCarthy N. R. (1985). Diagnosis and management of hereditary angio-oedema. *Brit. J. Oral Maxillofac. Surg.*, **23,** 123–7

Amyloidosis

Babejews A. (1985). Occult multiple myeloma associated with amyloid of the tongue. *Brit. J. Oral Maxillofac. Surg.*, **23,** 298–303.

Chapter 45

Red, white and pigmented lesions

RED LESIONS

Causes include:

(a) geographical tongue,
(b) acute candidosis,
(c) chronic atrophic candidosis (denture-induced stomatitis),
(d) atrophic glossitis,
(e) median rhomboid glossitis,
(f) purpura,
(g) telangiectases,
(h) haemangiomas,
(i) Kaposi's sarcoma,
(j) erythroplasia.

Geographical tongue (Erythema migrans)

Clinical features

1. Commonly asymptomatic but may cause soreness
2. Irregular depapillated areas which change in shape and size
3. Typically affects the dorsum of the tongue
4. Fissured (scrotal tongue) is often affected by erythema migrans

Diagnosis

1. History
2. Examination

Management

Reassurance.

Acute atrophic candidosis

Clinical features

1. Diffuse erythema and soreness
2. Typically follows antibiotic or corticosteroid therapy
3. Typically affects the dorsum of the tongue

Diagnosis

1. History (note recent drug therapy and exclude immune defect, e.g. HIV)
2. Examination
3. ± Gram-stained smear or saliva culture

Management

1. Stop any offending medication
2. Antifungal (e.g. nystatin pastilles, 100 000 i.u. dissolved in mouth, four times a day)
3. Refer if possible immune defect.

Denture-induced stomatitis (denture sore mouth)

Clinical features (see also Chapter 35)

1. Diffuse erythema limited to denture-bearing area (candida-associated)
2. Typically found beneath a complete upper denture
3. Asymptomatic but there may be an associated angular stomatitis.

Diagnosis

1. History
2. Examination

Management

1. Improve denture hygiene: clean and store overnight in 1% hypochlorite or 0.2% chlorhexidine
2. ± antifungals (mainly required where there is also angular stomatitis)
3. ± attention to dentures.

Atrophic glossitis

Clinical features

1. Red, smooth and usually sore tongue
2. May be associated with angular stomatitis and/or mouth ulcers due to deficiency of iron, folic acid, and/or vitamin B_{12}, or candidosis

Diagnosis

1. History (note especially diet, blood loss or gastrointestinal symptoms)
2. Examination (including skin and cardiovascular)
3. Haematological (full blood picture; haematinic assays)

Management

1. Identify and treat cause of deficiency
2. Replacement therapy
3. Benzydamine oral rinse

Median rhomboid glossitis

Clinical features

1. Depapillated, rhomboidal usually asymptomatic area in the centre line of the dorsum of tongue, anterior to circumvallate papillae.
2. Usually the patient is a smoker.

Diagnosis

1. History
2. Examination
3. Biopsy rarely needed

Management

1. Stop the patient smoking
2. ± antifungals (may be related to candidosis).

Purpura

There are many causes of purpura. Commonly the cause of oral purpura is local trauma or suction, but platelet deficiency or defect should always be excluded by history (of bleeding tendency or bruising), examination (for purpura) and investigation (full blood picture, white cell count and differential, and platelet count). A medical opinion should be sought.

Telangiectases

Telangiectases are dilated capillaries that may reflect a congenital condition (e.g. hereditary haemorrhagic telangiectasia) or may appear in, for example, systemic sclerosis, or may follow radiotherapy.

Haemangiomas

Clinical features

Typically a red or blue fluctuant lesion that blanches on pressure.

Diagnosis

1. History (usually present from birth)
2. Examination
3. ± aspiration

Management

Depends on size, site and symptoms. May often be left alone but may be treated with cryosurgery, sometimes with argon laser, or rarely by ligation of feeding blood vessels.

Kaposi's sarcoma

Clinical features

1. Usually a red, blue or purple macule or nodule
2. Typically seen in the palate
3. Classically a manifestation of secondary immune deficiency such as HIV infection

Diagnosis

1. History (especially note high-risk group for HIV; or any immunosuppression)
2. Examination (particularly for skin lesions, or other oral lesions suggestive of HIV infection)
3. Serology (HIV antibodies, after counselling)
4. Biopsy

Management

1. Refer to physician with interest in AIDS
2. Radiotherapy or vinblastine

Erythroplasia

Clinical features

1. Red velvety lesion level with, or depressed below, the mucosa
2. Typically in elderly patients
3. Most commonly on the floor of mouth/ventrum of tongue, or soft palate
4. High premalignant potential (80% +)

Diagnosis

1. History
2. Examination
3. Biopsy

Management
Excision.

WHITE LESIONS

Causes include:

   (a) Congenital lesions such as white sponge naevus;
   (b) keratoses (leukoplakias);
   (c) neoplasms (some papillomas and carcinoma);
   (d) immunologically-mediated disorders (lichen planus and lupus erythematosus);
   (e) infections (candidosis mainly);
   (f) others.

White sponge naevus

Clinical features

Asymptomatic, persistent white lesions in mouth and sometimes genital mucosa. Rare.

Appearance usually noted since childhood: may be positive family history.

Diagnosis

1. History (especially family)
2. Examination
3. ± biopsy

Management

Reassurance.

Keratoses

Keratoses can be classified as:

   (a) primary (idiopathic);
   (b) secondary—
      (i) smoker's keratosis,
      (ii) frictional keratosis,
      (iii) syphilitic keratosis,
      (iv) candidal leukoplakia,
      (v) keratosis in chronic renal failure,
      (vi) hairy leukoplakia.

Clinical features

Smoker's keratosis. Common in the palate in pipe smoker, or on lower lip or elsewhere in cigarette smokers. Rarely premalignant.

Frictional keratosis. Tends to be found in the buccal mucosa at the occlusal line, or on edentulous ridges. Rarely premalignant.

Syphilitic keratosis. Leukoplakia of the dorsum of the tongue with a fairly high premalignant potential.

Candidal leukoplakia. This is typically speckled and at the commissures and has a highish premalignant potential.

Hairy leukoplakia. This is typically hairy or corrugated, at the lateral margins of the tongue, and in HIV-positive persons. It is not known to be premalignant.

In general, keratoses tend to be uniform white plaques (*homogeneous leukoplakia* — most common in the buccal mucosa and of very low premalignant potential). Speckled leukoplakias have a much higher premalignant potential. Leukoplakias of the floor of mouth/ventrum of tongue have probably the highest premalignant potential (20–50% in some studies).

Diagnosis

1. History (especially note habits such as tobacco use)
2. Examination
3. Biopsy (to assess degree of dysplasia)

Management

1. Remove or treat predisposing cause
2. Severely dysplastic keratoses — surgery, then follow-up
3. Mildly dysplastic keratoses — observe.

Neoplasms

Some papillomas and some carcinomas present as white lesions.

Lichen planus (LP)

Clinical features

1. Commonly asymptomatic
2. Lesions are white papules, striae and/or plaques
3. Typically bilateral in buccal mucosa and/or tongue

Diagnosis

1. History (note drug usage, and lesions on skin or mucosae)
2. Examination (note especially lesions on other mucosae or skin or appendages)
3. Biopsy (to exclude keratosis, lupus erythematosus and neoplasia)

RED, WHITE AND PIGMENTED LESIONS

Management

1. If possibly drug-induced (e.g. by non-steroidal anti-inflammatory agents), request physician to consider changing medication.
2. Asymptomatic LP — reassure
3. Symptomatic LP — initially try benzydamine oral rinse, then corticosteroids
4. *Follow-up*, particularly erosive LP (small chance of malignant change)

Lupus erythematosus (LE)

Clinical features

White lesions similar to LP but may have a dense brush-like border surrounding a speckled atrophic area.

Diagnosis

1. History
2. Examination
3. Biopsy
4. Urinalysis (to exclude proteinuria of systemic LE)
5. Haematology (full blood picture)
6. Serology (for anti-DNA antibodies)

Management

1. Topical corticosteroids for oral lesions
2. Refer to a physician for systemic LE.

Candidosis ('thrush')

Clinical features

Scattered white papules and plaques that can be wiped off using gauze.

Thrush signifies either changes in local flora because of antibiotics, corticosteroids or cytotoxic agents, or xerostomia, or systemic disease such as leukaemia or HIV. However, healthy neonates may also contract thrush!

Diagnosis

1. History (especially of drug use, HIV infection or leukaemia)
2. Examination (note any lymphadenopathy)
3. Urinalysis (for diabetes)
4. Haematology (full blood picture and white cell count)
5. ± serology for HIV after counselling

Management

1. Identify and treat predisposing cause
2. Antifungals.

PIGMENTED LESIONS

Causes of localized pigmented lesions include:

(a) amalgam tattoo;
(b) naevi;
(c) melanoma;
(d) Kaposi's sarcoma.

Causes of generalized pigmentation include:

(a) racial;
(b) smoking;
(c) Addison's disease;
(d) others.

Amalgam tattoo

Clinical features

1. Blue or black, localized submucosal pigmentation
2. Typically in mandibular gingiva or at apicectomy site
3. Sometimes radiopaque

Diagnosis

1. History
2. Examination
3. ± radiography

Management

Reassurance.

Naevi

Clincial features

1. Brown or black, asymptomatic macule
2. Typically on vermilion or palate

Diagnosis

1. History
2. Examination (see below)

RED, WHITE AND PIGMENTED LESIONS

Management

Reassurance.

Malignant melanoma

Clinical features

1. Brown or black lesion usually
2. Features suggestive of malignancy include rapid increase in size, change in colour, ulceration, pain, the appearance of satellite lesions, or regional lymph node enlargement

Diagnosis

1. History
2. Examination
3. Biopsy at time of definitive operation

Management

Surgery.

Racial pigmentation

Clinical features

1. Most oral hyperpigmentation is racial, even in those with white skins
2. Brown pigmentation is usually symmetrically distributed over gingiva and palate

Diagnosis

1. History
2. Examination (note skin and hair colour)

Management

Reassurance.

Addison's disease

Clinical features

1. Hyperpigmentation in areas normally pigmented (e.g. genitals) and sites of trauma (e.g. skin flexures)
2. Mucosal patchy pigmentation
3. Hypotension, weakness, weight loss, nausea
4. Usually a female patient

Diagnosis

1. History
2. Examination (especially for low blood pressure, weight loss and pigmented skin)
3. Plasma cortisol levels (reduced)
4. Synacthen test (reduced cortisol response to injection of adrenocorticotrophic hormone).

Management

1. Refer to physician
2. Hormone replacement needed
3. Defer dental treatment.

FURTHER READING

Red, white and pigmented patches — general

Scully C., Cawson R. A. (1986). White, red and pigmented patches. *Med. Int.*, **2**, 1138–42.
Scully C., Flint S. (1989). *An Atlas of Stomatology* London: Martin Dunitz.

Geographical tongue

Brooks J. K., Balciunas B. A. (1987). Geographical stomatitis: review of the literature and report of five cases. *J. Am. Dent. Assoc.*, **115**, 421–4.

Candida-related lesions

Odds F. C. (1987). Candida infections: an overview. *CRC Crit. Rev. Microbiol.*, **15**, 1–5.
Samaranayake L. P. (1989). *Oral Candidosis*. Guildford: Butterworths.
Scully C. (1986). Chronic atrophic candidosis (leading article). *Lancet,* **ii,** 437–8.
Scully C., Porter S. R., Millard D., Mason D. K. (1989) Candidosis. In *World Workshop on Oral Medicine*. Chicago: Year Book Publishers.
Wright B. A., Fenwick F. (1981). Candidiasis and atrophic tongue lesions. *Oral Surg.*, **51**, 55–61.

Purpura, telangiectasia, angiomas

Colvin B. T. (1985). Thrombocytopenia. *Clin. Haematol.*, **14**, 661–81.
Flint S. R., Keith O., Scully C. (1988). Hereditary haemorrhagic telangiectasia. *Oral Surg.*, **66**, 440–4.
Stal S., *et al.* (1986). Haemangioma, lymphangioma and vascular malformations of the head and neck. *Otolaryngol. Clin. North. Am.*, **19**, 769–96.

HIV-related lesions

Greenspan J. S., Greenspan D. (1987). Oral aspects of the acquired immune deficiency syndrome (AIDS). In *Oral Mucosal Diseases: Biology, Etiology and Therapy*. (Mackenzie I. C., et al., eds.). Copenhagen: Laegeforeningens forlag, pp. 65–9.
Porter S. R., Luker J., Scully C. et al. (1989). Orofacial aspects of a group of British patients infected with HIV-I. *J. Oral Pathol.* **18,** 47–8.
Schiodt M., et al. (1987). Clinical and histologic spectrum of oral hairy leukoplakia. *Oral Surg.*, **64,** 716–20.
Scully C., Porter S. R. (1988). Orofacial manifestations of HIV infection. *Lancet*, **i,** 976–7.

White sponge naevus

Ciola B., et al. (1976). White sponge naevus of the oral mucosa. *J. Conn. State Dent. Assoc.*, **51,** 122–6.

Keratosis and premalignancy

Banoczy J. (1982). *Oral Leukoplakia*. Budapest: Akademica Kiado.
Eveson J. W. (1983). Oral premalignancy. *Canc. Surv.*, **2,** 403–24.
Silverman S., Gorsky M., Lozado F. (1984). Oral leukoplakia and malignant transformation. *Cancer*, **53,** 563–8.

LP and LE

Schiodt M. (1984). Oral manifestations of lupus erythematosus. *Int. J. Oral Surg.*, **13,** 101–47.
Scully C., Elkom M. (1985). Lichen planus: review and update on pathogenesis. *J. Oral Path.*, **14,** 431–58.

Pigmented lesions

Batzakis J. G., et al. (1982). The pathology of head and neck tumours: mucosal melanomas. *Head and Neck Surg.*, **4,** 404–18.
Buchner A., Hansen L. S. (1980). Amalgam pigmentation (amalgam tattoo) of the oral mucosa: a clinicopathological study of 268 cases. *Oral Surg.*, **49,** 139–47.
Dummett C. O. (1980). Overview of normal oral pigmentation. *J. Indiana Dent. Assoc.*, **50,** 13–18.
Dummett C. O. (1985). Pertinent considerations in oral pigmentation. *Brit. Dent. J.*, **158,** 9–12.
Lamey P. J., Carmichael F., Scully C. (1985). Oral pigmentation, Addison's disease and results of screening. *Brit. Dent. J.*, **158,** 297–305.

Chapter 46

Pain and neurological disease

OROFACIAL PAIN

Causes include:

(a) local disease (mouth or ENT),
(b) neurological disease,
(c) psychogenic disorders,
(d) vascular causes
(e) referred pain (rarely).

Local disease

Most orofacial pain is odontogenic in origin. Antral causes are less common; ENT or eye causes rare.

Neurological disease

Neuralgia in trigeminal area is usually *idiopathic* but disorders such as disseminated sclerosis or tumours must be excluded (see p. 403 for herpetic neuralgia).

Clinical features of idiopathic trigeminal neuralgia

Usually middle-aged or older patient. Lancinating, unilateral, severe orofacial pain in a division or branch of trigeminal nerve, ± trigger point. *No other neurological symptoms or signs.*

Diagnosis

1. History
2. Examination —
    (a) oral
    (b) cranial nerves
    (c) ± skull radiography

Management

1. Carbamazepine (monitor full blood picture and blood pressure)
2. Cryosurgery or other neurosurgery, if unresponsive or adverse drug effects excessive, e.g. ataxia

Refer to relevant physician if not 'idiopathic'.

Psychogenic disorders

Presentations include: oral dysaesthesias and atypical facial pain; and possibly TMJ pain–dysfunction syndrome.
Oral dysaesthesias include:

   (a) burning mouth syndrome (glossodynia: glossopyrosis);
   (b) atypical facial pain.

Burning mouth syndrome — clinical features

Middle-aged or older female usually. Persistent burning sensation — usually in tongue. Patient may admit anxiety about cancer. No organic lesion detectable.

Diagnosis

1. History (also exclude possible causal drugs e.g. captopril, and other psychogenic complaints)
2. Examination —

   (a) oral
   (b) cranial nerves
   (c) haematology (full blood picture; ferritin; folate; vitamin B_{12} levels to exclude deficiency states)
   (d) urinalysis (to exclude diabetes)

Management

1. Treat any organic lesions
2. Reassurance
3. ± psychiatric assessment for depression
4. ± antidepressants (or refer).

Atypical facial pain — clinical features

Middle-aged or older female — persistent dull ache, usually in maxilla. Pain not confined necessarily to one anatomical area nor awaking patient from sleep. Patient may or may not admit depression. No organic lesion detectable.

Diagnosis

1. History (also exclude other psychogenic complaints)
2. Examination —

(a) oral
(b) cranial nerves
(c) ± ENT
(d) radiography: especially antral and chest
(e) haematology: (see burning mouth syndrome, above)

Management
1. Treat any organic lesion
2. Reassurance
3. ± psychiatric assessment for depression
4. Antidepressants (or refer).

Vascular causes

These include migraine, migrainous neuralgia and giant-cell (cranial/temporal) arteritis.

Clinical features, diagnosis and management (Table 46.1)

Table 46.1
Clinical features, diagnosis and management of orofacial pain of vascular origin

	Migraine	Migrainous neuralgia	Giant-cell arteritis
Prevalence	Common	Uncommon	Rare
Age	Young or middle-aged adult	Young or middle-aged adult	Middle age +
Sex	Female mainly	Male mainly	Either sex
Main site of pain	Headache	Circumorbital	Temple
Type of pain	Intense throb	Intense throb	Burning
Timing	Daytime	Early morning (2 am)	Daytime
Duration	Hours	Minutes/hours	Minutes/hours
Known precipitating factors	None, or stress, or foods, e.g. bananas	None, or alcohol	None
Other features	Fortification spectra Nausea/vomiting Photophobia	Lacrimation Nasal congestion Facial flushing	Tender over temporal arteries
Diagnosis	History	History	History ESR Biopsy (refer)
Treatment	Refer	Refer	Give systemic corticosteroids because of danger of eye involvement. Refer

Referred causes

Angina or lung cancer (both rare). Refer such patients.

OROFACIAL SENSORY LOSS

Causes include:

(a) peripheral trigeminal lesions,
(b) central lesions.

Either form may have traumatic, inflammatory, neoplastic, or other causes. *Orofacial sensory loss, unless of obvious local traumatic cause, is often of serious portent Refer the patient.*

Peripheral lesions

These include:

1. *Trauma*—especially from lower third molar surgery (to lingual or inferior alveolar nerve); mandibular fractures or osteotomies (inferior alveolar nerve).
2. *Inflammatory*—especially osteomyelitis (not dry socket).
3. *Neoplastic*—usually metatastic disease or leukaemia but also primary oral squamous carcinoma invading bone, antral carcinoma, nasopharyngeal carcinoma.

Central lesions

These include:

1. *Trauma*—head injury or surgery.
2. *Inflammatory*—basal meningitis, disseminated sclerosis, sarcoid, HIV, connective tissue disease.
3. *Neoplastic*—especially cerebellopontine angle tumours or metastases.
4. *Other*—idiopathic trigeminal sensory neuropathy;
    —drugs.

Diagnosis of orofacial sensory loss

1. History
2. Examination—
    (a) oral
    (b) cranial nerves
    (c) ± full neurological examination (dependent on possible cause)
    (d) radiography: mandibular, maxillary, antral and skull as indicated

Management

Refer to relevant physician or surgeon.

FACIAL PALSY

Causes include:

(a) Stroke (cerebrovascular accident; CVA);
(b) Bell's palsy (idiopathic but may be viral);
(c) *Rarely* — trauma, neoplasms, inflammatory lesions.

Clinical features

1. *Stroke* (upper motor neurone lesion): unilateral palsy — mainly of lower face — sometimes with monoplegia, hemiplegia or other features of stroke. Hearing and taste normal. Usually an older patient.
Rare causes include: disseminated sclerosis, HIV infection, brain tumours.

2. *Lower motor neurone lesion* (e.g. Bell's palsy): complete unilateral facial palsy with or without loss of taste and/or hyperacusis. Usually young or middle-aged adult.
Rare causes include: trauma to facial nerve (e.g. assault or salivary gland surgery), parotid or other neoplasms, brain tumours, otitis media, sarcoidosis, Lyme disease, herpes zoster.

Diagnosis

1. History (enquire also for hearing change, tinnitus, vertigo suggestive of ear or more central disease)
2. Examination —

    (a) inability to smile, whistle, or open eyelids against resistance
    (b) cranial nerve examination (especially corneal reflex and taste, dependent on cause)
    (c) ± full neurological examination
    (d) ear and hearing
    (e) blood pressure (may be hypertension)
    (f) urinalysis (may be diabetes)

Management

1. Eye pad to protect cornea
2. Other treatment depends on cause:

    (a) *Bell's palsy*: immediate systemic corticosteroids aid those 20% who will not recover spontaneously
    (b) *other causes*: refer to relevant physician/surgeon.

LOSS OF, OR DISTURBED, SENSE OF TASTE

Causes include:

(a) olfactory disorders;

(b) disorders of nerves involved in taste sensation, e.g. damage to chorda tympani or facial nerves, or CNS disease;
(c) dry mouth;
(d) psychogenic;
(e) malnutrition/vitamin/zinc deficiency;
(f) drugs;
(g) irradiation of tongue/face.

Diagnosis

1. History
2. Examination —

    (a) oral
    (b) test taste (sweet, salt, sour, bitter)
    (c) cranial nerve examination (especially I, V, VII, XI)
    (d) salivary function (to exclude dry mouth)

Management

Refer to relevant physician.

FURTHER READING

General aspects

Scully C., Cawson R. A. (1987). *Medical Problems in Dentistry* 2nd edn. Bristol: John Wright.

Orofacial pain, migraine and neuropathy

Browning S., Hislop S., Scully C., Shirlaw P. J. (1987). The association between burning mouth syndrome and psychosocial disorders. *Oral Surg.*, **64,** 171–4.
Feinmann C., Harris M. (1984). Psychogenic facial pain. *Brit. Dent. J.*, **156,** 165–9, 205–9.
Lecky B. R. F., Hughes R. A. C., Murray N. M. F. (1987). Trigeminal sensory neuropathy. *Brain*, **110,** 1463–85.
Loesser J. D. (1985). Tic douloureux and atypical facial pain. *Can. Dent. Assoc. J.*, **12,** 917–23.
Remick R. A., Blasberg B. (1985). Psychiatric aspects of atypical facial pain. *Can. Dent. Assoc. J.*, **12,** 913–16.
Scully C. (1986). Orofacial manifestations of disease. 6. Neurological, psychiatric and muscular disorders. *Hospital Update*, **6,** 135–9.

Facial palsy

May M. (1980). Bell's palsy: diagnosis, prognosis and treatment. *Surg. Rounds*, **38,** 60.

Scully C. (1989). Neurological disorders. In *The Mouth in Health and Disease* (Scully C., ed.). Oxford: Heinemann Medical.

Loss of taste and smell

Schiffman S. S. (1983). Taste and smell in disease. *N. Engl. J. Med.*, **308,** 1275–9, 1337–43.
Scully C. (1989). Disorders of taste. In *The Mouth in Health and Disease* (Scully C., ed.). Oxford: Heinemann Medical.

Chapter 47

Emergencies in practice

Occasionally the provision of dental treatment can result in some form of medical emergency. This may occur in a fit, or apparently fit patient, or one who has a known systemic problem. Many patients today would seem to look perfectly fit and well, but this appearance may result from modern drug therapy masking, perhaps, quite serious systemic problems.

It is of paramount importance that each patient has a full, updated medical history taken to avoid such problems. In any areas of doubt, contact could be made with the patient's medical practitioner. Often a quick telephone call, rather than a letter, is the best form of contact.

IMPORTANT DRUGS

There is a number of drugs a patient may be taking which might cause problems in routine dental treatment. These include:

1. *Corticosteroids*. Taken for conditions that include rheumatoid arthritis, allergic disease, skin complaints. Such treatment can suppress the natural activity of the adrenal cortex, and during times of stress, apprehension or infection will lessen their capacity to meet the body's increased demand for steroids. The result of this adrenocortical insufficiency would be collapse, with weakness, nausea, vomiting and potentially fatal hypotension.

Treatment of collapse requires intravenous steroids — hydrocortisone sodium succinate, 100 mg. To avoid such an eventuality, further information should be sought where a patient has had steroid treatment within the past 2 years. Where a patient is on this therapy, an increased dose should be administered the day before, the day of, and the day after treatment, for all but very minor dental treatment. The patient on corticosteroids should carry a *blue warning card*.

2. *Anticoagulants*. These are used to prevent a recurrence of thrombosis and embolism. Treatment such as dental extractions can result in prolonged bleeding. Close liaison with the patient's general medical practitioner should result in an agreement about any alterations to drug therapy which may be needed before extractions.

3. *Diabetes*. A patient may be taking oral hypoglycaemic drugs or self-dosing with insulin. Usually these patients present no problems when well controlled, but treatment is best carried out at a time of day when the patient is stable. It is advisable not to delay meal times.

Such patients could enter a hypo- or hyperglycaemic coma. Poorly controlled diabetics, or those taking large amounts of insulin should be treated after consultation with the patient's physician.

4. *Hypnotic or sedative drugs.* The use of sedative agents is not recommended in patients with a history of liver or kidney disease, or those already taking such drugs. The hypnotic effect may be prolonged, and the rate of excretion of the drug is retarded.

5. *Anti-depressants.* Depressed patients may be taking monoamine oxidase inhibitors or polycyclic antidepressants. Nowadays, there is not thought to be a problem in using adrenaline-containing local anaesthetic, as long as it does not directly enter the blood stream (hence self-aspirating syringes for the administration of local anaesthetic solutions; Chapter 42). Commonly, these patients tend to have a dry mouth.

UNEXPECTED COLLAPSE

Unexpected collapse of a patient may still result despite all precautions being taken. These may be in the form of:

1. *Vasovagal attack* (faint). Lay the patient flat, with the legs higher than the head, and loosen clothing around the neck.

2. *Angina or cardiac arrest.* For angina, the patient may be carrying glyceryl trinitrate, which can be taken as directed. For cardiac arrest, cardiopulmonary resuscitation should be started, and an ambulance summoned.

3. *Hypersensitivity or anaphylactic shock.* True anaphylactic shock may result, for example, from the administration of penicillin to a susceptible patient. Symptoms include vomiting, dyspnoea, convulsions, collapse and death. Time of onset depends upon the route of administration, but generally, the sooner the symptoms appear, the worse the reaction will be. Treatment is by 1:1000 adrenaline (0.5 ml, intramuscular) and hydrocortisone sodium succinate, at least 100 mg intravenous, plus ventilation with oxygen. Call for an ambulance.

4. *Epilepsy.* The patient may have an 'aura' of an impending attack, or a fit may occur without warning. The patient should be placed on the floor in an area where they are prevented from self-damage. Prolonged attacks before consciousness is regained may indicate the more serious condition of *status epilepticus*, which will need specialized treatment.

5. *Hypoglycaemic coma.* Such a condition may develop where a patient takes a dose of insulin, but omits a meal. This can be controlled by sucking a sugary sweet or, if the patient loses consciousness, intravenous dextrose solution.

6. *Respiratory obstruction.* Usually as the result of a foreign body in the airway, or laryngeal spasm. This might begin with crowing or croaking on inspiration, combined with a violent respiratory effort. It leads to cessation of breathing and increasing cyanosis.

Respiratory failure can also be caused by an overdose of anaesthetic or hypoxia.

Treatment of these involves maintaining a good airway and the administration of oxygen under pressure, or, alternatively, mouth-to-mouth resuscitation.

In the case of a foreign body lodged in the lower respiratory tract, an alternative airway may need to be established.

7. *Strokes*. Lodgement of a clot in the brain may result in some sort of loss of function, depending on the size of the vessel affected and its site in the brain. It may result in loss of consciousness and muscle weakness of a specific area, such as an arm and leg on one side. Treatment involves hospitalization.

8. *Asthma*. An asthmatic patient should be asked to bring all drugs, such as inhalers, to any treatment session. In this way they can treat themselves, should an attack occur.

An attack in the surgery might be a result of anxiety or exposure to allergens. The patient will become breathless and wheeze on expiration. Should this happen, the patient should not be laid flat, but allowed to use the inhaler and given oxygen.

9. *Haemorrhage*. This may follow an extraction, or other form of minor oral surgery, assuming the haemorrhagic diseases have been previously ruled out. The patient is best cleaned up, the socket sutured and packed under a local anaesthetic, using a haemostatic pack. The patient is retained in the surgery until bleeding has ceased. Where this is not possible, or large amounts of blood have been lost, the patient should be hospitalized.

Chapter 48

HIV infection

BACKGROUND

Human immunodeficiency virus (HIV) is an RNA-containing virus whose origins remain obscure. Until recently it was considered to have passed from the monkey population into man, since native and some captive monkey colonies had a non-pathogenic virus that bore some similarities to HIV. However, it has been now found that HIV and its possible simian counterparts are only very distantly related, thus any simian-to-human transfer of HIV must have taken place many generations ago (if at all). HIV has then slowly evolved along with humans.

The precise reason why HIV infection emerged in Africa or the USA in the 1960s is also unclear; however, increased availability of air travel and sexual promiscuity have been important factors in the rapid worldwide spread of the virus in the 1980s.

ROUTES OF TRANSMISSION

HIV can be found in almost all body fluids; however, only semen and blood have sufficient concentrations of virus to permit infection.

Saliva, tears and nasal fluids also contain HIV, but they do not seem to permit viral transmission since household members of HIV-infected individuals only become infected through sexual contact. At present there is one unconfirmed case of HIV transmission via a human bite; the recipient of the bite may have been infected via sexual intercourse during a 'one-night stand'.

Social contact with HIV-infected individuals does not result in infection and, to date, healthcare workers have only become infected after intimate contact with blood or faeces from HIV-seropositive individuals.

EPIDEMIOLOGY

Since HIV is transmitted by sexual intercourse — both anal and vaginal — or via intimate contact with blood, the individuals who are most likely to become infected are those who are sexually promiscuous and/or who experience direct blood-to-blood contact; for example, intravenous drug misusers, individuals with haemophilia or recipients of blood transfusions. The virus can pass across the placenta so children may become infected in utero if the mother is HIV-infected.

Thus the patients in whom HIV has been most frequently detected, and who therefore form the groups at greatest risk of HIV infection are:

(a) male homosexuals or bisexuals;
(b) intravenous drug misusers;
(c) haemophiliacs receiving blood products;
(d) recipients of blood transfusions;
(e) new-born children and sexual partners of the above groups.

In the UK there are distinct variations in the risk groups of infected individuals. In England and Wales the majority of HIV-infected individuals have been male homosexuals or bisexuals. However, in Scotland the majority of infected individuals are intravenous drug misusers resident on the east coast.

Infected individuals live in all parts of the UK, but the greatest number of cases has been recorded in and around London. Some of these patients live elsewhere and only come to London for medical treatment.

PATHOGENESIS

Human immunodeficiency virus destroys the body's defence — the immune system — and impairs neural function. It achieves this by being able to enter and reproduce within specific cell types. Principally it attacks monocytes and to a lesser extent cells important in defences against fungal and viral infections and in controlling antibody production — the T4- (or CD4-) lymphocytes. Monocytes seem to be the main reservoir of HIV and are not themselves destroyed by HIV, but merely impaired in their role as phagocytes and processors of antigens. The groups of T4-lymphocytes infected by HIV are mainly involved in cell-mediated immunity; thus affected patients have an increased susceptibility to fungal, mycobacterial (for example, tuberculosis) and viral infections. Monocytes and T4-lymphocytes are also involved in the generation of antibodies, so affected patients also risk infection by microbes other than viruses and fungi.

The infection of the immune system is a slow process and may take many years; however, ultimately most components of the immune system begin to fail (Table 48.1) and affected individuals develop clinical illness.

Human immunodeficiency virus probably infects the central nervous system of all infected individuals. The exact means by which HIV crosses the blood–brain barrier is unclear. It is known that HIV does not greatly affect the grey matter but seems to infect and destroy glial cells (for example, astroglia and oligodendroglia-cells, similar to Schwann cells of the peripheral nervous system). Affected individuals develop cognitive, sensory and motor abnormalities, collectively termed HIV encephalitis.

CLINICAL ASPECTS OF HIV INFECTION

Infection with HIV does not immediately give rise to infection; indeed, most individuals do not develop severe problems in the first few years of infection.

Six to eight weeks after acquisition of HIV, individuals may suffer a glandular fever-like illness comprising night sweats, transient generalized lymph-node enlargement, weight loss, malaise, diarrhoea and oral candidosis.

After this, infected individuals usually return to normal health but may then develop enlargement of lymph nodes at several sites of the body. The nodes may be greater than 1 cm in diameter and can remain enlarged for several months. This stage of HIV disease is termed *persistent generalized lymphadenopathy* (PGL). The lymph node enlargement is due to marked proliferation of lymphoid tissue.

PGL may occur on its own or be accompanied by a number of other clinical problems such as:

(a) weight loss,
(b) persistent night sweats,
(c) persistent oral candidosis,
(d) other transient opportunistic infections.

This stage of disease is collectively termed AIDS-related complex (ARC).

The increasing illness is due to a progressive failing of the immune system. Eventually immunodeficiency causes increased susceptibility to severe opportunistic infections and the development of certain tumours. This is the stage of acquired immune deficiency syndrome — AIDS.

The syndrome is clinically characterized by severe opportunistic infections, tumours and occasional autoimmune phenomena (Table 48.2).

Table 48.1
Immunologic abnormalities of HIV infection

Characteristic abnormalities

Depletion of CD4- and T-lymphocytes
Decreased lymphoproliferative responses to soluble antigens
Impaired *in vivo* delayed-type hypersensitivity reactions
Decreased gamma-interferon production in response to antigens
Polyclonal B-cell activation with increased spontaneous proliferation and immunoglobulin production
Decreased primary humoral response to immunization

Consistently detected abnormalities

Lymphopenia
Decreased poliferative responses to T-cell mitogen and alloantigens
Decreased proliferative responses in autologous mixed lymphocyte reaction (AMLR) and to T3 antigens
Decreased proliferative responses to specific B-cell mitogens
Decreased interleukin-2 production
Decreased cytotoxicity to virally infected cells
Increased immune complex formation
Decreased natural killer (NK) cell activity
Decreased monocyte chemotaxis
Decreased MHC class II antigen expression on monocytes and macrophages
Increased acid-labile alpha-interferon levels

Table 48.2
Clinical consequences of HIV infection

Opportunistic infections

Respiratory
Pneumocystis carinii
Aspergillosis
Candidosis
Zygomycosis
Strongyloidosis
Toxoplasmosis
Atypical mycobacterioses
Legionella
Klebsiella
Pseudomonas aeruginosa
Staphylococcus aureus
Streptococcus pneumoniae
Haemophilus influenzae
Cytomegalovirus

Oral and oesophageal
Candida albicans
Histoplasmosis
Cryptococcus neoformans
Atypical mycobacterioses
Klebsiella pneumoniae
Geotrichosis (rare)
Cat-scratch bacillus (rare)
Herpes simplex
Herpes zoster
Cytomegalovirus
Epstein–Barr virus
Papillomavirus
ANUG
Periodontal diseases

Lower gastrointestinal
Mycobacterium avium intracellulare
Cryptococcosis
Giardiasis

Lower gastrointestinal—
Continued
Isospra belli
Salmonella typhimurium
Campylobacter fetus

Neural
Polyoma JC virus
Toxoplasma gondii
Papovavirus
Cryptococcus neoformans

Cutaneous
Candida albicans
Histoplasmosis
Papillomavirus
Herpes simplex
Herpes zoster
Pox virus
Cryptococcus neoformans
Amoebiasis
Staphylococcus aureus
Typical and atypical
  mycobacterioses

Ocular
Cytomegalovirus
Toxoplasmosis

Disseminated
Atypical mycobacterioses
Cryptococcus neoformans
Histoplasmosis
Epstein–Barr virus
Cytomegalovirus
Adenovirus
Coccidiomycosis

Neoplasms
Kaposi's sarcoma
Non-Hodgkin's and Hodgkin's lymphoma
Squamous cell carcinoma (e.g. of mouth (rare) and of anus)
Small cell carcinoma
Malignant melanoma
Embryonal cell carcinoma

Neurological disease
Subacute encephalitis
Peripheral neuropathies (including cranial)
Vascular myelopathy
Aseptic meningitis

Other
Seborrhoeic dermatitis
Granuloma annulare-like eruptions
Thrombocytopenic purpura
Drug eruptions

The *infections* are severe, often atypical in presentation, can be persistent and difficult to manage. A spectrum of infections can arise, however most notable are candidal infection, *Pneumocystis carinii* pneumonia (PCP) and oral/oesophageal candidosis.

Kaposi's sarcoma (KS) is the most frequent *tumour*. This can present on any cutaneous surface but more frequently it occurs on the face, trunk and upper extremities. The sarcoma can affect the viscera and can rapidly metastasize. Lymphomas, both Hodgkin's and non-Hodgkin's, are other tumours commonly associated with AIDS.

During the PGL, ARC and AIDS stages, HIV infection of the neural system may cause HIV encephalitis. HIV encephalitis has a spectrum of manifestations that include personality changes, loss of memory and severe motor impairment.

To summarize the clinical consequences of HIV infection:

1. HIV acquisition may follow sexual intercourse with an infected individual or direct blood contact with infected blood or blood products.
2. Infected individuals usually develop a glandular-fever-like illness 6–12 weeks after HIV acquisition.
3. Persistent generalized lymphadenopathy or AIDS-related complex may then develop.
4. Finally, patients develop AIDS (acquired immune deficiency syndrome).
5. At any stage of infection, other than the acute illness, patients may also manifest features of HIV encephalitis.

INCUBATION PERIOD

The mean incubation period of HIV is 7–8 years. This is the average time from acquisition of HIV to initial manifestations of AIDS. Depending upon cofactors it may take up to 15 years before AIDS develops in some infected individuals, but it is now thought that at least 99% of all infected patients will develop AIDS. Almost all patients die 2–3 years after developing initial manifestations of AIDS.

MANAGEMENT OF HIV INFECTION

The management of AIDS follows conventional lines, namely *antimicrobial* and *antitumour therapy*. Many of the infections are severe and atypical and may not respond to conventional antimicrobial measures — indeed, in some cases there is no available antimicrobial. Localized tumours can be managed by surgery, local radiotherapy or laser therapy; when the tumours are disseminated, chemotherapy has to be considered.

Immunomodulation — bucking up a failing immune response — has been limited to only a few patients; it can have severe side-effects and has generally only caused transient improvement.

'Specific' *virustatic drugs*, such as azidothymidine (AZT), are the mainstay of therapy for many patients. These drugs are given at any stage of infection. They can limit or reverse neurological and immunological disease, but they have many side-effects and do not result in complete recovery; most patients still develop AIDS.

At present there is no *vaccine* available for HIV infection. There have been several attempts to produce a suitable vaccine but there have been no detailed clinical trials of any putative vaccine. It is unclear if a vaccine will ever be developed because HIV infection is caused by more than one virus. In addition, HIV undergoes changes within infected individuals such that any vaccine will need to recognize all variants of HIV. The brain is a major reservoir of HIV: it is not known if a vaccine-induced immune response could destroy infected neural tissue. Although infected patients have antibodies specific for HIV, the infection persists and progresses, and thus a vaccine that simply generates a specific humoral response would be of little effect. There is evidence to suggest that some putative vaccines may enhance HIV infections later rather than limit the disease. These are only some of the problems that remain to be overcome before a suitable anti-HIV vaccine becomes available (summarized in Table 48.3). It is unlikely that any vaccine will become available for many years (if at all). Thus, at present, the only means of tackling HIV infection is to limit its continued spread. There have been several reports of reduced sexual promiscuity amongst groups of male homosexuals and the use of barrier techniques of contraception has increased amongst homosexuals and prostitutes.

There have been several publicity campaigns directed towards limiting the sexual and blood-borne spread of HIV. The likely benefits of these projects have been questioned and there is little evidence to suggest that they have changed the sexual or drug addiction habits of most individuals.

It is estimated that 1% of UK individuals in their third or fourth decade of life may die from HIV-related infection. The number of known infected individuals is continuing to rise in all countries of the world; these persons only account for a fraction of the true numbers of the HIV-infected. In view of the lack of any effective treatment and the only slight change in sexual habits, the outlook is therefore bleak.

Table 48.3
Difficulties in the development of HIV-specific vaccine

Wide viral heterogeneity
Viral components may be inaccessible to the immune response
Lack of suitable animal model
Generated antibodies do not have neutralizing activity *in vivo*
HIV infection may be enhanced by various components of the immune response
Ethical difficulties in human trials

DENTAL ASPECTS OF HIV INFECTION

The aspects of HIV infection that are relevant to dentistry include:
(a) recognition of oral manifestations of HIV infection;
(b) risk of HIV cross-infection during dental treatment;
(c) assessment of HIV risk status of patients.

Oral manifestations of HIV infection (Table 48.4)

There are many oral manifestations, but of these, several are extremely uncommon while others are almost pathognomonic of HIV infection. Oral disease is a frequent feature of HIV infection. Many dentists treating infected individuals may be the first clinician to recognize one or more of these disorders. Because medical practitioners may be unable to recognize the more subtle oral changes of HIV, the dentist has an important role in the recognition of early HIV disease.

Common oral problems

Common oral features of HIV infection include candidosis, herpetic infection, hairy leukoplakia and Kaposi's sarcoma. In addition, cervical or submandibular lymphadenopathy may be a feature of at least 95% of all HIV-infected patients at some stage of their infection.

Oral candidosis may be present in over 75% of infected individuals and may occur at any stage of infection; in AIDS it is most severe.

Thrush, or *pseudomembranous candidosis* is the most common presentation of oral candidosis in HIV disease and *Candida albicans* is the most frequently isolated species. Pseudomembranous candidosis presents as white or creamy curds on the palate, posterior buccal mucosa and fauces. The pseudomembrane can be wiped away to leave a red, ragged ulcer — it is a surprisingly painless lesion.

Angular cheilitis is another recognizable candidal complication of HIV infection. It may present at any stage of infection, and in HIV infection is not associated with reduced vertical face height or any haematinic problem. Angular cheilitis in a young non-denture wearer is unusual and always warrants further investigation.

Other uncommon forms of oral candidosis associated with HIV infection include:

Chronic atrophic candidosis. This may also be referred to as erythematous candidosis. If this affects the mid-dorsal area of the tongue it may form a median rhomboid glossitis.

Chronic hyperplastic candidosis. This appears as adherent white plaques that have the same histological features as chronic hyperplastic candidosis in non-HIV-infected individuals. If there are plaques on several surfaces the term chronic multifocal oral candidosis may be applicable.

Herpetic infections in and around the mouth can develop in the ARC and AIDS stages of HIV infection. Causative viruses are usually herpes simplex or herpes zoster. Infection manifests as severe, painful orofacial vesiculation

Table 48.4
Oral lesions associated with HIV infection

Fungal infections
Candidosis:
   pseudomembranous
   erythematous
   hyperplastic
   angular cheilitis
Histoplasmosis
Cryptococcus neoformans
Geotrichosis

Bacterial infections
HIV ANUG
HIV gingivitis
HIV periodontitis
Myobacterium avium intracellulare
Klebsiella pneumoniae
Enterobacterium cloacae
Escherichia coli
Sinusitis
Exacerbation of apical periodontitis
Submandibular cellulitis

Viral infections
Herpetic stomatitis
Cytomegalovirus
Hairy leukoplakia
Varicella zoster
Papillomavirus lesions:
   verruca vulgaris
   condyloma acuminatum
   focal epithelial hyperplasia

Neoplasms
Kaposi's sarcoma
Squamous cell carcinoma
Non-Hodgkin's lymphoma

Neurological disturbances
Paraesthesia
Facial palsy

Unknown aetiology
Recurrent aphthous ulceration
Progressive necrotizing ulceration
Toxic epidermolysis
Delayed wound healing
Idiopathic thrombocytopenia
Salivary gland enlargement
Xerostomia
HIV embryopathy (disputed)
Hyperpigmentation

followed by ulceration. Zoster may affect any one or more of the trigeminal divisions.

Hairy leukoplakia. Until recently, this lesion was regarded as pathognomonic of HIV infection.

Hairy leukoplakia has been observed in HIV-infected individuals from all risk groups. It usually affects the lateral borders of tongue, but it may commonly involve dorsal and ventral surfaces of the tongue, and the floor of the mouth. Hairy leukoplakia typically presents as a raised white patch which has a hairy appearance due to epithelial hyperplasia.

Hairy leukoplakia is not a manifestation of candidal infection since antifungal therapy does not result in its regression. A viral cause presently seems most likely: Epstein–Barr virus (EBV) is present in the tissue and acyclovir prescribed for severe herpetic infection can cause coincident regression of the leukoplakia.

Hairy leukoplakia is almost always asymptomatic; occasionally it causes mild oral or pharyngeal irritation due to the extreme lengths of the hair-like epithelial projections. This can be managed by simply cutting the projections without local anaesthetic. Antiviral treatment of hairy leukoplakia is *not* indicated.

Hairy leukoplakia has recently been observed in non-HIV-infected immunosuppressed individuals. Hence this lesion is an oral marker of immunosuppression.

Oral *Kaposi's sarcoma* only occurs in the AIDS stage of HIV infection. In one report as many as 44% of individuals with AIDS-associated Kaposi's sarcoma had intraoral lesions. Oral Kaposi's sarcoma presents as red, blue or purple macules, papules or nodules, and most commonly affects the hard and soft palates. The gingiva is another frequently affected oral site. Lesions can often be painful especially if near palatal nerves or if there is associated ulceration. The tumour may cause erosion of underlying bone; indeed, there have been cases where severe alveolar destruction has resulted in teeth being retained by sarcomatous tissue alone.

Small, isolated, oral Kaposi's sarcoma lesions can be managed by local excision or cryosurgery; larger isolated lesions require local external radiotherapy. To minimize resultant mucositis, radiotherapy beams are kept as narrow as possible. Chemotherapy is indicated where oral lesions are large or associated with systemic Kaposi's sarcoma. Recently intralesional vinblastine has proved successful for some oral Kaposi's sarcoma.

The common oral disorders of HIV infection have been found to be of *prognostic* importance: for example, severe oral candidosis, especially when associated with oesophageal infection, can be a marker of poor prognosis. Similarly, individuals with severe orofacial herpetic infection or hairy leukoplakia have a poorer clinical course than other HIV-infected patients who do not suffer these orofacial problems. Oral Kaposi's sarcoma is a marker of AIDS; thus affected individuals have a very poor prognosis.

Periodontal aspects

Gingivitis, often manifesting as acute ulcerative necrotizing gingivitis (ANUG), is a recognized complication of HIV infection. For example, at the

Royal Dental School in Copenhagen, 20 patients who consecutively presented with ANUG were all found to be infected with HIV.

Severe ANUG has also been noted in American, German and British HIV-infected patients. Aside from ANUG, a more non-specific gingivitis may arise. This may have a distinct halo of red inflammation about the marginal gingiva and has been termed HIV gingivitis. The exact causative organisms associated with this disorder are not yet known.

Severe periodontal destruction has also been noted in some infected patients. This manifests as a generalized, rapid destruction of alveolar bone with subsequent development of deep true pockets and periodontal abscesses. This disorder is termed HIV periodontitis. Gingival and periodontal disease are common in HIV infection although no detailed investigation of these has as yet been undertaken. The severity of these problems appears to be not commensurate with local levels of plaque.

Other tumours

Nine individuals with AIDS have been reported to have squamous cell carcinomas of the mouth. While the prevalence of oral carcinoma is sufficiently high to suggest that its occurrence in HIV-infected patients may be coincidental, the young age of the affected patients does suggest a possible aetiological association between HIV infections and oral squamous cell carcinoma.

Unlike oral carcinomas, oral lymphomas have been observed in a considerable number of HIV-infected individuals — these can manifest as maxillary and mandibular radiolucencies, oral ulcers and papules. Confusingly, oral lymphomas may occasionally manifest as epulides.

Other oral disorders

A spectrum of rare oral disorders can arise in HIV infection.

Several *infections* other than herpes and candida have been observed. Oral ulceration or red erosions have been found to be due to a variety of infectious agents including:

(a) cytomegalovirus,
(b) chickenpox,
(c) histoplasmosis,
(d) *Cryptococcus neoformans*,
(e) geotrichosis,
(f) *Enterobacterium cloacae*,
(g) *Escherichia coli*,
(h) *Klebsiella pneumoniae*.

However, only a handful of patients have been reported to be infected with one of these agents; thus these problems should *not* be regarded as oral markers of HIV infection.

Dry sockets after simple uncomplicated extractions have been observed in German and British HIV-infected patients. The exact frequency of this problem requires further investigation. Osteomyelitis and actinomycosis are other rare, non-specific oral complications of HIV infection.

A variety of oral disorders of unknown aetiology has been observed; most are not specific to HIV infection.

Xerostomia (dry mouth) has been reported in some infected individuals. However, the salivary flow rates of affected patients have not been assessed in detail so it is not known if xerostomia is a true sign. Parotid enlargement, unrelated to xerostomia, has been noted in children affected with HIV; the enlarge ment is frequently bilateral. The cause of either salivary problem is not known.

Recurrent oral ulceration is an uncommon complication of HIV infection. The ulcers may sometimes be similar in appearance to minor or major aphthae, but it is not known if the ulcers have the same periodicity as recurrent aphthous stomatitis (RAS). Some patients suffer severe oral ulceration which can rapidly spread into the fauces, pharynx and epiglottis; this painful complication can be managed with thalidomide.

Purpura and petechiae of the palate can arise as a consequence of HIV-associated *thrombocytopenia*. The purpura can be clinically indistinguishable from Kaposi's sarcoma. It is also important to remember that male homosexuals frequently develop petechiae as a consequence of oral sex.

Hyperpigmentation of the gingiva and buccal mucosa has been observed in British and German HIV-infected patients. The pigmentation may be secondary to adrenal cortical hypofunction or a side-effect of ketoconazole or clofamazine therapy. However, at present the aetiology of the pigmentation of three affected individuals is unknown.

Orofacial consequences of HIV encephalopathy may include trigeminal neuralgia and paraesthesia, and VIIth nerve palsies.

Toxic epidermolysis (Lyell's syndrome) is a very rare oral complication of combination drug therapy. It has been observed in one German HIV-infected patient.

Risk of HIV infection during dental treatment

Much has been written on the possible risk of HIV being transmitted during routine dental treatment. However, present evidence indicates that HIV cross-infection is minimal in dentistry.

HIV *has* been isolated from saliva, but it is present in very small amounts and it has proved difficult to culture HIV taken from saliva specimens; this may be due to the HIV-inhibitory activity of saliva—particularly submandibular or sublingual secretions.

Further evidence indicating that saliva is not a major means of HIV transmission comes from an analysis of HIV epidemiology. If salivary spread could lead to HIV transmission, coughing and sneezing would also permit spread of HIV infection—this does not occur. Similarly, reports of salivary transmission between lesbians or via human bites remain unconfirmed. Transmission of HIV within families of infected individuals only occurs via sexual intercourse and direct blood-to-blood contact; sharing of eating utensils does *not* cause spread of HIV within families. However, in view of the possible risk of blood-borne transmission the sharing of toothbrushes and razors is not advised.

Table 48.5
Occupational risk of HIV transmission to dental staff

Country	Number of tested dental staff	Number proved HIV-positive	Year
Denmark	961	0	1986
USA	1309	1	1988
USA	1195	0	1988
Germany	1087	0	1988
Various	167	0	1988

HIV was present in the North American community years before AIDS was known about, yet to date there is only one recorded case of a dentist becoming infected with HIV during routine dental practice. The dentist did not routinely wear rubber gloves during dental treatment although it is unclear if he belonged to an HIV at-risk group. Many dentists in the USA, Denmark and Germany have been tested for HIV infection and, aside from this one individual, none has been found to be infected with HIV (Table 48.5).

No hygienist has been found to be infected: thus airborne spread of HIV via an ultrasonic scaler within a dental environment may not occur. This observation highlights the low transmissibility of HIV, since the poor periodontal status and severe gingivitis of some HIV-infected individuals might be expected to permit easy transmission of HIV from blood to the dental operator.

There may be a very small risk of HIV being transmitted during dental treatment, but it seems only likely to occur as a result of needlestick injuries. Therefore, provided the practitioner and staff take particular precautions against this possibility and limit transmission risk by other means, the probability of HIV transmission between patient and staff would appear to be close to zero.

Assessment of HIV risk status of patients

Some individuals will immediately reveal that they are infected with HIV. However, others are unwilling to do so in view of the knowledge that some HIV-infected individuals have been refused treatment by dentists, despite a previously good patient–dentist relationship.

It can be difficult to assess the risk status of most patients, but a variety of factors can aid the identification of such individuals as follows.

1. *Recurrent attendance at a genito-urinary medicine (GUM) clinic.* Promiscuous male homosexuals and prostitutes more frequently have sexually transmitted diseases; however, questioning about such matters must be tactful — many individuals attend GUM clinics for the diagnosis and management of non-infectious genital problems. In addition, there has been a recent fall in the incidence of sexually transmitted diseases in male homosexuals, so recurrent attendance at GUM clinics may *not* be as useful a marker as once believed.

2. *A history of viral hepatitis or chronic active hepatitis.* In a young individual this may be an indication of HIV high-risk status. However, it must be remembered that while the transmission routes of HIV and hepatitis viruses are similar, the risk groups of the viral infections are slightly different.

3. *Unexplained weight loss, night sweats, and enlargement of the lymph nodes in the neck and elsewhere.* All these warrant further questioning.

4. *Oral candidosis.* Thrush is uncommon in non-diabetics, individuals without xerostomia, or those not receiving antibiotic or corticosteroid therapy. Thrush is a manifestation of immunodeficiency; HIV infection and leukaemia are probably the most common causes of immunodeficiency in young adults.

5. *Oral Kaposi's sarcoma.* This is a very strong indication of HIV infection. Aside from haemangiomas, red, purple or blue oral lesions are generally uncommon and are usually suggestive of neoplasia, Kaposi's sarcoma probably being the most common one.

6. *It is unwise to judge patients by their dress or demeanour.* Similarly, regardless of whether patient consent has or has not been obtained, patients must *not* be tested for HIV by a dentist. If HIV infectivity is suspected an individual should be treated just as any other patient except when operative dentistry is undertaken. If a patient has an oral disorder that may be suggestive of HIV infection, he or she should be referred to the local oral surgery or oral medicine unit for further evaluation. General medical practitioners do not give details of their patients' HIV status. Oral surgeons and oral physicians do not test such patients; instead they are referred to a GUM clinic for pre-test evaluation and counselling. The patient can refuse to be investigated further, but if he or she does 'have the test', further counselling will be given when the result is known.

Dentists and hygienists have the right to refuse to treat any individual, but in view of the very low risk of HIV infectivity, the known reluctance of some clinicians perhaps seems unfounded.

Other reasons why dentists or hygienists may be unhappy to care for HIV-infected individuals may include:

(a) loss of regular patients;
(b) reputation of being homosexual;
(c) inability to cope with the concerns of ancillary staff;
(d) possible high costs of treatment.

To date, there is no evidence that any of these reasons are true. In London, there are cost-effective dental practices and clinics where HIV-infected individuals are regularly treated along with non-infected individuals. Education of the dental profession regarding aspects of HIV is still required. Studies in the USA have shown that even in areas such as San Francisco there is still ignorance and prejudice within the dental community regarding the dental treatment of HIV-infected persons. This may be overcome by labour-intensive health education.

FURTHER READING

Porter S. R., Luker J., Scully C. et al. (1989). Orofacial aspects of a group of British patients infected with HIV-I. *J. Oral Pathol.* **18,** 47–8.
Porter S. R., Luker J., Scully C. et al. (1990). Orofacial manifestations of HIV disease. *Dent. Update*, (in press).
Porter S. R., Scully C., Cawson R. A. (1987). AIDS: Update and guidelines for dental practice. *Dent. Update*, **14,** 9–17.
Porter S. R., Scully C., Greenspan D. (in press). Secondary immunodeficiency. In *Oral Manifestations of Systemic Disease* (Jones J. H., Mason D. K., eds.). London: Bailliere Tindall.
Scully C., Porter S. R. (1988). Orofacial manifestations of HIV infection (leading article). *Lancet*, **i,** 967–8.

Chapter 49

Oral surgery for the general dental practitioner

As the emphasis on the various practical branches of dentistry changes, oral surgery is receiving more attention from the dental practitioner. Most general practitioners have little experience of oral surgical procedures and, as a result of this, lack confidence to carry out procedures which would be regarded as commonplace in Minor Oral Surgery departments of hospitals. Familiarity with these procedures brings confidence and enables one to work faster and without stress, both of which are ultimately of advantage to the patient as reflected in the improved healing of the more skilfully handled tissues. Oral surgery is already becoming an important part of a few practices where the practitioners have either been House Officers or SHOs in Oral Surgery departments or have been clinical assistants to consultants in hospitals for one session a week for extended periods (say, 15–20 weeks). This is recommended as a means for a practitioner to extend his or her dexterity and his or her knowledge and confidence in a busy department carrying out a great deal of oral surgery under local anaesthetic.

Fundamental to this learning process is a knowledge of a few basic principles and it is the aim of this chapter to present these in a simple form.

RADIOGRAPHS

Adequate and detailed radiographs must be available for every oral surgery case involving bone, e.g. apicectomies of upper premolars, to establish the number and form and position of their roots. Canines buried in the palate should also have parallax views. Wisdom teeth should have an intraoral view with the film tight against the lingual mucosa and the central ray directed between the lower first and second molar so that there is no overlap of contact points, and there should also be exact coincidence of the buccal and lingual cusps. It is contraindicated medico-legally to attempt to remove a lower wisdom tooth without a film which shows the area of bone behind and below the tooth. This is revealed on an orthopantomogram or lateral oblique film. Root detail is generally better on the intraoral film and this is helpful with the more complex root forms.

A view of the bone around the tooth ensures that the mandibular canal is visible and also the lower border of the mandible. The operator will therefore know whether the mandible is dangerously thin and whether the canal is likely to be damaged with a bur. Other structures whose relationship to the operative site must be established preoperatively are the maxillary antrum and the mental foramen.

SCOPE OF WORK UNDER LOCAL ANAESTHESIA

No patient should be subjected to an operation under local anaesthetic which is estimated to take longer than 20 min. Sedation will ease this stricture to a slight extent but the rule is a good guide to practice and does not include the time for the local anaesthetic to take effect. Experience and ability enable one to make accurate estimates of operative times and it is best to play safe by overestimating while gaining experience. Never get into the situation where the patient's reserves run out and the operation has to be abandoned.

Children are a special case. Operations should be short, local anaesthetic paste should be used prior to injection, and previous pleasant experience in the dental chair will help cooperation. If there is a risk of permanently putting off the child, it is better to use general anaesthesia, thus preserving the carefully laid-down confidence that may be instilled in preparing the patient for dentistry later in life.

DIAGNOSIS

Usually the question of diagnosis in oral surgery occupies a chapter on its own but if the practitioner has any problem with the diagnosis he or she would best refer the patient. However, like the surgery itself, experience helps one's diagnosis to be more accurate. We are all familiar with the pain associated with acute pericoronitis of the lower wisdom tooth. It occurs in a particular age group and is associated with limitation of opening and sometimes with lymphadenitis; the patient may well be febrile. Local examination will reveal the inflamed gum flap and antibiotics should be administered if there is lymphadenitis and febrility, together with possible extraction of the associated upper third molar or grinding of the upper second molar to relieve trauma. Hot salt mouth baths should be prescribed. However, other common causes of pain in the jaws are referred pain from the muscles around the temporomandibular joint, sinusitis, pulpitis of other teeth and it is important that one should look for these alternative diagnoses. The character of the pain and the initiating factors are also clues to the diagnosis, e.g. acute pulpitis is likely to respond to thermal and osmotic stimuli within the mouth.

MEDICAL HISTORY

A frank and reassuring talk with the patient will help you to decide whether he or she is psychologically suited for surgery under local anaesthesia, with or without sedation in the adult.

The physical state of the patient has then to be assessed to decide on their suitability for treatment in the dental surgery.

Assessment

Local factors

1. *Infection*. Surgical intervention should not be carried out in the presence of acute infection, which should be brought under control with antibiotics and/or surgical drainage beforehand. The danger lies in spreading the infection in the bone during the process of bone removal, leading to osteomyelitis. This is an infection in the mandible that can produce severe pain and fever with possible sensory disturbance in the distribution of the mental nerve and ultimately serious loss of part of the bone as a sequestrum

2. *Calculus and gingivitis*. These are contraindications to surgery in that in their presence wounds are more likely to become infected. Scaling and polishing should be carried out thoroughly, and at least 7 days left for the level of organisms to settle prior to operation.

The presence of acute Vincent's infection (necrotizing ulcerative gingivitis) will cause breakdown of blood clots and promote bleeding. Here again the infection should be brought under control before operating but, where urgent treatment is required, at least 24 h of antibiotic treatment should precede surgery.

3. *Pathology in relation to surgical site*. This includes swellings, ulcers and haemangiomas. All swellings in the mouth should be regarded with suspicion until proved benign. All ulcers of more than 3 weeks duration, particularly if they are indurated, should be biopsied to include normal tissue and sent to a pathology laboratory. Alternatively they should be referred to hospital for treatment.

Any sign of bluish/red discoloration of the mucosa should be referred because of the danger that the lesion may be a cavernous haemangioma. Even a local anaesthetic injection could prove fatal in such circumstances.

General factors

1. *Infection*. Most obvious of these is the risk of the patient having hepatitis B or HIV infection (Chapter 48) which can be transmitted to the operator or his assistant and also, of course, to other patients if full precautions are not taken.

The British Dental Association and the Department of Health have issued guidelines on the handling of these known or suspected cases, which will be regularly updated.

Every health worker should be vaccinated against hepatitis B, which is the most infective of the diseases, but careful precautions should be taken with all patients as there are many unknown carriers and a patient, in any case, may give a misleading history.

The best method of sterilization is the autoclave and, because protein interferes with the process, instruments should be ultrasonically cleaned before sterilization.

2. *Acute fevers.* Surgery should be avoided wherever possible on a patient who has the acute phase of an infection, e.g. glandular fever. He or she is quite likely to be infectious and will have a low tolerance to treatment both physically and mentally.

3. *Anticoagulant therapy.* Some patients are on warfarin in order to reduce the ability of their blood to clot. This is usually following myocardial infarction, but may be for other reasons. The patient will carry a card which gives you some idea of his or her blood clotting capability, given as the INR (International Normalized Ratio), which replaces the old prothrombin index.

For the removal of one tooth we are happy to accept a ratio of less than 2, but precautions would have to be taken, which would include an absorbable pack in the socket, a silk mattress suture, and great care on the part of the patient postoperatively. The ratio would have to be lower for more extractions and for the lifting of a flap, otherwise bleeding would be difficult to control postoperatively.

On some occasions, the physicians do not wish to withdraw completely the warfarin and we have to proceed in the face of higher INRs. In general these cases are better handled in the hospital as patients' responses to warfarin are very variable and out-patient attendance at hospital enables us to take the patient straight from the laboratory to surgery without delay.

4. *History of rheumatic fever, scarlet fever or valvular heart disease.* Unless these patients have been specifically told otherwise by medical advisers (and this should be checked), they will need prophylactic antibiotics to combat the inevitable bacteraemia of tooth removal or any form of oral surgery. It is common practice to administer oral amoxycillin 3 g, 1 h before operation, provided the patient is not allergic to penicillin and has not had amoxycillin or related substances within the last 4 weeks. A suitable alternative where the patient is allergic to amoxycillin is to give erythromycin stearate by mouth, 1.5 g 1 h before operation followed by 500 mg orally 6 hours later.

The patient's medical adviser should be consulted because, in certain high-risk cases, these prophylactic measures are inadequate and the patient would have to be referred to hospital for further assessment and treatment.

5. *Hypertension.* Many sufferers from hypertension are rendered relatively normal by the carefully balanced hypertensive drugs which they take. These patients will look normal and will walk into the surgery in the normal way and will not be breathless. There is no reason why they should not have small doses of xylocaine (2%) with adrenaline (1:80 000) provided these are given slowly. For patients whose fitness is in doubt and who walk slowly and are breathless, it is much safer to use prilocaine (Citanest) 3% with octapressin (Felypressin; 0.03 iu/ ml).

Care should be taken with these patients to raise them from the horizontal slowly, otherwise they may become dizzy or faint having suffered from cerebral anoxia.

6. *Diabetes.* Diabetes varies in its severity and mild cases can be treated by controlled diet and oral drugs such as chlorpropamide. These cases are not usually a problem for mild surgery, but should have antibiotics after treatment to help prevent infection.

More severe diabetics will be on injections of insulin on a regular schedule and controlled dosage. Those who have no problems with instability in their diabetic control can have minor oral surgery under local anaesthesia provided they have adhered to their recommended diet and drug regimen. If the patient should become unwell and show signs of anxiety and sweating with a raised blood pressure and strong and rapid pulse, a glucose drink should be administered as they are suffering from hypoglycaemia. The opposite condition of diabetic ketosis is less usual and would indicate a missed dose of insulin or excessive stress. The state of diabetic ketosis and unconsciousness is more slow in onset than hypoglycaemic coma and is less likely to occur in the dental surgery after a careful history. If there is no response to the glucose drink, medical help should be called.

The more severe and unstable diabetic is best treated in hospital and should be referred for oral surgery.

7. *Steroid therapy*. Patients who have had prolonged steroid therapy for conditions such as arthritis or chest complaints may have adrenal cortical atrophy in which they lose their ability to respond to stress. This is more likely to occur if the dosages have been high and prolonged. Surgery under local anaesthesia is carried out with an indwelling needle in place in the arm so that in case of vascular collapse they can be given 100 mg of hydrocortisone hemisuccinate. This, together with placing the patient in a horizontal position, is usually enough to revive them but if there is doubt about the dosage of steroids the patient's medical adviser should be consulted. If there is any further doubt the patient should be referred to hospital where conditions are undoubtedly better for resuscitation.

8. *Bleeding disorders*. If it is evident from the patient's history that there is a problem with bleeding after any operation they should be referred to a haematological department for assessment. If it is established that the patient has a coagulation defect then they should be referred to hospital for treatment where the Haematology and Oral Surgery departments can work together. These bleeding diseases are very numerous; they include haemophilia and Von Willebrand's disease.

9. *Allergies*. Should the patient inform you that they are allergic to a number of substances, leading questions should be asked to ascertain if they are allergic to antibiotics such as penicillin and to any other drugs that are likely to be used dentally. Although allergy to local anaesthesia is rare there are established cases and if the patient has an allergic history they are more likely to be in danger from the administration of any foreign substance. All drugs should therefore be given slowly and with care, and every dental surgery should have the appropriate drugs to deal with an allergic or anaphylactic reaction. The latter will manifest itself as severe shock with a fall in blood pressure and difficulty in breathing, and there may be oedema of the face and neck and an urticarial rash. Immediate treatment is required and also an immediate call for medical help. One millilitre of 1:1000 adrenaline solution should be injected slowly intramuscularly.

An important medicolegal principle is involved in the above comments — that one should be *au fait* with the possible complications of any procedure which one carries out and should have the means and ability to deal with those complications.

ORAL SURGERY FOR THE GENERAL PRACTITIONER

INSTRUMENTS FOR MINOR ORAL SURGERY

The following kit of instruments, sutures and materials is required; these can be autoclaved together on a wrapped metal tray. Most local hospitals will advise on instrumentation.

Handpiece
American sucker end and stillette
No. 3 Bard Parker scalpel handle
Periosteal elevator (Fickling)
Gillies' tissue forceps
Left and right Warwick James' elevators
Ash straight root elevator
Left and right Cryers elevators
Coupland's chisel No. 1 and No. 2
Ash surgical burs — round and fissured
Pkt. irrigation tubing
Hand towel
Metal galipot
Angled tongue depressor
Austin retractor
Howarth's raspatory
Cross-action towel clip
Kilner cheek retractor
Gauze swabs, 10 × 10 cm (4)
Curette (double-ended), Ash 86
Excavator, Ash 127/128
Curved Mosquito artery forcep
Spencer Wells' artery forceps
Fickling's forceps — plain and toothed
Kilner needleholder
Straight pointed scissors, 5 inch
Suction tubing
Dressing towel (disposable; as patient's bib)

A selection of forceps should also be available.

Sutures are contained in sterile packs and the recommended suture for all circumstances is the 3/0 Mersilk W577 with a 22 mm cutting needle (see Suturing below).

Instruments are available from a dental or surgical supply company.

BASIC ORAL SURGERY TECHNIQUES

General principles

1. Never ignore the history of difficult extractions.
2. Never use chisels on the conscious patient.
3. Remember the principle that an ulcer of 3 weeks duration should have a biopsy taken.

4. Roots which are broken can be left under the following circumstances.

(a) If their removal is likely to involve structures such as the mental or mandibular nerve and the antrum, provided they are:
- (i) smaller than a third of the root length;
- (ii) free of infection;
- (iii) have not been moved.

(b) An X-ray must be taken and, if a root has moved in the socket, it must be removed. Severe pain can follow the retention of a displaced root.

5. Do not operate in the presence of acute infection except to produce drainage.

6. Do not contaminate yourself with blood. Wear gloves at all times. Protective spectacles should also be worn at all times as blood-borne infection has been known to enter the body via the conjunctiva.

Abrasions and cuts on any exposed area should be covered with protective dressings and a facemask should be worn. Disposable gowns, although at present expensive, are the best way to deal with body and clothing protection. Accidental damage to the skin either by needlestick or otherwise should be treated immediately by placing under running water and allowing the wound to bleed. Betadine should be applied and the wound covered with a suitable dressing if necessary. Medical advice should be sought. If the operator is vaccinated as recommended, hepatitis B should be no problem and, even by needlestick injury, HIV is known to be difficult to transmit (see Chapter 48).

7. While you still have difficulty estimating the duration of an operation, arrange your appointments so that surgical patients are on the end of a list.

Basic flap design and handling

1. The flap should be based on the blood supply.
2. Its base should be broad so that the inevitable trauma of lifting the flap does not jeopardize its vitality.
3. Incisions should be made at right angles to the bone so that neither side of the wound is shelving. This makes elevation of the mucoperiosteum and suturing easier.
4. Incisions involving the gingival margins should be made axially down the gingival crevice.
5. Use a No. 15 blade on a No. 3 handle. The margins of the flap should be chosen after anticipating the amount of bone removal that is going to be necessary to carry out the surgical operation because it is desirable that the edges of the flap be returned to a bony shelf and not be sutured over the blood clot. The chances of primary healing are much higher in these circumstances.
6. A sharp periosteal elevator such as the Fickling type is a useful instrument as not only does it have a sharp blade but also a handle which can be gripped easily. To lift the gingival margin it is best to approach it from slightly beneath the gingival margin, and to strip away the unattached mucoperiosteum and

work towards the gingival margin, pressing hard on the bone so that the soft tissue is lifted cleanly without tearing. Any tearing which occurs will jeopardize the healing of the flap.

Bone removal

An autoclaved handpiece should be used for bone removal, with adequate cooling of the bur. Cooling is best supplied by a plastic bag of sterile saline, as used for transfusion purposes, connected by an infusion set to the handpiece preferably via an electrically operated switch which allows the saline to run when the drill is actuated. The coolant supply must be adequate at all times and directed towards the bur tip. The best burs to use are the self-clearing surgical burs which remarkably have only three teeth. These burs are tungsten carbide and were designed by Toller specifically for surgery.

Overheating must be avoided at all costs as it is known that moderate heat will kill osteocytes. This does not mean that high speed cannot be used provided that cooling is more than adequate. Many special electrical engines and handpieces are on the market for use in oral surgery. These are very reliable and the handpieces are autoclavable. Speeds vary between 12–20 000 revolutions per min. After the operation has been performed any sharp edges which are likely to perforate the flap should be removed and this can be easily done with the bur.

Immediate treatment of broken root

Radiography will probably reveal the cause of the breakage and the root can be approached accordingly. It may well be that elevation will be sufficient to remove the root, as for example in the retained root of the lower molar which can be elevated via the empty socket using the Cryer's or hospital curved elevator. This can also be carried out in the upper molar sockets, but care must be taken that the antrum does not lie between the roots. Any attempt to elevate from one socket to the next may then involve the antrum or even push the offending root into it. It may then be necessary to make a buccal flap. This buccal flap should follow the above principles and this may mean that the flap has to be extended around the gingival margin of the next tooth. The relieving incisions vertically should be directed at 45°; this improves access and fulfils the principle of a broad-base flap. The upward extent of these incisions should be to the sulcus. The gingival margin will have to be incised at its attachment to the bone in the same way as if the tooth were present; and bone can be removed rapidly with the drill carefully to expose the root if this is in a buccal position. This is easily done until such time as sufficient of the root is exposed to elevate it with a small elevator or probe.

Palatal roots are more of a problem, especially as the antrum may be very low into the trifurcation, but bone can usually be removed medially or distally to the root with a fair degree of safety. This will allow the gentle application of an elevator or probe to displace the root, care being taken not to push it upwards or to involve the trifurcation.

Single roots that are broken are given the same treatment but care must always be taken when removing bone to avoid involvement of the roots of other teeth which, if severe, can result in pulp death and, if minor, may be followed by root resorption.

Where the flap is in relation to the mental nerve area, it is better to extend the flap forward to the distal of the lower canine so that, with a 45° flare forwards, the mental foramen will be well behind the base of the incision. It is then wise to elevate the periosteum gently towards the mental foramen when the mental nerve will become apparent through the intact periosteum. It can then be gently protected with a retractor so that the bur will not accidentally run into it.

Should the antrum be involved to a minor degree in the root removal at the base of a deep socket, all that is necessary is to suture the socket and allow a blood clot to form. The hole should not be probed. Advise the patient to take the usual precautions to preserve the clot and give them a 5-day course of antibiotics, telling them not to blow their nose and to try and suppress sneezes for the next 4–5 days. Usually this is sufficient. Should the hole be very large or the socket shallow the integrity of the clot is more at risk and the buccal flap should be turned away from the bone, using a pair of Gillies' tooth forceps, and an incision made above the reflection horizontally to incise the periosteum from one end of the flap to the other. This will give immediate relief as the inelastic periosteum is severed and the elastic mucosa will allow the flap to be pulled over the socket. Closure should then be made with vertical mattress sutures to induce eversion of the flap edges, and precautions taken as above.

A special warning about retained roots applies to the rarely occurring lingual root of the lower wisdom tooth. If present, this often breaks off and is retained in the socket. Removal of this root is quite tricky as sometimes the lingual plate is deficient at its apex or very thin, and the root is easily displaced into the submandibular space. It should be left in situ (again provided there is no local infection), unless it is obviously easy to remove bone mesial and distal to it and to elevate it with a probe, small elevator or excavator without involving the mandibular nerve, which may run lateral to it.

Suturing

Many different kinds of materials have been used for suturing in the mouth but the one which is most commonly used is braided silk. A small cutting needle is required and the thickness of the silk should be 3/0. A sterile pack should be used, e.g. Mersilk W577, which has a needle 22 mm in length. There has been a vogue recently for absorbable sutures but they tend to shred, encourage retention of food material and ultimately microorganisms, and sometimes prematurely fall apart, thus leaving the wound to its own devices. There is a great economic advantage in not having to bring the patient back for removal of sutures, but one has to review the patient and 7–10 days is a quite satisfactory time to see them for this purpose and to remove the sutures.

The type of suturing commonly used in oral surgery is the interrupted suture, where each stitch is a separate entity and is simply inserted by taking a bite of the free flap about 2–2.5 mm from the edge and then passing the needle through the more or less fixed flap before tying it using a simple surgeon's twist with one lock-twist to fix it. On occasions where primary healing is important and the suture line is not supported by bone, a mattress suture should be used, e.g. in oroantral fistula closure. This may be either horizontal or vertical but essentially it is passed from the free flap to the fixed flap and then back through the fixed flap to the free flap again. The effect being one of eversion of the edges of the wound when it is tightened, thus producing a more watertight junction. The vertical mattress has its two strands above one another whereas the horizontal has them side by side.

ASSESSMENT OF WISDOM TEETH

1. As a guide to the kind of wisdom tooth that should be tackled in the dental surgery, the tooth should either be partially erupted or palpable. As experience increases, somewhat deeper teeth can be tackled but it is said that the difficulty increases as the square of the depth, which is probably an exaggeration but indicates that problems can increase rapidly with deeper teeth.
2. The position of the tooth — (a) vertical, (b) mesioangular, (c) distoangular, (d) inverted, (e) transverse across the ridge — in the latter case the crown is usually on the lingual side.
3. Age of patient: this dictates the bone density and also the brittleness. The radiograph will have told you how much bone there is beneath the roots but the patient who is over 55 years of age and female may have osteoporosis, increasing the problem of jaw fracture; if male he will certainly have a more dense bone, increasing the difficulty of removal.
4. Density of bone: are there sclerosed areas involving the tooth which might make bone removal difficult and certainly might induce overheating of the bur?
5. If there is an enlarged follicle space? Although this may indicate the possibility of infection or a cyst, it does also mean that some of the bone removal has already been done for you.
6. Root form of the adjacent second lower molar. If the root is conical there is a danger of accidental elevation of this tooth and this danger must be borne in mind at operation.
7. Presence or absence of the first molar: this tooth will act as a buttress to a second molar with an unfavourable root form.
8. Relationship of root to mandibular canal: if your radiograph shows the shadow of the canal passing across the root there is a danger that they are closely related. The darker the shadow over the root of the tooth, the more likely the root is to be grooved — this is usually on the lingual side. The depth of this groove is also indicated by the disappearance of the so-called tramlines which represent the lamina dura of the mandibular canal. If the groove is deep, the nerve is actually against the tooth substance and does not have lamina dura between itself and the root. If the nerve goes through the root of the third molar, the radiographic signs are as follows:

(a) narrowing of the shadow of the canal;
(b) darkening of the shadow of the canal;
(c) disappearance of the lamina dura.

Accurate determination of this relationship can be established by parallax using a lateral oblique film and an intraoral, periapical film of the area.

Removal of lower wisdom teeth

The incision starts posteriorly, just medial to the ascending ramus, 2–2.5 cm behind the distal surface of the second molar, depending on the anticipated difficulty. If the wisdom tooth is partially erupted the incision passes downward and medially to meet the exposed part of the crown at a point where the crest of the ridge would be. The incision is then continued around the buccal gingival crevice to the distal of the second molar. If the wisdom tooth is unerupted the incision is brought forward to the centre of the distal surface of the second molar. The incision is then continued downward and forward at 45° from the distal surface of the second molar without involving the buccal gingival margin and stopping short of the sulcus. Incisions must be made deliberately down to bone so that the flap can be lifted cleanly. Healing is poor if incisions are made in the middle of the buccal gingival margin. The buccal flap is lifted in the recommended way and the periosteal elevator is carried under the lingual periosteum behind the tooth and brought forward, so as to lift the lingual periosteum and mucosa and allow insertion of a Howarth's raspatory (periosteal elevator) inside the periosteal sac to avoid trauma to the lingual nerve. Care should be taken that the edge of the raspatory does not involve the lingual nerve and the periosteum should remain intact. The operator should now be able to see the bone clearly lingually and distally to the tooth and a bur can be used without involving the soft tissues. An Austin retractor is used to hold back the buccal flap.

Inspection of the bone in relation to the tooth will then indicate how much bone needs removal and, using the radiographs as a guide, the round bur is used to produce a channel on the buccal side of the tooth and also distally, care being taken when distolingual bone is removed. A point of application is made by inserting the bur in front of the crown of the wisdom tooth, while carefully avoiding the root of the second molar. Taking the root form and position of the tooth as a guide, one must visualize the path of withdrawal of this tooth and bone must be removed accordingly. For example, a distoangular tooth will require more bone removal distally and extra care with the provision of a point of application since its root will be closer than that of a vertical wisdom tooth to the root of the second molar. Another problem with bone removal in distoangular wisdom teeth is the relative proximity of the inferior dental canal behind and below the crown of the tooth and care must be taken not to involve the nerve at this point.

If the tooth has a favourable angulation and the crown is free of bone, it may be possible to elevate it directly at this stage. However, attempts at elevation may result in the tooth quickly becoming impacted against a bony overhang—experience will tend to reduce the occasions when this happens, as one's anticipation of how much bone is to be removed improves with time. The tooth should be pushed back fully into its socket and the additional bone removal carried out before elevation takes place. With horizontal impactions and some mesioangular impactions, it is necessary to remove the crown. Occasionally this will also occur with distoangular impactions, as removal of the crown can produce an economy in bone removal. The crown of the horizontal or mesioangular tooth is removed by cutting through at about the cervical margin. This is not easy to do and care must be taken that the bur does not protrude at the other side of the tooth and damage the mandibular nerve in its canal. The angle of cut is important as the fragment of crown removed must not have a wider base than its superior end or the crown will become a wedge which cannot be elevated. On occasions where there are difficulties it is often helpful to turn to a No. 7 or 8 standard fissure bur to carry out the section, so that a wide gap is developed when the crown is cut off; this allows disimpaction backwards of the third molar crown where it is tightly impacted against the second molar.

Attempts should not be made to elevate a mesioangular or horizontal tooth with great force because the nerve is in medullary bone and the roots are relatively streamlined so they will be pushed back onto the nerve as the tooth finds itself tight against the back of the second molar.

As far as the distoangular tooth is concerned, elevation is difficult because of the previously mentioned lack of space between the root of this tooth and the second molar. It is a good general rule not to decoronate a distoangular impacted tooth until the tooth has been loosened, otherwise visibility and access to the roots will be found to be difficult.

Special care must be taken with the patient who has a horizontally impacted wisdom tooth against the posterior surface of a distoangular second molar. These teeth are particularly difficult to disimpact.

Removal of all the tooth fragments should be followed by saline irrigation and a further search for debris. The tooth follicle should be removed; a curette is usually used for this. Where a distal pocket has been present behind the second molar, the distal surface of this tooth must be curetted to ensure that there is no calculus present, which would certainly interfere with re-attachment. The wound is closed with simple interrupted sutures, and it may be necessary, where the tooth has been partly erupted, to advance the flap so as to close the socket completely and protect the blood clot. One suture is used directly behind the second molar and a second suture posterior to this. It is not necessary to suture the buccal incision.

Postoperative instructions are given to the patient and precautions to prevent bleeding are explained. Analgesics are recommended where required. There is still debate about whether antibiotics should be prescribed.

We tend to use antibiotics postoperatively in wisdom teeth cases where:

(a) there has been chronic pericoronitis;
(b) the clot and therefore the socket is unusually large and will tend more easily to break down;
(c) it has been necessary to use more than usual local anaesthetic with vasoconstrictor;
(d) there is a history of dry socket.

This is all somewhat unscientific but is based on clinical experience. One of the few things that is known about dry socket is that it is more common in cases where teeth have been removed under local anaesthesia.

Phenoxymethylpencillin, i.e. pencillin V, is prescribed 250 mg q.d.s. for 5 days. A good alternative is metronidazole (Flagyl) 400 mg, 8.00 am and 8.00 pm for 5 days. Erythromycin is another alternative but tends to produce sickness or nausea in a number of patients.

Removal of upper wisdom teeth

The incision starts posteriorly behind the tuberosity short of the sulcus, drops over the centre of the tuberosity to the centre of the back of the second molar if the upper wisdom tooth is unerupted. If it is partially erupted the incision passes around the buccal gingival crevice of the wisdom tooth to the distobuccal papilla of the second molar and then at 45° upwards and forwards to the sulcus.

The same principles of bone removal apply as for lower wisdom teeth — sufficient bone must be removed to allow the tooth to be delivered and a point of application must be established. Often the bone can be removed with a chisel held in the hand without using the bur. The bone is often soft enough to allow the elevator to make its own point of application when sufficient bone has been removed.

Upper wisdom teeth are generally much easier to remove than lowers because the roots are more favourable and the bone softer. However, access is difficult and one must remember that the antrum is usually in close relationship. Care must be taken that the tooth is not pushed upwards. When elevating, a finger must be held under the tooth so as to prevent it shooting down the throat. Care must be also taken that it is not lost behind the tuberosity under the flap. As before, bone fragments and follicle are removed from the socket and the wound sutured.

One suture across the crest of the ridge is usually sufficient, but some surgeons do not suture at all.

APICECTOMY AND RETROGRADE ROOT FILLING

The following are the possible indications for apicectomy in dead teeth.

1. Cyst or large apical area involving apex
2. Multi-rooted teeth
3. Complicated root canal forms
4. Obstruction in canal, e.g. secondary dentine, pulp stones
5. Open apex
6. Broken instrument in canal
7. Hooked root
8. Fracture of apical third
9. Foreign material in apical region
10. Failed root-canal therapy

Most of these indications represent difficult or impossible circumstances for cleaning out the contents of the root canal. To this list may be added the coronal restoration, the removal of which may commit the tooth to extraction.

Having said this the ideal apicectomy would be carried out on a tooth which had been orthograde root-filled beforehand, for two reasons: firstly there is more chance of preservation of the tooth simply because lateral canals would be to a certain extent sealed; and secondly, condensation of the retrograde root filling would be easier with a firm base in the canal. In wide canals the amalgam would not pass down the canal and interfere with future post-crowning.

All forms of teeth have been apicected and retrograde root filled satisfactorily but the prognosis for single-root teeth is undoubtedly better than for multi-rooted teeth, and posterior tooth root access can be difficult. It is therefore recommended that, under local anaesthesia, these operations be confined to the 12 anterior teeth or possibly the premolars, if one is prepared to deal with the added complication of the mental nerve and antrum, and the possibility of multi-roots on the upper premolars. In general, if the area of operation is to be large, needing good access, then a gingival incision should be made which includes the gingival margin of the tooth on either side. This will give access to a lesion which extends almost to the gingival margin. For smaller lesions the so-called semilunar flap is easier to handle and suture and is less likely to cause recession.

The flap is lifted and quite often there is a sinus with granulations coming through the surface of the bone. If this is not so then the radiograph must be consulted and the bur used gently to remove a window of cortical bone to expose the apex. If this does not expose the apex, then deeper drilling should be carried out above where the root is thought to be, approaching it from above. The aim of this is to avoid damage to cementum remaining behind. When the apex is identified a fissure bur is used to cut it off at an angle so that the root surface will be visible and the canal identifiable for root filling. A retentive cavity is then prepared to receive the amalgam retrograde root filling. It is important to remember in lower incisors that the canal is often slit-like, and the whole of the canal should be opened from labial to lingual so as to ensure that the final seal is good. A No. 2 or 3 round bur can be used in a straight handpiece, provided the cut surface of the root has been angled satisfactorily. The cavity is then washed and dried. Granulation tissue is removed, although to reduce bleeding this can be left until after the tooth has been filled with amalgam. The cavity must be dry and this is sometimes difficult.

On occasions the bone cavity is packed with Surgicel to reduce bleeding and possibly collect fragments of amalgam. Warm dry air is used in a chip syringe to dry out the cavity before the insertion of the amalgam. Zinc-free amalgam is inserted and condensed in the usual way to excess, and the condensed amalgam is trimmed down and very lightly burnished. The amalgam is inserted into the retentive cavity using a very fine orthodontic-tubing carrier and there should be no excess pieces of amalgam around the cavity, which will show as shrapnel on the final X-ray. The Surgicel is then removed if it has been applied, the cavity washed out with saline, and the flap carefully sutured into position. Antibiotics are usually given for 5 days and the patient is told not to eat anything hard on the tooth for 6 weeks to allow time for regrowth of bone and firming up of the tooth support. A postoperative X-ray must be taken, partly for medicolegal reasons to confirm that all is well, and secondly as a baseline for the X-ray that will be taken 6 months later for a check-up of bone regeneration. After 6 months the patient is discharged and asked to return should there be any further trouble, provided that the X-ray at that time shows satisfactory bone regeneration and the tooth is symptomless.

Amalgam has been shown experimentally to make a good seal in the root surface but the fact is that some apicectomy cases fail for no apparent reason. There is room for research on this subject and other materials have been tried. Recent work involves a composite filling material, but the question of toxicity is being studied.

As far as the more difficult apicectomies are concerned it is usually possible to fill palatal roots of upper first and second premolars via the buccal wound, but this entails involving the antrum on occasions. However, provided one does not fill the antrum with amalgam, all seems to go well and the antral floor will regenerate over the apex of the tooth if the apicectomy is successful. When dealing with lower premolars in relation to the mental foramen, one exposes the nerve and protects it as mentioned previously; but one does not cut under the apex to expose the tooth but rather makes a window above the apex at the level of the proposed root section so that the apex can be cut off and then delivered upwards out of the cavity; in this way there is no interference with the nerve. If this is done, care must be taken when using an excavator to remove granulations from the bottom of the cavity.

ORTHODONTICS AND ORAL SURGERY

The oral surgeon of today spends much of his or her time cooperating with the orthodontist. This is a relationship which has developed in recent years to our mutual advantage and certainly it is of utmost importance in cooperation with the planning of osteotomy surgery. However, there are joint clinics at which we discuss problems other than osteotomies and I will mention a few of these which may come your way because of orthodontic recommendations.

Exposure of a tooth

The reasons why some teeth erupt as far as the mucosa but will not actually come through it are unknown and this is an interesting field for research. However, certainly those that are within 3 years of their normal eruption date and still buried can be helped by the removal of the overlying mucosa. The tissue is excised widely around the tooth in what is termed a 'saucerization' so as to illustrate that the removal of tissue should be wide. If there is bone overlying the tooth, some means of removal other than the bur or chisel should be used in case of damaging the tooth — a Coupland's chisel is usually not an extremely sharp instrument and can be used gently to remove bone up to the follicular space without actually involving the tooth.

When this exposure has been carried out, one must have in mind the path of eruption of the tooth and the intention of the direction it will take after it has been exposed, but bone must be removed away from the crown so as to allow this eruption. The mucosa must also be trimmed accordingly. As far as possible, gingival margins are preserved and, if the tooth is on the labial side, the gingival margin of the exposed tooth is preserved as much as possible. If it is trimmed right back, one may find that the labial gingival margin will be permanently raised when the tooth has come down into position. Having reached this stage of the operation it is necessary to insert a pack. Coepack can be used and sutured into position, or gauze impregnated with Whitehead's varnish.

It is our practice to keep these packs in position for 2 weeks before removing them and sometimes the orthodontists will wish to apply a bracket at this stage if at all possible. Another way of maintaining the opening over the exposed tooth is to use a plate to cover the pack. In deep cases a simple clear acrylic base plate fitting around the gingival margins is made preoperatively and extends into an edentulous area where necessary. It is held in place by cribs on the first molars. In a sense this is a more satisfactory method, in that it pushes the pack into the wound, which is the opposite direction to the way that sutures tend to pull the wound edges inwards. Economically it is not favoured, but it is a very useful technique if a removable appliance already exists.

Removal of unerupted palatal upper canines

The necessity for removal will no doubt have been explained to the patient or parents, but, if not, it should be. The problem with removing these teeth is the proximity of other teeth. The necessary X-rays should be taken beforehand and these include parallax intraorals and a naso-occlusal. This should tell one whether the root form is satisfactory and will confirm the position from the parallax views — the tooth in the palate moving with the tube in relation to the other teeth in the arch.

A gingival flap is used in the palate and extends from, and includes, the second premolar on the side of the tooth to the canine on the other side. This flap is lifted and, if necessary, incisive canal vessels are cut and clipped so as to free the flap completely. It is then quite likely that the tooth will be visible, or at least the follicle will be visible and bone can be removed in the usual way with the round bur using a Howarth's raspatory as a retractor. Care must be taken to avoid the root of the first premolar and, in attempted elevation, care must be taken of all the related teeth. Usually a Coupland's gouge is a satisfactory instrument for elevation, but it is important that bone is removed about halfway down the root to be sure of the easy removal. It may be necessary to remove the crown, but the tooth should be loosened first before this is done, using a fissure bur. When the tooth has been removed, the follicular remnants and loose pieces of bone are removed with an excavator, and sharp edges of bone must be smoothed. The wound is closed with interdental sutures and pressure must be applied to the flap with a damp swab for 5 minutes to avoid formation of a palatal haematoma, which is a problematical complication possible in these cases.

Unerupted labial canines

Extraction of unerupted labial canines is usually easy as they only have thin labial bone over them. The incision is usually gingival or semilunar, according to the height of the tooth. Care must be taken to avoid trauma to other teeth during elevation and, as far as possible, to return the flap margins to a bony shelf. Again, if the tooth proved difficult to disimpact, then the crown should be removed first, taking care not to damage the other teeth on either side with the bur.

Labial fraenum

If the labial fraenum needs removing it is usually a fleshy fibrous band extending from the incisive papilla into the lip, such that when the lip is pulled forwards the papilla moves. It is this sort of anatomy which tends to maintain a midline diastema against the efforts of the orthodontists to close the space. It is much easier to remove before the orthodontists have attempted closure of the space. The operation is difficult to describe, but relatively easy to carry out. This is usually in children and anaesthetic paste should be applied before local anaesthetic is injected. As soon as the injection has been made, a damp swab should be pressed into the area, squeezing the fraenum first to stop or reduce ballooning of the tissues that tends to mask the identity of the fraenum and make accurate excision difficult. First, a tranverse cut is made at the anterior end of the incisive papilla. Forward, parallel cuts are then made from this on each side of the fibrous fraenum and avoiding the mesial gingival margins of the centrals, thus excising the fibrous band as one passes forward between the teeth. These parallel incisions are kept to the side of the fraenum as one passes forward into the soft tissue of the lip. The web is then dissected from the lip by turning the scalpel into a horizontal position, inserting it through both parallel incisions with the lip held out, and bringing it forward until the fibrous band is completely excised. The most important suture to be inserted is one at the height of the sulcus, which is stitched through the mucosa of one side of the wound, then through the periosteum against the bone in the midline, then out through the other edge of mucosa. When this is tied you will notice that the mucosa is pulled tightly against the mucoperiosteum at the height of the sulcus; this is known as the 'anchor' suture, because it tends to stop the scar 'tenting' between the lip and the ridge, thus replacing the original fraenum with a fibrous band. Once this anchor stitch has been inserted, other simple interrupted stitches can be applied as necessary.

Impacted lower second premolar

The impacted lower second premolar is quite a common problem and is made more difficult if the associated first premolar and first molar are close to each other or even in contact. Adequate radiographs are important and it may be necessary to have a larger film to show the apex. Again, care must be taken not to damage the associated teeth. Eventually exposure will show that the tooth is tightly engaged with the associated teeth and the only way to remove this is to take a generous slice out of the cervical margin using a fissure bur and going completely through the tooth. This allows disimpaction of the crown and delivery of the root.

Instanding lower second premolar

With instanding lower premolars, radiographs are also important to detect the shape of the hook due to displacement of the path of eruption of the tooth. If the tooth is completely excluded from the arch with the first premolar and molar together, it is usually quite easy to grip it with a pair of upper Reed forceps from the other side of the mouth and with care, to wiggle the crown so as to dilate the socket, in the meantime keeping a careful eye that other teeth are not damaged. Sometimes this will be achieved better with a straight pair of narrow forceps, particularly when some withdrawal has already been achieved.

If the tooth is not completely excluded from the arch, then narrow lower-root forceps can be used to remove it in the lingual direction — again with care being taken not to damage the other teeth. Most of these teeth require gentle prolonged rocking to dilate the socket and help their removal, bearing in mind that mandibular bone is quite dense. Matters can be helped along by a gentle tapping from the buccal side, using a slightly upward angulation of a 'knock thro'' instrument between first premolar and molar, engaged at the cervical margin. This is a modified dental instrument, the working part of which is 3 cm long and tapers from the base at 2.2 mm to the hemispherical tip at 1.8 mm.

This procedure often saves one from a difficult situation where one cannot get a grip on the tooth without damaging the surrounding teeth. Obviously extreme care must be used with the 'knock thro'' instrument as it is very easy to get it between two teeth and damage them or push them out. Eventually one gets the feel of it, and it should be applied to the tooth so it is lifted out of its socket as well as pushed to the lingual side. A change in note will be heard as one taps and the tooth comes loose.

If the instanding lower second premolar is covered with mucosa, the added depth can raise problems. This case should be referred to the hospital for removal; here it may be necessary to raise a lingual flap, which depends very much on patient cooperation and may need a general anaesthetic.

PREPROSTHETIC SURGERY

The surgical preparation of the denture-bearing areas or dentures involves many kinds of pathology (see also Chapter 35). These may be fibroepithelial polyps, undercuts, flabby ridges and so on. Buried teeth and roots are also included, and radiographs should be taken to check on the presence of these before dentures are made. It must always be remembered that edentulous patients, especially in the older age group, have brittle bone and possibly also thin mandibles. In some cases radiographs may show that the teeth occupy practically the whole thickness of the jaw and these would, of course, be hospital cases. There are, however, many minor procedures which can be carried out in practice under local anaesthesia.

The flabby ridge

This is usually a problem associated with the upper or lower anterior region of the jaws and is easily dealt with by excision of an elongated 'melon slice' with its apex on the crest of the ridge and its lateral extensions as far as is necessary to reduce the flabby area. Care should be taken not to run into the premolar region in the atrophic mandible as the mental foramen may be located in that position. Excision is followed by interrupted suturing of the defect.

The sharp ridge

This is usually in the lower anterior region and the problem it presents to the patient can be easily detected by applying pressure with the finger to the crest of the ridge, when immediate pain will be elicited. This is easily reduced by making an incision vertically at the crest of the ridge to more than cover the area of sharpness and carefully reflecting buccal and lingual flaps. This has to be done with care as the ridge is often quite fibrous over the sharp ridge and tightly bound down. When the bone is exposed, bone nibblers, followed by a large round bur, are used to smooth down the ridge, and the buccal and lingual mucoperiosteum are then sutured together. It may be necessary to excise a little mucoperiosteum, but usually the insertion of mattress sutures will produce a protective pad over the ridge and this will fibrose down to make a good denture base.

The undercut ridge

The area of undercut is generously exposed using a mucoperiosteal flap based in the usual way. Exposure of the undercut will then allow it to be removed with a large round bur. A preoperative radiograph will be needed in the maxillary region to be sure that the removal of an undercut does not involve the antrum and, of course, the mental foramen must be properly located before removing an undercut in this region so as to protect it. The area can again be covered temporarily with tissue conditioner after suturing, until healing has taken place and the denture can be relined.

Denture-induced hyperplasia

This condition (Chapter 35) is fairly common. For treatment planning, the patient should not wear the denture for about 6 weeks. This will reduce the size of the hyperplasia, which will have been inflamed and may be ulcerated. If this seems impossible or inadvisable, then the flange of the denture should be reduced considerably to take away irritation from the area. In some cases the hyperplasia will disappear and will need no treatment, or at least will be so small that the denture can be made over it. In a situation where hyperplastic tissue still remains, which is usually in the lower incisor region labially, the overgrowth is gripped in Gillies' forceps and lifted. It can then be easily excised flush with the surface. It is not necessary to suture it, in fact it is inadvisable, and the denture should be re-inserted with tissue conditioner underneath it, when the area will heal well. The excised tissue should be sent for pathological investigation. Larger denture-induced hyperplasias are best dealt with in hospital, where appliances may be needed to treat them properly and possibly skin grafting in extreme cases.

CHRONIC OROANTRAL FISTULA

The acute oroantral fistula and its closure has been discussed above, but the chronic oroantral fistula is a different problem. Quite often the connection between mouth and antrum may not be obvious at the time of the initial surgery and it is unwise to test for fistulae by passing a probe into the antrum as this may well breach the intact antral lining. The best way to check for a fistula is to ask the patient to blow their nose, when bubbles should emerge from the hole. Sometimes this does not happen if the lining is intact or if there is a polyp protecting the hole, but symptoms will eventually develop where-by tea or some other liquid taken into the mouth comes down the nose. These cases should be referred to hospital and clear details should be laid out in the letter as to how the fistula came about and particularly if there is a root missing. If there is, the practitioner should state whether this is likely to be in the antrum or not. It is a help if the practitioner sends along the crown and the rest of the roots of the tooth, so that it is easy to match the size of the missing root with the various shadows on the X-rays and thereby locate the root.

As antral surgery is involved as well as the closure of the fistula, these patients will be dealt with under a general anaesthetic in hospital, when some surgeons will also carry out a nasal antrostomy to allow drainage into the nose.

FRACTURED TUBEROSITY

Fracture of the maxillary tuberosity occurs most commonly when the first or second molar have been lost some time previously so the antrum has expanded down towards the crest of the ridge. This weakens the tuberosity, and if the tooth to be removed, which is usually the second or third molar, has fairly complex roots, it is quite likely that the tuberosity will fracture. It is important that bone should be preserved at all oral surgery operations, not least for preprosthetic reasons, and the tuberosity is no exception. The problem for the practitioner is detecting that the tuberosity has fractured. If the proper grip is used for removing upper molars—the index finger in the palate on the right side and the thumb in the buccal sulcus on the right side and on the left side with the index finger in the sulcus and the thumb in the palate—it is possible to grip the tuberosity as the tooth is being removed. If the tuberosity starts to move with the tooth, then the operation should be immediately abandoned; obviously the tuberosity has fractured and it is very important at this stage not to proceed with the extraction or the mucosa will be torn and it will make repair difficult. It is quite possible that when this patient is referred to hospital, which should be done urgently, we will proceed to operation quickly because healing is likely to be best within the first 24 hours after the accident. The oral surgeon will decide whether to dissect out the tuberosity if it is small, or whether to splint it and preserve it and remove the tooth surgically later if the fragment is large. It is important that the mucosa is intact for this surgical closure to be carried out satisfactorily.

INFECTIONS

As mentioned above, infections should be treated by first taking bacteriological swabs to confirm exactly which organism you are dealing with and its particular sensitivity. Sometimes, because we are concerned about the consequence of the infection, we will start treating infection empirically until such time as we receive confirmation of the sensitivity of the organism, when we will then change the antibiotic or antibiotics as necessary.

Probably the most common infection which the dental surgeon will see, apart from the acute apical abscess, is the pericoronal infection. It has already been said that this should be treated with antibiotics if the patient is febrile and if there is lymphadenitis. However, on occasions this infection can spread in various directions as follows.

1. Into the buccal space, so that the cheek is swollen.
2. Under the medial pterygoid into the so-called pterygoid space, which will result in severe trismus.
3. It can also track into the submasseteric space, which will also result in trismus. From there it has been known to track upwards to the temporal space, which is more difficult to treat, but of particular danger is the spread backwards into the pharynx via the lateral pharyngeal space, which is continuous with the retropharyngeal space. It is at this stage that the infection may spread downwards and produce airway problems, and it is for this reason that these infections must not be treated lightly. Certainly, marked trismus is a sign that things are not going well and the patient should be referred.
4. Lower molars that are apically infected can spread their infection to the buccal side or to the lingual and, if their root apices and the point of discharge through the bone is below the mylohyoid ridge, this passes directly into the submandibular space and can produce a large swelling under the jaw, which will certainly need some form of hospital treatment.

Upper molars and premolars can discharge apical abscesses into the antrum, or show on the buccal side and spread to the buccal space, producing a large swelling of the cheek. Usually treatment is sought before this stage. The upper incisors usually produce labial abscesses except for the upper lateral where the root is set back into the palate and will often produce a palatal abscess. Sometimes these labial and buccal abscesses, in their early stages when they are fluctuant, can be treated by incision under ethyl chloride spray or even local anaesthetic in the mucosal surface when the palate is involved. It must be remembered that a simple incision in a domed swelling in the palate is not sufficient because as soon as the thick mucosa collapses the wound will close. It is therefore necessary to excise an ellipse of tissue to avoid this happening. All these procedures should be followed by rigorous hot salt mouthbaths and empirical antibiotics; pus should be sent for bacteriological investigation.

POSTOPERATIVE ANALGESIA (see also Chapter 38)

Patients should be warned of the possibility or even probability of postoperative pain and some oral surgeons believe that the patient should take two paracetamol tablets (500 mg) about the time the anaesthesia is expected to wear off, and then two more tablets can be taken 4-hourly if required. We find this is quite an effective analgesic with most patients. As an alternative we prescribe codeine phosphate tablets (50 mg, one or two, 4-hourly). This is a more effective analgesic but unfortunately is constipating. Soluble aspirin is probably the best all-round analgesic in those who do not suffer from gastric ulcers. There is a possibility that it will interfere with haemostasis but this is rare. It must not be administered to children under 12 years of age. Each tablet is 300 mg and the dose can be one or two, 4-hourly. It is wise to ask the patient to return if pain continues, especially on the second or third day.

The wound in this case is quite likely to be losing, or to have lost, its clot by lysis, in which case it should be gently irrigated to remove the remaining lysing clot and food debris, and dressed with a mix of oil of cloves and zinc oxide, impregnated on 0.5 inch ribbon gauze and lightly packed in the wound. This will bring welcome relief as a rule but should be augmented with a change in antibiotics or initiation of antibiotics if the patient is not on them already and the symptoms are severe.

REFERRAL OF A PATIENT TO HOSPITAL

If it is desired to refer a patient to a hospital consultant, the most important preparation is the letter. The letter must have the patient's full details including name and address and date of birth. It must include all details of the medical history and any special comments, e.g. particular nervousness or anxiety, disabilities.

The letter should then go on to describe the patient's condition on presentation and any action which has been taken, e.g. attempted removal of a tooth, fractured tuberosity, and should describe any action which the dental surgeon has taken after the incident. If there is a question of a retained root or an oroantral fistula or fractured tuberosity, the relative specimen should be inserted with the letter (see above). If the referral is for some non-urgent condition it is sufficient to send the letter to the consultant concerned at the hospital. However, if there is urgency, as in one of the above accidents, a phone call should be made to the hospital to contact the consultant or a member of the junior staff to make urgent arrangements for a consultation.

The letter should state clearly who is referring the patient, as quite often we have a problem knowing who actually referred because the signature is unrecognizable and there are perhaps six names printed on the top of the notepaper.

MEDICOLEGAL ASPECTS

The medicolegal implications of all types of surgery are becoming more serious and it is important that you warn your patients of the possible hazards of your operations before you start them. For example, if you are carrying out surgery near mandibular or mental nerves, then you must warn the patient of possible numbness of the lip and chin. For removal of lower wisdom teeth the warning should be that there could be numbness of the mental distribution and of the tongue as the lingual nerve may be involved. It is very easy to play down the effects and say there may be a 'touch of pins and needles' after the operation, but this leaves one in a rather difficult position if there is numbness, and it is better to be truthful about the extent of the possible hazards.

We know that recovery of the mandibular nerve, and possibly the mental as well, is good and quite often complete, but with the lingual nerve recovery tends to be slower and quite often incomplete. Particularly in the neurotic patient this can be a source of irritation which they may well feel needs some compensation. If they have a clear picture of the possible hazards beforehand they are less likely to be able to have a successful claim. It is for this reason that ultimately it will be necessary to have specific written consent for this kind of operation and more and more discussion is taking place with the Defence Societies about these aspects. For the same reason, radiographs must always be adequate. Remember also that if the numbness should persist the patient should be warned very strongly about biting the lip accidentally. This can produce ulceration and swelling which it is even more difficult for the patient to avoid biting. This alerting of the patient to the hazards of operation should be done with a witness present. No longer can we assume that the patient presenting themselves in the surgery and allowing us to carry out operations on them is a form of consent and records of all warnings should be made in the notes.

Part Five
Examination Techniques

Chapter 50

General preparation

THE MGDS EXAMINATION

Always try to make sure that you have made adquate preparation for any part of the examination. Read the latest papers in the journals, and follow those papers and articles which specifically refer to any aspect of a case you may be presenting. It is also advisable, as far as possible, to be aware of the identity of your Examiners, and know which topics interest them most. You can be sure that your 'viva' or written question may include some topic along the Examiner's favourite lines!

Keep abreast of the current journals, especially the *British Dental Journal*, *Dental Update*, and *Dental Practice* — all have topical ideas and articles. Make sure your reading list has covered the undergraduate texts and papers suggested by individual departments and, if you have time, look a little further afield and broaden your ever-increasing knowledge.

For external examinations, the scope widens but, as stated in the last section, check out the Examiners and their interests. Prepare for the external examinations by attending a recognized course, e.g. one of the Regional MGDS courses, because here you will be given guidance about the examination. For instance, if you are attempting to sit for the MGDS examination, it may well be a few years since you undertook any formal study in the way that will be required at this level. A Course Tutor will advise you with regard to the Regulations, which books to read, and at what level. He or she will possibly provide some past papers, and even a small 'mock' examination. In this way, you can find out whether the idea of taking the examination actually appeals, or whether it would be a waste of time. Answer some essays, and try to get them looked at by someone on the course. This will give you practice in 'keeping to time', and give you an idea about your present standard. This can also be very useful for undergraduates who are experiencing difficulties in a particular subject. Try to find a sympathetic member of that department, and arrange for a few essays to be set and marked. It is surprising how this method of learning helps to increase your knowledge of a subject.

Chapter 51

The written papers

All examinations have some element of writing in their content, so it is important to be prepared and to remain cool and calm about the proceedings, even if it has been years since you wrote under examination conditions!

Several types of written examinations are used today. The old favourite is the 3-h essay paper, where the candidate has to answer five or six questions in this time. This is the sort of paper that has always been popular, and those coming back into the system after several years will no doubt be familiar with its workings.

Secondly, there is the Multiple Short Answer (MSA) paper. Here, for instance, the candidate has 2 h in which to answer 20 questions. A broader spread of knowledge is required, but possibly not so much detail. With only 5 min to answer each question, lists, small diagrams and charts may well explain things in much quicker and better terms, and put over more facts than writing in conventional sentences. In fact, some questions of this format simply ask for a list of five or six reasons why a particular event may occur.

The third form of paper is the Multiple Choice Questionnaire (MCQ). This can be the nasty one if a penalty system for guessing is used — and it usually is! Do not guess — you may end up losing a mark you gained in the previous question. Read the original question very carefully so as to avoid being caught out by the tricky wording of the statement. Some of these papers seem to have a mathematical answering system with, say, five statements, of which either two or three will be true or false. Once you have done a few of these questions on the paper, look back to see if this is so. However, beware, because if you have not correctly 'cracked the code' this could be equally dangerous.

Back to the essay question papers; these can be the biggest stumbling blocks for all examinees. Let us go right back to basics: first, leave yourself time to get to the Examination Centre. If this is away from your home town, consider the possibility of an overnight stay just to be sure. Take with you your Examination Card and Number. Keep a case with a couple of spare pens, ink, pencils, erasers, colours for diagrams, etc. The pen you are using will inevitably go wrong at the least opportune moment. In other words, arrive early and be fully prepared!

Read the entire paper, and make sure you understand the basic instructions. Some papers may be in more than one part, with only one question to be answered from that part. Then all the remaining questions may have to be answered. Sometimes four out of five questions have to be answered, so do not waste valuable time answering five where four will do; you will not gain marks, and will almost certainly lose some because of the effort put into the four principal contenders!

Having decided upon the format of the paper, decide upon the order of answering the questions. Read them all very carefully, making sure you understand the emphasis the Examiner is trying to make. So many candidates just do not answer the set question, yet a lot of thought at the Examiners' meetings, where the questions are set, goes into getting the wording and phrasing of the question as near to perfect as possible. The ambiguous question rarely reaches the final paper.

Start with a question you find relatively easy — if you can! Plan your answer along the subdivisions you intend to pursue. You can then expand your text under these headings as you proceed with the essay. Keep an eye on the clock — do not get carried away with this nice first question for the first hour! You will not have time to catch up later!

Layout is important. First impressions count. When an Examiner picks up a paper to mark, remember that he or she might have a pile of 50 to wade through, and so give him or her a neat, legible, well-structured and factually correct essay. This is the examiner's dream! Imagine you have to mark your own work at the end of a busy, tiring day. It may make you want to give more thought to presentation! You will then keep your answers short and to the point. It makes it easier for you and cuts down on the amount of writing.

Subdivide, underline, use new paragraphs, but do not use lists or tables unless you justify their use in the text. Use the last 10 min of the examination time to check through the odd spelling mistake, or the doubtful sentence which seemed to make sense when you wrote it!

Note the special terms in the question. Some will be of a definite clinical nature, with terms such as differential diagnosis, aetiology, clinical findings, etc. Aetiology means *causes*, so do not give a long treatment plan unless asked for in a later part of the question.

If the question is split up into several parts, allow equal time for each part, as the marks will usually be divided by the number of parts to the question.

Variations in question style include: 'give an account of'. Here the situation or condition must be seen through from aetiology, pathology, signs and symptoms, and finally treatment and prognosis. If you are asked to 'discuss' a topic, pick out the controversial and the important aspects, and compare and contrast. When a 'differential diagnosis' is required, there should be in your mind a list of possible alternative diseases or conditions, and these alternatives should be mentioned along with the clinical, radiological, pathological or biochemical and surgical methods of arriving at this differential diagnosis.

When faced with a basic science question, do not immediately think 'What can I draw on this paper to fill up this half-hour?', because essentially you will find that somewhere, unless you are very unlucky, the emphasis will be on the practical applications of the topic.

'Finals' for the undergraduate is the University's way of seeing whether a student is fit to practise dentistry unsupervised, not to see if you are potentially the world's greatest biochemist!

Examinations like the MGDS are designed to see how you can cope with life in practice, or the general practicalities of dentistry. Do you know your limitations, are you well versed on current trends, do you keep your working environment up to date? These are some of the questions the Examiners will wish to know.

So, to summarize, always look for the practical side of the question, and be prepared, not only with pens and pencils, but by adequate revision. Try to obtain some of the past papers. Sit down and work through the essays in the allotted time. Get them marked if possible to find out if and where you are going wrong. This latter point is of particular value to those who have not sat a written paper for many years, and are out of practice with the timing and structure of essays.

The rest is between you and the Examiner!

Chapter 52

The clinical case

As an undergraduate, you will often have to present a clinical case as part of your examination. This may take the form of presentation of notes, models and a treatment plan, along with results and outcome. It may take the form of a specific piece of work performed on a patient, such as a full-coverage crown, or a molar endodontic case. The patient will usually be examined before your 'viva' but at the same visit.

The main essential here is to know your patient/case thoroughly and to have planned and looked at the case before you start. For the MGDS examination, the Log Diary assessment is a valuable and large part of the examination, and great emphasis is placed on patient selection. The work must be adequate and sensible, and the outcome satisfactory after your plan of treatment.

Let us return to the undergraduate case where, for example, a single crown performed on a patient is being presented to the examiners. The candidate must know the entire history of that patient—past and present. Medical history goes without saying, but dental history is of equal importance. The mouth must not only be worthy of such a restoration, but the patient must understand the implications of being an 'examination case' and that this may involve them in attendance for a visit purely for inspection only. The patient must be available for this at the time scheduled in the examination time-table, otherwise all is in vain!

Patient assessment is paramount. Oral hygiene should be good–excellent. This will make any subsequent restorative work easier, if nothing else. Radiographs and models will show what is going on elsewhere in the mouth, because the patient is much more than just 'an upper right six'!

Make a very careful diagnosis. Note existing and potential restorations, and check for attrition, abrasion, erosion, etc. Check for periodontal problems and note pocketing and any sinuses present in your general examination of the soft tissues. Note any teeth missing from the arch, and determine their fate, or whether they were ever present in the first place. The results of all these tests may well influence your treatment plan. Along with periodontal treatment, some dietary advice may be required. If this is the case, then you may have picked your patient unwisely. Now is the time to think again—carefully!

Check the soft tissues for signs of denture stomatitis, ulceration, or anything that strikes you as unusual. If seen, find out the reason or cause because the examiner will probably use it as a talking point, even if not directly related to the clinical task in hand.

Recheck the radiographs and compare/contrast them within the clinical picture you have now obtained. Try not to miss obvious secondary caries, overlooked in the mouth but obvious on the bitewings!

You should now be in a position to know virtually all the relevant information regarding the case and then to proceed or otherwise. Let us change theme now and consider the MGDS patient. This patient will be seen by a pair of Examiners in the candidate's practice environment (Royal College of Surgeons of England Regulations). The Examiners will have seen the completed Log Diaries before arrival, and will have formulated an idea of the case, and a line they may wish to pursue in the 'viva'. They will inspect the patient for 10–15 min and then question the candidate, not in the presence of the patient, who by this stage has usually left the premises.

This is obviously more complex than the undergraduate case, but again, all the points made earlier are valid, and the treatment must be deemed to be appropriate under the circumstances. In complex cases there will be plenty of room for discussion, and the candidate should have several alternative treatment plans lined up for this 'viva'. Presentation here counts for a lot. The Examiners may be seeing a complex case, so the Log Diary should be written up to help them understand the course/s of treatment, the 'whys and wherefores', and any viable alternatives. Radiographs and models are required also. The cases do not have to be very complex, and most candidates present slightly 'out of the ordinary' NHS cases, such as restorative/periodontal/oral surgery combinations. There is no requirement to present 32 bonded crowns with occlusal equilibration—and if you do, not only will you have to be very accurate, but very good at justification!

The Diary must be A4 size, and in a folder. The precise details can be obtained from the appropriate Royal Colleges. The pages should be protected with plastic sleeves, and the use of double-pack radiographs is recommended, so that the originals can be left in the patient's notes. The Diary has to be typed—or 'word-processed' nowadays—and, of course, this aids clarification for the Examiners.

Going back to the undergraduate presenting his/her crown case, if the student has access to a typewriter, then why not use it! Present the case with all the categories lined up. Start with the usual—name, date of birth, hospital number, etc. Continue with medical and dental history, original complaint, and then work through the sequence in logical order as you would in a Primary Care Unit. Finally arrive at your diagnosis and treatment plan, even if it is only for this one tooth. It must fit in with any other treatment the patient should or is prepared to receive, and must be examined in context.

By doing this you will have a presentation which will impress the examiners, and by typing out this treatment pattern and arranging it thus, you will certainly know the patient and their problems thoroughly. Again, present your sheets in a folder, and you will have a head start over the others. Do not, however, write a companion volume to *War and Peace*, because in a 10-min presentation, there is no time to read a novel, but the point is there to be taken.

Know your materials, what you have used and why, and what your alternatives may have been. The example which springs to mind here is the cement used to secure the aforementioned crown—'I used the cement I usually use' is a little lacking somewhere!

Again, for the MGDS, know what you used and why, and a little about the chemistry — or at least what the materials contain.

For all presentations, be smartly dressed; you will feel better if you are clean and tidy. Use clean instruments, neatly laid out on the tray. Have some articulating paper and some floss to hand, along with anything else special to the case such as models, radiographs, etc. If you are presenting a patient to the examiners, then always introduce the patient. He or she must come first, because without their dentition — or lack of it — you would not be having the 'viva'!

Chapter 53

The 'viva' examination

Here, our candidate comes face-to-face with a pair of Examiners for somewhere between 10 min and half an hour. Both Examiners may 'chip in' with questions, or one will question whilst the other listens to the proceedings so that a final judgement may be drawn up after the 'viva'. Models, radiographs or a presentation of a completed case (without the patient) are the usual starting points. The case may be one brought along for discussion by one of the Examiners, or it may be a case treated and nominated by the Examinee.

Let us look at the nominated case. Always have some means of presentation ready, usually in the form of some typed sheets for clarity. Have your models ready, labelled along with the series of radiographs, and all in order! This sequence is very important, especially in something like a molar endodontic assessment.

Introduce the case, if required to do so, but in a brief way, indicating the really relevant points such as name, age, medical and dental status. Then make a start on the particular dental problems of the case if no further peripheral areas deemed important remain.

Prepare to be stopped in full flight, and asked questions — time is short, and the Examiner has to make sure you know the basis of the case. In most cases which the candidate presents, he or she will already know the tricky areas, where things are a little amiss, and should be able to talk around some of them. A possibility here would be the discussion of alternative treatment plans so, again, know your case thoroughly because the Examiner's eye will go straight to the area you wish to avoid — be prepared!

If you are given 10 min to examine a prepared case brought in for examination purposes, start by reading the card often supplied along with the models/radiographs/photographs. Nothing will be there which is irrelevant — so use it all if you can. Make notes on your pad, and try to ascertain what it is that the Examiners are after. It should be a fairly straightforward case, but may have one or two hidden 'bonus' points which will need to be searched out. The subsequent line of questioning will allow you to reveal this. Never jump in with the rare conditions. Always start with the common problems and disorders and work your way up. Most clinical cases will be reasonably straightforward, either a prosthetic problem or a conservative/restorative problem, such as the patient who repeatedly fractures crowns and/or other restorations. There will usually be the popular attrition/erosion/abrasion case in there somewhere!

With the radiographs and models, count the teeth — there may be more or less than expected! Look for apical areas on the radiographs, along with caries and other abnormalities, the latter especially if faced with an orthopantomogram. Look for areas on the lower first molar, for example, as this is a more common source of pain than pericoronitis associated with the 'buried' wisdom tooth also shown on the X-ray! Look for caries rates and previous restorations in the patients. This may give you a guide to forming a treatment plan for discussion. Bone loss shown on the radiographs should also be noted.

List the points that you see quickly, formulate a brief treatment plan and await your fate!

A standard 'viva' can hinge around any subject which the Examiner cares to nominate, so tread warily at first until you can judge the depth of knowledge required, and the spread of subjects to be covered in the time. Aim for the easy, common topics as the discussion broadens out, and try to let the 'viva' go the way you want it to later on. Take a few seconds to structure your answer, rather than just jumping in — you may hit a topic about which you know nothing bar the name, and it can be all down hill from there! Try to answer each question exactly, and keep to the point. Do not make too much of it, otherwise you may lead yourself off at a tangent, open to unprepared topics.

'Viva' technique is something that the candidate has to learn but, fortunately, should not have too much practice.

Chapter 54

Causes of failure

The main cause of failure in any examination is inadequate preparation. This is really self-explanatory, and the only cure is more work, or redirection of one's efforts in the right direction. After most examination results, someone is at hand to explain the reasons for failure, and where the candidate went wrong or where there were gaping holes in knowledge. Often the cause can lie a little deeper, and none of us are very good at expressing ourselves at oral examinations. Try to discuss selected topics with others on your course, be it in discussion groups on postgraduate courses, or just with your flat-mates if you are still an undergraduate. It all helps, and gives you a yardstick by which to measure your own depth of knowledge. It can work both ways — if you try this with some of your undergraduate colleagues, you may become despondent, but before this happens, think about their answers because they may be totally irrelevant. Always try to answer the questions in a straightforward, simple way. The common things are common, so do not be blinded by science; think about clever answers, they may be too clever!

Whenever answering questions, start with the easy bits, and work upwards to the rare and odd conditions or forms of treatment. Your treatment plan for clinical cases should be as simple as possible — do not forget, although you may be discussing the case purely from models and radiographs, what would happen if you had actually to treat the patient with your treatment plan. — Could you, or would you, wish you had thought of something easier? Treatment plans should follow a logical and orderly sequence of events, listing correct items in order.

Do not argue with the Examiner: it never pays, and usually leads to failure! Try to stay calm; say you do not know the answer to the question, and, if necessary, ask the Examiner to move on to another topic! This does not mean you have to be humble, but always be polite and try to carry out a 'conversation' about the topic although, under examination conditions, this is easier said than done!

Index

Abscess, dental, 410
Acid etching, 237
Acid etch-retained composite resin, 163–4
Acyclovir, 326–7
Addison's disease, 423–4
Adrenaline, 389, 390–1, 393
Advanced tooth wear, 270–5
  aetiology, 270
  clinical presentation, 270
  effects, 274–5
  mechanism, 270
  patient evaluation, 270–2
  post-treatment problems, 275
  treatment options, 272–4
  treatment planning, 271–2
AIDS, *see* Human immunodeficiency virus infection
Allergy, 310, 392, 454
Alveolar bone, 338–9
Amalgam, 107, 163, 209–16
  alloy components effects, 210
    copper, 210
    silver, 210
    tin, 210
    zinc, 210
  amalgamation reaction, 212
    properties of phases, 213
  composition, 209
  high-copper alloys, 210
  non-gamma-2 alloy, 214–16
  particle size/shape, 211–12
    advantages of spheres over filings, 212
Amalgam tattoo, 422
Amelodentinal junction, 8, 18
Amoxycillin, 323, 356
Amphotericin, 326
Ampicillin, 322
Amyloidosis, 413
Analgesics, 327–32
  centrally acting, 330–1
  local, 331–3

peripherally acting, 327–30
Anaphylactic shock (hypersensitivity), 434, 454
Anexate (flumanezil), 333, 383–4
Angina, 434
Angina bullosa haemorrhagica, 405 (table), 406
Angio-oedema, 412–13
Angular cheilitis (stomatitis), 307, 309, 442
Anterior (greater) palatine nerve, 27
Antibiotics, 322–5, 369–70
Anticoagulant, 15, 434, 453
Antidepressants, 434
Antifungal agents, 325–6
Antimicrobial therapy, 355–6
Antiviral agents, 326–7
Aphthae (recurrent aphthous stomatitis), 308, 398–9, 446
Apicectomy, 462–4
Articulators, 293–4
Aspirin, 14, 328
Asthma, 435
Atrophic glossitis, 416
Atypical facial pain, 427–8
Augmentin, 323, 356
Auriculotemporal nerve, 29–30

Balancing extractions, 62–5
Barnsley N_2O monitor, 376
Bell's palsy, 430
Bennett angle, 279–80
Bennett movement, 279–80
Benthamine penicillin, 322
Benzodiazepines, 332–3
Benzylpenicillin, 322
Betadine, 456
Bleeding disorders, 15, 454
Blood coagulation, 14–15
Bondent Pins, 207
Bone removal, 457
Bowen's resin (dimethylacrylate), 253
Branchial arches, 6

Branchial arches – *continued*
  derivatives, 6 (table)
Breathing difficulties, 16–17
Broken root, 457–8
Brufen (ibuprofen), 330
Buccal abscess, 37
Buccal space, 37
Burning mouth syndrome (glossodynia; glossopyrosis), 427

Calcium hydroxide base linings, 240
Calcium hydroxide cement, 232
Candidal leukoplakia, 420
Candidosis (thrush), 311, 415–16, 421–2, 442
  chronic atrophic, 442
  chronic hyperplastic, 442
  HIV associated, 442
  pseudomembranous, 442
Canine fossa, 39
Canines, 57–9
  deciduous, exfoliation by erupting permanent lateral incisor, 56
  maxillary deciduous, successors ectopically placed, 58–9
  misplaced, treatment, 57–8
    interception, 58
    late referral, 58
  serial extraction, 56
Carcinoma, oral, 308
Cardiac arrest, 434
Caries, *see* Dental caries
Castable ceramics, 242–3
Cast ceramic, 163
Cast gold, 163
  bevelling, 168
Cast gold post, 220, 228–9
Cavity preparation, 155–74
  adjustment of cavity walls/margins, 167–8
  bevels for cast gold restorations, 168
  bevels for composite resin restorations, 168–9
  caries removal at enamel-dentine junction, 157
  carious, unsupported enamel removal, 157–9
  chemical treatment of enamel/dentine, 171
  deep caries removal, 169–70
  design to restore cuspal enamel, 163–4
  direct attachment, 166
  extension of cavity, 159–62
  gaining access to caries, 157
  near-parallelism, 166
  replacement restorations, 171–4
    improving cavosurface angle, 173
    root-treated teeth, 173–4
  shaping cavity, 162–3, 164
  undercuts, 164–6
  washing/drying preparation, 171
Cellulitis, 392
Cements, 230–3
  accelerated zinc oxide-eugenol, 230
  Bowen's resin (dimethacrylate), 233
  calcium hydroxide, 232
  copper phosphate, 231
  EBA (ethoxybenzoic acid), 230–1
  glass-ionomer, 232
  resin-bonded zinc oxide-eugenol, 230
  temporary luting, 233
  zinc oxide-eugenol, 230
  zinc phosphate, 231
  zinc polycarboxylate, 231
  zinc silico-phosphate, 231
Cementum, 339
Cephalosporins, 323
Cermets, 256
Charlton post, 220–2, 227
Cheeks, sensory innervation, 33
Cimetidine, 333
Cleft lip, 3, 7
Cleft palate, 5, 7
Cloxacillin, 322
Codeine, 331
Coeflex, 194
Coeliac disease, 404
Collapse, unexpected, 434–5
Committee of Enquiry into Unnecessary Dental Treatment Report (1986), 176–9
Compensating extractions, 65
Complete dentures:
  complaints, 282–5
    angular stomatitis, 284
    cheek biting, 284
    difficulty keeping clean, 285
    fracture, 285
    generalized pain under, 283
    localized pain under, 283–4
    loose dentures, 282–3
    pain in masticatory muscles, 284
    retching, 284
    saliva excess, 285
    speech disturbance, 284
    tongue biting, 284
  duplication, 304–5
  impression technique, *see under* Impression techniques

occlusion and 280–1
Composite resins, 107
  bevelling, 168–9
Consent to sedation, 375
Copper phosphate cement, 231
Corticosteroids, 433, 434
Coumarin, 15
Coumarin-like substances, 15
Coxsackie virus infection, 403–4
Crohn's disease, 404
  oral, 411
Crossbites, 52–4, 93–4, 95–6
Cusps:
  guiding, 278
  supporting, 278
Cyanosis, 11

Deciduous dentition, 47
Dental abscess, 410
Dental caries, 119–80
  cavity preparation, see Cavity preparation
  clinical appearance of early lesions, 121–2
  dental plaque, 120
  descriptive status, 130
  dietary carbohydrate involvement, 120
  dentine caries, 124–6
  enamel caries, 123–4
  incidence, 128
  individual variation, 128
  preventive management, 131–6
    defective restorations, 135–6
    fissure lesions, 133–4
    fissure sealant, 134–5
    pit lesions, 133–4
    smooth surface lesions, 132–3
  process, 121
  progression, 130–1
  pulpal response, 127
  radiography, 122–3
  restorative treatment, 137–47
    caries management problems, 137–8
    criteria, 143–5
    dental services-related problems, 139–40
    patient-related problems, 142–3
    preventive resins, 146–7
    restoration replacement problems, 138–9
    restorative materials problems, 142
    restorative procedures problems, 140–2
    sealant restorations, 145–6

short durability of restorations, 143
risk factors, 128–9
susceptible tooth surface, 120
timing of causal interactions, 121
way forwards in management, 175–80
Dental plaque, 120
Dental Strategy Review Group (1981), 175
Dentine:
  caries, 124–6
  development, 8
  hydrodynamic mechanism, 19
  mineral content, 8
  nerves, 18
  sensitivity, 18–19
  tubule, hydrodynamic mechanism, 19
Dentine bonding agents, 235–6
  glutaraldehyde/hydroxyethyl methacrylate systems, 236
  phosphonate derivatives, 235–6
Denture-induced hyperplasia, 309, 468
Denture-induced mucosal problems, 310
Denture-induced stomatitis (denture sore mouth), 308, 416
Dextrapropoxyphene, 330
Diabetes mellitus, 433–4, 453–4
Diazepam (Diazemuls; Valium), 333, 375, 379
Dicor, 242
Dicoumarol, 15
Diflunisal, 329
Digit sucking, 50
Dihydrocodeine, 330
Dimethacrylate (Bowen's resin), 253
Dispersalloy, 210
Distalgesic, 330

EBA (ethoxybenzoic acid) cement, 230–1
Echovirus infection, 403–4
EDTA (ethyldiaminetetracetic acid), 255
Embden-Myerhof glycolytic pathway, 121
Emergencies, 433–5
  drug-induced, 433–4
  unexpected collapse, 434–5
Enamel bonding agents, 234–5
Enamel caries, 123–4
Endodontics, 181–92
  access, 183
    preparation of openings, 186–7
    accessory canals, 183, 184 (table)
  aims of treatment, 181
  anatomy:

Endodontics, anatomy – *continued*
  individual teeth, 183–5
  pulp space, 183
  average working distance of teeth, 183 (table)
  canal filling, 190–2
  canal preparation, 187–90
  clinical examination requirements, 182
  radiographic examination requirements, 182
Epilepsy, 392, 434
Epithelansatz (Gottlieb), 337
Epulides, 412
Erythema migrans (geographical tongue), 414
Erythema multiforme, 405 (table), 406
Erythromycin, 324
Erythroplasia, 418–19
Extrude, 195

Face bow, 294
Facial development, 3–6
Facial nerve, chorda tympani branch, 31
Facial nerve palsy, 395, 430, 446
Factor XII, 15
Faint, 10–11
  emotional (vasovagal syncope), 10, 434
  postural (postural syncope), 11
Felypressin, 332, 391
Fibroepithelial polyp, 412
Filpin, 207
Fissure sealing, 100–2, 134–5
Flexipost, 226–7, 228
Floor of mouth, sensory innervation, 33
Flucloxacillin, 322
Flumanezil (Anexate), 333, 384
Fluoride, 97–9
  topical, 98–9
Foreign body in airway, 434–5
Fraenum, upper lip, abnormally large, 54–5
Fuji, 107

Gentamicin, 325
Geographical tongue (erythema migrans), 415
Giant-cell arteritis, 428 (table)
Gingiva, 335–8
  connective tissue, 338
  interdental papilla, 338
  junctional epithelium, 336–7
  outer epithelium, 335
  sensory innervation, 32–3
  sulcular epithelium, 336

Gingivitis:
  acute ulcerative, 311
  acute (ulcerative) necrotizing (Vincent's disease), 346–7, 444–5
  chronic, 340–1
  HIV, 445
Glass-ionomer cements, 107, 232, 254–61
  adhesion, 255
  biocompatibility, 255–6
  cariostatic effect, 257
  contraindications, 258
  indications, 257–8
  laminates, 260
  microcavities, 260
  light-cured, 260–1
  metal reinforcement (cermets), 256
  opacity, 256
  powder liquid form, 254
  radiopacity, 256
  sandwiches, 260
  setting reaction, 255
  storage, 257
  strength, 256
  tunnel restoration, 260
  use, 258–60
  water-hardening (anhydrous) form, 254
  water loss/gain, 257
Glossitis:
  atrophic, 416
  median rhomboid, 417
Gluma, 236
Glossodynia (glossopyrosis; burning mouth syndrome), 427
Greater (anterior) palatine nerve, 27
Guiding cusps, 278

Haemangioma, 417–18
Haemophilia, 15, 454
Haemorrhage, 435
  recovery after, 20–2
Haemostasis, 14–15
Hairy leukoplakia, 420, 444
Hand, foot and mouth disease, 403
Herpangina, 403
Herpes labialis, 402
Herpes simplex virus infection, 402, 442–4
Herpes varicella-zoster virus infection, 402–3, 442–4
Homogeneous leukoplakia, 420
Human immunodeficiency virus (HIV) infection, 436–48
  clinical aspects, 437–40

dental aspects, 442–8
  assessment of patient risk status, 447–8
  risk of HIV transmission, 446–7
 epidemiology, 436–7
 immunologic abnormalities, 438 (table)
 incubation period, 440
 management, 440
 oral manifestations, 442–6
 pathogenesis, 437
 persistent generalized lymphadenopathy, 438
 transmission routes, 436
 vaccine, 441
Hydrocolloids, 197–9
 irreversible (alginate), 198
 reversible, 198
Hyperglycaemic coma, 434
Hyperplasia, denture-induced, 309
Hypersensitivity (anaphylactic shock), 434, 454
Hypertension, 453
Hypnotics, 434
Hypnovel (midazolam), 333, 379, 381–3
Hypolgycaemic coma, 434
Hypoxia, 11–14
 anaemic, 12–13
 hypoxic, 12
 stagnant, 13
 tissue susceptibility, 13–14

Ibuprofen (Neurofen; Brufen), 330
Impacted lower second molar, 466–7
Implantology, 315–17
 biological response, 315–16
 endosseous, 315, 316–17
 osseointegration, 316
 subperiosteal, 315
 transosteal, 315
Impregnum, 197
Impression materials, 193–204
 classification, 192
 distortion on removal from mouth, 200
 duration of storage, 200
 elastomeric, 194–5
  polyethers, 196–7
  polysulphides, 194–5
  silicones, 195–6
 factors affecting accuracy, 194
 hydrocolloids, 197–8
  irreversible (alginate), 198
  reversible, 198

properties requirements, 193
 rigid (non-elastic) materials, 201–4
  plaster, 202–3
  waxes, 203
  zinc oxide-eugenol paste, 204
 storage conditions, 200
Impression techniques, 199–200, 286–92
 complete denture, 286–9
  flabby upper ridge, 288
  functional impression, 289
  neutral zone impression, 288–9
  preliminary impression, 286–7
  trays, 287–8
 partial denture, 289–92
  altered cast technique, 291
  chairside reline, 291–2
  laboratory reline, 292
  preliminary impression, 290
  working impression, 290–1
Infections, 470–1
Inferior alveolar nerve, 30 (fig.), 31–2
 block, 23
Inflammatory papillary hyperplasia of palate, 308–9
Infraorbital nerve, 26
Infratemporal space, 39
Instanding lower second premolar, 467
Insulin, 433–4
Intercuspal position, 276
Interdental papilla, 338
Iron deficiency, 306–7

Jaw movement, 277–80
 Bennett angle, 279–80
 Bennett movement, 279–80
 determinants, 278 (fig.)
 in natural dentition, 279–80
 see also Occlusion

Kaposi's sarcoma, 418, 440, 444
Keratoses, 419–20
 frictional, 420
 smokers', 420
 syphilitic, 420
Ketacfil, 107
Ketokonazole, 326
Krebs tricarboxylic acid cycle, 121
Kurer post, 222–3, 227

Labial fraenum, 466
Laboratory-cured composite resin, 163
Lactic acid, 121
Laryngeal spasm, 434–5
Lateral pterygoid nerve, 29

Left lateral occlusion, 276
Lesser (posterior) palatine nerve, 27
Leukoplakia:
  candidal, 420
  hairy, 420, 444
  homogeneous, 420
Lichen planus, 308, 405 (table), 406, 420–1
Light-activated resins, 237–41
  factors influencing curing, 239
  moderate to highly filled systems, 236
  setting of composite materials, 238–9
  ultraviolet, 237
  unfilled/lightly filled systems, 238
  visible, 237
Light-activating systems, 237–41
  light-activated, see Light-activated resins
  posterior composites, 239–41
Lignocaine, 389
  + adrenaline, 331–2
Lingual nerve, 30–1
Link Plus, 205, 206, 207
Lips, sensory innervation, 33
Local analgesia, 15–16, 385–96
  complications/precautions, 390–3
    allergy, 392
    bleeding disorders, 391–2
    cellulitis, 392
    epilepsy, 392
    local, 394–5
    monoamine oxidase inhibitors, 392–3
    overdosage, 390
    poor blood supply, 391
    sepsis, 392
    tricyclic antidepressants, 392–3
    vasoconstriction, 39–40
  drug mode of action, 387–90
  failure to obtain, 393
  intraligamentary, 395–6
  psychological effects, 394
Ludwig's angina, 392
Lupus erythematosus, 421
Luting cements, 258, 259–60
Lyell's syndrome (toxic epidermolysis), 446
Lymphangioma, 409–10
Lymphoma, oral, 445

Macroglossia, 413
Macrostomia, 7
Malignant melanoma, 423
Malocclusion, 43–5

  mandibular displacement on closure, 44
  traumatic overbite, 44
Mandible:
  displacement on closure, 44, 45 (figs.)
  midline cleft, 7
  nerve supply, 28 (fig.), 31–2, 385–7
Mandibular facial dysostosis (Treacher-Collins syndrome), 7
Mandibular incisors, 55
  central, lingually erupting, 56–7
  developmentally absent, 55
  supplemental, 55
Mandibular nerve, 27–32
  buccal branch (long buccal nerve), 29
  meningeal branch (nervous spinosus), 28
Mandibular rest position, 17–18
  tissue elasticity, 18
  tonic muscle activity, 17–18
Mandibular tori, 409
Markley pin, 208
Masseteric nerve, 29
Master post, 224 (fig.), 225, 227
Maxilla, nerve supply, 24 (fig.), 25–6, 385–7
Maxillary air sinuses, 39–40
Maxillary canines, deciduous, successors ectopically placed, 58–9
Maxillary central incisors, 47–51
  avulsed, 48–9
  digit sucking effect, 50
  dilacerated maxillary central incisors, 48
  permanent, non-eruption, 47–8
  traumatic loss, 49
  unerupted blocking supernumerary tooth, 47
Maxillary lateral incisors, 50–2
  developmental absence, 50–1
  supplemental, 51–2
Maxillary molar block, 387, 392
Maxillary nerve, 24 (fig.), 25–7
  ganglionic branches, 25
Maxillary tori, 409
Maxillary tuberosity fracture, 469–70
Medial pterygoid nerve, 29
Median rhomboid glossitis, 417
Mefenamic acid (Ponstan), 330
Meningeal nerve, 25
Mepivicaine, 332, 389
Mercury, 212
  handling, 216
  vapour, 216

Mesiodens, 54
Methadone, 330
Methylparabens, 392
Metronidazole, 324–5, 356
MGDS examination, 475–484
  causes of failure, 484
  clinical case, 479–81
  viva examination, 482–3
  written papers, 476–8
Miconazole, 326
Midazolam (Hynovel), 333, 379, 381–3
Migraine, 428 (table)
Migrainous neuralgia, 428 (table)
Mixed dentition, 47–71
  abnormally large fraenum of upper lip, 54–5
  analysis, 105–6
  avulsed maxillary central incisors, 48–9
  developmentally absent mandibular central incisor, 55
  developmentally absent maxillary lateral incisors, 50–1
  digit sucking effects, 50
  early radiographic screening, 45–7
  exfoliation of deciduous canine by erupting permanent lateral incisor, 56
  lingually erupting madibular permanent central incisors, 56
  mesiodens, 54
  non-eruption of maxillary permanent central incisors, 47–8
    dilacerated maxillary central incisors, 48
    unerupted blocking supernumerary tooth, 47–8
  one or more incisors in crossbite, 52–4
  serial extraction, 55–6
  supplemental mandibular incisor, 55
  supplementary maxillary lateral incisors, 51
  traumatic los of maxillary central incisors, 49
Molars, 67–73
  first permanent, of poor prognosis, 67–71
  impacted first permanent, 67
  removal of second permanent, 72
  removal of third by lateral trepanation, 72–3
  submerging deciduous, 62
  submerging first permanent, 67
Monoamine oxidase inhibitors, 392–3
Morphine, 330

Mouth:
  lymphatic drainage, 34–6
  sensory innervation, 22–34
Mouth lumps, 408–13
  developmental, 409–10
  inflammatory, 410–11
  neoplasia, 412; *see also* Squamous cell carcinoma
  trauma-related, 412
Mouth ulcers, 397–406
  associated conditions, 401–6
    gastrointestinal diseases, 404–5
    infections, 401–4
    skin diseases, 405–6
  causes, 397
  drugs, 400–1
  clinical features, 396
  diagnosis, 397
  management, 398
Mucosal problems:
  chemical/physical trauma induced, 311
  denture induced, 310

Naevi, 422–3
  white sponge, 419
Nalbuphine (Nubain), 330
Nasopalatine nerve, 27
Near-parallelism, 166
Neoplasia of mouth, 399–400
Neurofen (ibuprofen), 330
Nichrome crown, 109
Nitrous oxide + oxygen, 375–8
  advantages, 376
  contraindications, 376–7
  disadvantages, 376
  essential advice to patient, 377
Non-gamma-2 alloy, 214–16
Non-steroidal anti-inflammatory drugs (NSAIDs), 329–30
Noradrenaline, 392–3
Nubain (nalbuphine), 330
Nutritional deficiencies, 306–7
Nystatin, 325–6

Oblique facial cleft, 7
Occlusion, 276–81
  bilateral balanced, 280–1
  centric (intercuspal position; tooth position), 277
  complete dentures, 280–1
  definitions, 276
    intercuspal position, 276
    left/right lateral occlusion, 276
    protruded position, 276

Occlusion, definitions – *continued*
  retruded contact position, 276
  natural dentition, 278
  see also Jaw movement
Odontoblasts, 18–19
Oedema, 19–20
Oral cavity, *see* Mouth
Oral hygiene, 350–1
Oral hypoglycaemic drugs, 433–4
Oral surgery for general dental practitioner, 450–72
  apicectomy, 462–4
  basic techniques, 455–62
    bone removal, 457
    broken root, 457–8
    flap design/handling, 456–7
    suturing, 358–9
  chronic oroantral fistula, 469
  diagnosis, 451
  fractured maxillary tuberosity, 469–70
  impacted lower second molar, 466–7
  infections, 470–1
  instanding lower second premolar, 467
  instruments, 455
  labial fraenum, 466
  local anaesthesia, 451
  medical history, 451–4
    assessment, 452–4
  medicological aspects, 472
  orthodontics, *see* Orthodontic treatment
  postoperative analgesia, 471
  radiography, 450–1
  referral to hospital, 471–2
  retrograde root filling, 462–4
  wisdom teeth, *see* Wisdom teeth
Oral ulceration, recurrent, 446
Orbital nerve, 27
Oroantral fistula:
  acute, 458
  chronic, 469
Orthodontic treatment, 78–95
  Class I malocclusion, 91–4
    crossbites, 93–4
    crowding, 92
    rotations, 93
    spacing, 93
    treatment objectives, 91
  Class II, division 1 malocclusion, 79–88
    crowded teeth, 82
    dissimilar molar occlusion, 87
    mandibular arch treatment without appliances, 81–2
    maxillary arch treatment with removable appliances, 80–1
    overjet reduction stability, 79, 80 (fig.)
    space requirements assessment for overject reduction, 82–7
  Class II, division 2 malocclusion, 88–91
    crowded mandibular arches, 91
    maxillary central incisors position, 88–9
    uncrowded mandibular arches, 89–91
  Class III malocclusion, 94–6
    all maxillary incisors in crossbite, 95–6
    some maxillary incisors not in crossbite, 94–5
  timing, 44–5
  tooth exposure, 464–5
  unerupted labial canine removal, 465–6
  unerupted palatal upper canine removal, 465
Osseointegration, 316

Pain, orofacial, 426–9
  psychogenic, 427
  vascular origin, 428
Palate:
  inflammatory papillary hyperplasia, 308–9
  sensory innervation, 33–4
Paracetamol, 328–9
Parapharyngeal space, 38
Palatal union, 6
Parapost, 223–4, 227
Parotid space, 37, 38
Partial dentures, 295–303
  components, 296–7
  damage caused by, 297–8
  design, systematic, 300–3
    choice of materials, 302
    connectors, 302
    horizontal displacement prevention, 301–2
    information, 299–300
    retention, 301
    RPI system, 302–3
    saddles, 300
    support, 301
  necessity?, 298–9
  oral health associated, 295–6
  surveying, 299–300
Pemphigoid, 405 (table), 406
Pemphigus, 405 (table), 406

INDEX

Penicillins, 322–3
Pentazocine, 330
Percoronitis, 346, 451
Periodontal abscess, acute lateral, 348–9
Periodontal diseases, 340–9
  acute, 346–9
  chronic, 340–6
  treatment, 349–57
    acute disease, 349–50
    antimicrobial therapy, 355–6
    chronic disease, 350
    deposit removal, 351–5
    oral hygiene phase, 350–1
    splinting, 356–7
    surgery, *see* Periodontal surgery
Periodontal dressings, 369
Periodontal membrane, 339
Periodontal pocket, 337 (fig.), 342, 345
Periodontal surgery, 358–73
  aims, 359
  antibiotic treatment, 369–70
  contraindications, 359
  extractions, 365
  failure, 372
  flap raising, 362–4
  free gingival graft, 366–8
  healing, 371–2
    conventional gingivectomy, 371
    flap surgery, 371–2
    free gingival graft, 372
  indications, 358
  mucogingival, 366
  osseous recontouring, 365
  postoperative instructions, 370–1
  postoperative problems for patient, 370
  re-attachment procedures, 361–2
  repositioning procedures, 364
    apical, 364–5
  resection, 359–61
    conventional gingivectomy, 360–1
    electrosurgery, 360
  subgingival curettage, 365–6
  surgical tray contents, 373
Periodontitis:
  chronic, 342–5
  HIV, 445
  juvenile, 345
  prepubertal, 346
  rapidly progressive, 345–6
Periodontium, 335–57
  diseases, *see* Periodontal diseases
  health maintenance, 339–40
Peritonsillar space, 38

Permanent dentition, 72–3
  early treatment, 72–3
  later treatment, 73
Permlastic, 194
Pethidine, 330
Phenoxymethylpenicillin (pen V), 323
Phosphoric-acid etching, 255
Pigmented lesions, 415–25
  hyperpigmented, 446
  local, 422–4
  red, 414–19
  white, 419–22
Pins, 205–8
  factors affecting retention, 206–7
  indications, 205
  risks, 208
  tooth factors affecting placement, 207
  types, 207–8
Plaque, 120
Plaster, 202–3
Platelets, 14
Polyethers, 196–7
Polysulphides, 194–5
Ponstan (mefenamic acid), 330
Posselt's envelope, 277
Post crowns, 217–29
  anterior teeth, 217–27
    arguments against decoronation, 216–19
    cast gold post, 220
    Charlton post, 220–2
    criteria for post/core systems, 219–20
    Flexipost, 226–7
    Kurer post, 222–3
    Master post, 224 (fig.), 225
    Parapost, 223–4
    Radix-Anker post, 225–6
    Wiptam post, 222 (fig.), 223
  posterior teeth, 227–9
    cast gold post, 228
    Charlton post, 227
    Flexipost, 228
    Kurer post, 227
    Master post, 227
    Parapost, 227
    Radix-Anker post, 228
    Wiptam post, 227
  root-fractured tooth, 228 (fig.), 229
Posterior (lesser) palatine nerve, 27
Posterior superior alveolar nerve, 25–6
  block, 387
Posterior superior nasal nerve, 27
Postural syncope (vasovagal syncope), 10

Precision attachments, 312–14
  bar, 313
  extracoronal, 313–14
  intracoronal, 314
Pregnancy epulis, 410
Premolars, 59–62
  developmentally absent second premolars, 59–62
    crowded cases, 60–2
    uncrowded cases, 59
Preprosthetic surgery, 467–9
  denture-induced hyperplasia, 468–9
  flabby ridge, 468
  sharp ridge, 468
  undercut ridge, 468
Prescription writing, 321–2
President, 195
Preventive resin restoration (sealant restoration), 101–2, 146–7
Prilocaine, 389
  + felypressin, 332
Primary teeth conservation, 104–9
  cavity preparation, 106
  mixed dentition analysis, 105–6
  pulp treatment of primary molars, 107–9
  restorative materials, 107
  stainless-steel crowns, 109
Primary teeth injuries, 113–15
  avulsed teeth, 114
  complications, 114–15
    damage to underlying permanent tooth, 115
    pulp death, 114
  crown fracture, 114
  intruded teeth, 114
  loosened teeth, 113–14
  root fracture, 114
  treatment of non-vital anterior teeth, 115
Procaine penicillin, 322
Protruded position, 276
Provil, 195
Pterygomandibular space, 37–8
Pterygopalatine nerve, 24 (fig.)
Purpura, 417
Pyogenic granuloma, 410

Quinsy, 38

Racial pigmentation, 423
Radiographic screening, early mixed dentition, 45–7
Radix-Anker post, 225–6, 228

Recurrent aphthous stomatitis (aphthae), 308, 398–9, 446
Referral to hospital, 471–2
Reflect, 195
Removable appliances, 74–5
  maxillary arch, 80–1
Reprosil, 195
Resin-bonded bridges, 262–9
  advantages, 266
  bonding technique, 267–8
    rebonding failed bridges, 268
  contraindications, 265
  design features, 266–7
  disadvantages, 266
  failure rate/causes, 268
  indications, 265
  metal framework, 263–4
    chemical etching, 264–5
    electrolyte etching, 264
    non-perforated retainers, 264–5
    perforated retainers, 263
  tooth preparation, 267
  types, 262–3
    natural crown pontic, 263
    resin pontics, 262–3
Resin-bonded zinc oxide-eugenol cement, 230
Respiratory failure, 434
Respiratory obstruction, 434–5
Retrograde tooth filling, 462–4
Retruded contact position, 276
Rheumatic fever, 453
Right lateral occlusion, 276
Rubber dam, 148–54
  equipment, 149–52
  multitooth isolation, 152, 153
  removal, 153–4
  single tooth isolation, 152

Sarcoidosis, 411
Scarlet fever, 453
Scotchbond, 235–6
Sealant restoration (preventive resin restoration), 101–2, 146–7
Sedation, conscious, 332–3, 374–84
  consent to, 375
  inhalation (relative analgesia), 375–8
    advantages, 376
    contraindication, 376–7
    disadvantages, 375–8
    essential advice to patient, 377
  intravenous, 378–84
    advantages, 380
    contraindications, 380

disadvantages, 380
preoperative checks, 381
preoperative instructions, 380–1
see also Diazepam; Flumazenil; Midazolam
legal aspects, 374–5
oral, 375
Sedatives, 434
Sensory loss, orofacial, 429
Sepsis, 392
Serial extraction, 55–6
Shingles (herpes zoster infection), 402
Silicones, 195–6
addition-cured, 195
condensation, 195
Single-tooth denture as space maintainer, 49
Splinting, 356–7
Spontaneous space closure, 75–8
Squamous cell carcinoma, oral, 399–400
Stabilock pin, 207
Stainless-steel crowns, 109, 164
Stephan curve, 121
Steroids, 433, 434
Stomatitis (angular cheilitis), 307, 309, 442
Stomatitis, denture-induced (denture sore mouth), 308, 416
Streptococcus mutans, 121
Stroke, 435
Sublingual abscess, 37
Sublingual space, 37
Submandibular abscess, 37
Submandibular space, 36–7
Submasseteric space, 37
Submental space, 36–7
Sulphonamides, 325
Supporting cusps, 278
Suturing, 458–9
Swelling, 19–20
Sybralloy, 210, 211
Syphilis, 307–8
keratosis, 420

Taste disturbance/loss, 430–1
Teeth:
abnormalities of position, 9
development, 7–8
eruption process, 9
position, 43
root formation, 9–10
sensory innervation, 32
Teichoplanin, 325
Telangiectases, 417

Temazepam, 375
Temporal nerves, anterior/posterior, 29
Temporomandibular joint, effect of tooth wear, 274–5
Tetracyclines, 356
Threadmate system, 205
Thrombocytopenia, 446
Thrush, *see* Candidosis
Tissue spaces around jaws, 36–9
TMA Minim Double Shear pin, 207
Tongue:
development, 6–7
sensory innervation, 33
Tori, 409
Toxic epidermolysis (Lyell's syndrome), 446
Trauma to children's teeth, 110–15
assessment, 110
examination, 110–11
primary teeth, *see* Primary teeth injuries
treatment, 111–13
dentine-involved fracture, 111–12
loosened teeth, 112–13
no crown fracture, or of enamel only, 111
pulp-involved fracture, 112
root fractures, 113
Traumatic overbite, 44
Treacher-Collis syndrome (mandibular facial dysostosis), 7
Tricyclic antidepressants, 392–3
Trigeminal neuralgia, 426–7, 446
Trismus, 395
Tuberculosis, oral, 307
Tytan, 210, 211

Ulcerative disease, 404
Ulcerative gingivitis, acute, 311
Unerupted labial canine removal, 465–6
Unerupted palatal upper canine removal, 465
Unitek crown, 109
Unosil, 195
Urethane resins, 241

Valium (diazepam), 333, 375, 379
Valvular heart disease, 453
Vancomycin, 324
Vasovagal syncope (emotional faint), 10, 434
Veneers, 244–53
acrylic, 245–6
castable glass ceramic, 248

Veneers – *continued*
　cementation, 252–3
　composite, 244–5
　contraindications, 249
　impression of preparation, 251
　indications, 248
　porcelain, 246–8
　temporary coverage, 251–2
　tooth preparation, 249–51
Verril's sign, 379
Vincent's disease (acute necrotising [ulcerative] gingivitis), 346–7
Vitamin B deficiency, 306

Waldeyer's tonsillar ring, 36
Warfarin, 15
Water fluoridation, 97
Waxes, 203
　impression, 203
　inlay, 203

White sponge naevus, 419
Willebrand's disease, von, 454
Wiptam post, 222 (fig.), 223, 227
Wisdom teeth, 459–62
　assessment, 459–60
　radiography, 450
　removal of lower, 460–2
　removal of upper, 462

Xerostomia, 307, 445–6

Zinc oxide-eugenol cement, 230
　accelerated, 230
Zinc oxide-eugenol impression paste, 204
Zinc phosphate cement, 231
Zinc silico-phosphate cement, 231
Zinc polycarboxylate sement, 231
Zygomatic nerve, 25